A New Approach to Diagnosis and Treatment of Prostate Cancer

A New Approach to Diagnosis and Treatment of Prostate Cancer

Editor: Peter Hayes

AMERICAN
MEDICAL PUBLISHERS
www.americanmedicalpublishers.com

AMERICAN
MEDICAL PUBLISHERS
www.americanmedicalpublishers.com

Cataloging-in-publication Data

A new approach to diagnosis and treatment of prostate cancer / edited by Peter Hayes.
p. cm.
Includes bibliographical references and index.
ISBN 978-1-63927-849-7
1. Prostate--Cancer. 2. Prostate--Cancer--Diagnosis. 3. Prostate--Cancer--Treatment.
4. Prostate--Diseases. I. Hayes, Peter.
RC280.P7 N49 2023
616.994 63--dc23

American Medical Publishers,
41 Flatbush Avenue,
1st Floor, New York,
NY 11217, USA

ISBN 978-1-63927-849-7 (Hardback)

Contents

Preface

The prostate gland is a part of the male reproductive system. It is located slightly below the bladder and in front of the rectum. It produces a fluid which is a part of the semen. Prostate cancer is a condition that causes malignant cells to develop in the prostate tissues. The symptoms comprise frequent urinating or a weak urine flow. It is diagnosed through tests which examine the prostate and blood. A biopsy is performed to diagnose prostate cancer and determining the grade of the cancer. There are various treatments available for patients with this cancer including surgery, hormone therapy, immunotherapy, targeted therapy, radiation therapy and radiopharmaceutical therapy, bisphosphonate therapy, and chemotherapy. This book is compiled in such a manner, that it will provide in-depth knowledge about the assessment and management of prostate cancer. It aims to shed light on some of the unexplored aspects of this disease. This book will prove to be immensely beneficial to students and researchers in this field.

After months of intensive research and writing, this book is the end result of all who devoted their time and efforts in the initiation and progress of this book. It will surely be a source of reference in enhancing the required knowledge of the new developments in the area. During the course of developing this book, certain measures such as accuracy, authenticity and research focused analytical studies were given preference in order to produce a comprehensive book in the area of study.

This book would not have been possible without the efforts of the authors and the publisher. I extend my sincere thanks to them. Secondly, I express my gratitude to my family and well-wishers. And most importantly, I thank my students for constantly expressing their willingness and curiosity in enhancing their knowledge in the field, which encourages me to take up further research projects for the advancement of the area.

Editor

1

Bone Seeking Radiopharmaceuticals for Metastatic Bone Pain

Marnix G.E.H. Lam[1] and Bernard A. Zonnenberg[1,2]
[1]*Department of Radiology and Nuclear Medicine*
[2]*Department of Internal Medicine*
University Medical Center Utrecht
The Netherlands

1. Introduction

Prostate cancer is the most common malignancy in men in the Netherlands. The majority of patients with advanced prostate cancer develop skeletal metastases, with bone pain as a frequent symptom. This poses a significant medical problem. Amongst other treatments, bone seeking radiopharmaceuticals are used to palliate painful metastatic bone disease. Efficacy has been sufficiently proven, as well as safety and feasibility. Practical issues as well as new developments and future prospects will be discussed.

This chapter will discuss the treatment of metastatic bone pain in hormone-refractory prostate cancer patients with bone seeking radiopharmaceuticals. Two main issues will be discussed:

1. Bone seeking radiopharmaceuticals in clinical practice. Issues regarding radiation safety and a protocol for routine use of bone seeking radiopharmaceuticals will be discussed in order to improve routine clinical care.
2. Enhancement of efficacy of bone seeking radiopharmaceuticals.

But first a short introduction will be given on clinical relevance and bone seeking radiopharmaceuticals in general.

2. Prostate cancer and skeletal metastases

The incidence of malignancy in the Netherlands was 74.500 patients in 2005. This will increase to approximately 95.000 new cases in 2015. Because malignancy related death is decreasing and it is likely to decrease further the prevalence of cancer patients will increase to an estimated 692.000 patients in 2015, compared to 366.000 in 2000 (an estimated doubling time of 15 years) (Coebergh, van de Poll-Franse, and Alers 2004; Visser and van Noord 2005). One of the major causes of cancer related death in men is prostate cancer. These patients will be the focus of this chapter.

The incidence of prostate cancer is high worldwide. It is the most common malignancy in men in the Netherlands. Approximately 9000 men are being diagnosed with prostate cancer each year (Figure 1). The rising incidence may be attributed to the incremental use of screening methods using prostate specific antigen (PSA) to detect prostate cancer. This hypothesis is supported by the growing number of patients being diagnosed with early stages of prostate cancer. The incidence also increases with age. Consequently, with a growing number of old men in our society the incidence of prostate cancer will further increase. Fortunately mortality from prostate cancer is decreasing due to better diagnostic methods and treatments (Dijkman and Debruyne 1996).

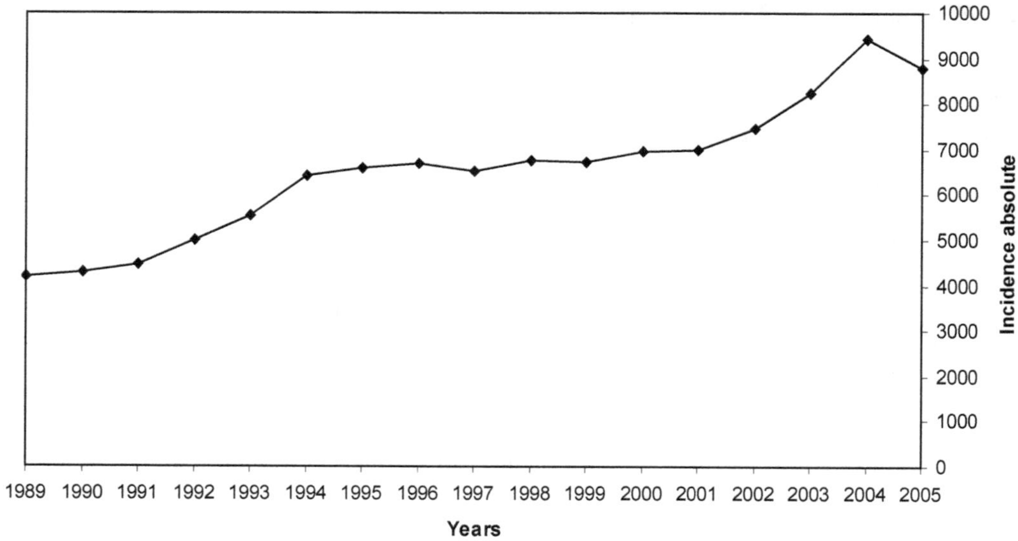

Fig. 1. Prostate cancer incidence between 1989 - 2005 derived from data on www.ikcnet.nl

A hallmark of metastatic prostate cancer is the development of osteoblastic bone metastases. Almost all patients with advanced prostate cancer eventually develop osseous metastases. In a majority of patients with prostate cancer, bone is the only site of clinical metastases. Many of the established prognostic factors for advanced prostate cancer (eg, performance status, alkaline phosphatase level, and haemoglobin level) reflect the clinical consequences of bone metastases. Hence, patients who develop widespread, progressive, or early bone metastases tend to suffer more from their symptoms and fare worse. Conversely, patients who develop limited, stable, or delayed bone metastases tend to experience less morbidity and have a less dismal clinical outcome. Conceivably, targeting the relevant bone metastases-associated factors may improve therapeutic results (Tu and Lin 2008). These factors consist of the main cells involved in bone metastasis (cancer cells, osteoblasts, osteoclasts, endothelial cells and stromal cells) and the numerous communicating substances (eg, interleukins, VEGF, RANKL, TNF-alfa, endothelins). They form a complex interaction and a microenvironment in which cancer cells may flourish (Tu and Lin 2008).

Frequently these skeletal metastases cause pain. Less common complications include myelum compression and pathological fractures (Dijkman and Debruyne 1996). Besides hormonal treatment most other treatment modalities in advanced prostate cancer patients are intended to palliate bone pain. Metastatic bone pain is a nociceptive somatic pain, initiated and maintained through local tissue injury. It is well recognized that chronic pain (including cancer pain) is a multidimensional phenomenon consisting of five dimensions (pathophysiological, sensory, emotional, cognitive, and behavioural). These five dimensions together form a complex pattern of relations (Quirijnen et al. 1996). Stress is a well known stimulus for nociceptive pain. The impression that pain may be uncontrollable produces stress for patients, which may lead to increased suffering and despair, and decreases the patient's performance (Chapman and Gavrin 1999). An effective pain management strategy requires breaking off this cycle using all available means. An effective pain control strategy, however, requires patients to take large quantities of opioids, often as much as 60 - 200 mg/day. This large dose may cause considerable side effects, including nausea, vomiting, constipation, and central sedation, all of which combine to a decrease in quality of life. Patients will have to take large doses of anti-emetics and laxatives to counteract nausea and constipation, respectively. Central sedation increases drowsiness, resulting in frequent falls, bone fractures, and driving accidents (Etches 1999). Supplemental therapy with local radiation, wide-field radiation, bisphosphonates, or bone seeking radiopharmaceuticals can significantly reduce the dose of opioids for most patients or may even completely eliminate the need for the medications in a few patients (Krishnamurthy and Krishnamurthy 2000).

Metastatic disease in prostate cancer may be treated first with hormonal therapy such as bilateral orchidectomy or medical first line hormone treatment (luteinizing hormone-releasing hormone agonist therapy). This androgen-deprivation therapy may be extended to maximal androgen blockade by adding anti-androgens (bicalutamide, flutamide, nilutamide). High risk prostate cancer patients may benefit from such a regimen even in the early stages of the disease (Klotz 2008). It is also recognized that discontinuation of an anti-androgen once hormone-refractory biochemical progression occurs is associated with a biochemical response in many patients. Anti-androgens may become agonistic due to a combination of androgen receptor over-expression and mutation (Kelly and Scher 1993; Small and Srinivas 1995). After a median of two years the prostate cancer cells generally become insensitive for hormonal treatment. In the case of hormone-refractory disease the patient may be treated by chemotherapy, local radiotherapy, systemic radiopharmaceuticals, bisphosphonates and analgesics, depending on the clinical status (Auclerc et al. 2000).

The clinical benefit of chemotherapy in hormone-refractory prostate cancer patients is limited. Some drugs showed potential as first-line treatment in hormone-refractory prostate carcinoma but were not sufficiently tested in clinical trials (Berthold, Sternberg, and Tannock 2005). Patients however may benefit from docetaxel chemotherapy in combination with prednisone. In a landmark study treatment with 75 mg/m^2 docetaxel i.v. every three weeks with 5 mg prednisone twice daily p.o. was compared with mitoxantrone 12 mg/m^2 every three weeks (Tannock et al. 2004). The median survival increased from 16.3 months in the mitoxantrone-group to 19.2 months in the docetaxel-group (Berthold et al. 2008). The group receiving docetaxel three weekly had a hazard ratio for death of 0.79 (95 percent confidence interval, 0.67 to 0.93; p=0.004) compared to the mitoxantrone-group (Berthold et al. 2008). Pain and quality of life improved significantly better in the docetaxel group and more patients (45% versus 32%; p<0.001) showed a 50% reduction of serum PSA levels (Tannock et al. 2004). However, docetaxel nor any other treatment will be curative in an advanced stage of prostate cancer.

Patients with hormone-refractory prostate cancer who have progressive disease after first-line chemotherapy may still benefit from several treatment options. At this stage of disease, patients can expect only a short duration of survival, and most patients become symptomatic. Most patients will cease docetaxel treatment because of progressive disease or unacceptable adverse events. To control symptoms after the cessation of chemotherapy should rely on optimizing medical therapy for palliation. This may be combined with radiotherapy applied to dominant painful bone lesions. External beam radiotherapy for painful skeletal metastases leads to a decrease of pain in 60 - 65% of the patients. In 33% of the patients a total remission of pain symptoms was observed (McQuay et al. 2008). Patients may be treated in one fraction (8 Gray). No difference has been found between such a single-dose regimen and multiple fractions (Hartsell et al. 2005; Kaasa et al. 2006; Roos et al. 2005). Furthermore, when needed, patients may be treated a second time with a reported response rate between 66% and 84% (Mithal, Needham, and Hoskin 1994; Van der Linden et al. 2004). Besides chemotherapy further hormonal manipulation with prednisone or dexamethasone may have some benefit as well. Glucocorticoids may lead to PSA response and/or relief of symptoms in patients with late-stage prostate cancer (Tannock et al. 1989). Some investigators have suggested that the superior results of regimens with taxanes may be due in part to the dexamethasone that is administered to avoid toxic reactions to these drugs. However, most patients have already received substantial treatment with glucocorticoids concurrent with first-line chemotherapy, so their potential benefit in later stages is probably minimal.

Other treatment options in the advanced stage of prostatic cancer include ketoconazole and estrogens. Inhibition of steroid synthesis by ketoconazole may increase the probability of an anti-androgen withdrawal response, although this did not translate into improved survival (Small et al. 2004). Estrogens may improve symptoms but caution must be used because of their ability to stimulate thrombosis and cardiovascular events. Estrogens were found to be equivalent to estramustine (which contains estrogen), probably as its activity is largely due to the estrogen component (Small et al. 2000). Transdermal administration of oestrogens through a patch avoids the entero-hepatic circulation and therefore it should not be associated with the same level of cardiovascular toxicity. Early data confirm the safety and efficacy of oestrogen patches as hormonal treatment in prostate cancer patients (Langley et al. 2008).

Currently new non chemotherapeutic options are studied such as endotheline antagonists (James et al. 2008) and abiraterone acetate, a potent, selective, small-molecule inhibitor of cytochrome P (CYP) 17, a key enzyme in androgen synthesis (Attard et al. 2008). Many other agents are being developed (Tu and Lin 2008).

3. Bone seeking radiopharmaceuticals

Bone seeking radiopharmaceuticals have proven to be useful for treatment of more generalized bone pain. All patients will finally progress to end stage disease with multiple skeletal metastases. These patients may receive bone seeking radiopharmaceuticals for generalized painful disease (Berthold, Sternberg, and Tannock 2005). The association of integrated cancer centres in the Netherlands (VIKC) developed an evidence based guideline on the diagnosis and treatment of pain in cancer patients. Radionuclide treatment of cancer patients with metastatic bone pain (so called bone seeking radiopharmaceuticals) was evaluated using all available literature (VIKC 2008). The conclusions are stated together with their level of evidence in Table 1.

Most of the patients who have participated in the mentioned trials were heavily pre-treated patients with previous radiotherapy, chemotherapy and/or hormone therapy. It was recommended that radionuclide treatment with bone seeking radiopharmaceuticals is indicated in patients with multifocal pain originating from osteoblastic skeletal metastases.

Repeated treatments are indicated after an initial response to treatment. The committee had the opinion that combined multimodality treatment should be performed in a trial setting. Further research in that field is warranted (VIKC 2008).
Radionuclide therapy with bone seeking radiopharmaceutical agents has been long used. It evolved from agents like ^{32}P-phosphate to newer agents like ^{188}Re-HEDP or ^{223}Ra (Table 2). Bone seeking radiopharmaceuticals consist of a radionuclide for the therapeutic effect and a carrier to reach the target site at the bone matrix level. Sometimes the carrier and the radionuclide are one and the same. This is the case for ^{32}P-phosphate, ^{223}Ra and ^{89}Sr. These radiopharmaceuticals behave as physiologic phosphate (^{32}P-phosphate) or Ca^{2+}-analogues (^{223}Ra and ^{89}Sr). They do not need a non-radioactive substance as a carrier to reach the target. Carriers like hydroxyethylenediphosphonic acid (HEDP in ^{186}Re-HEDP) and ethylenediaminetetramethylenephosphonic acid (EDTMP in ^{153}Sm-EDTMP) are being used in other bone seeking radiopharmaceuticals. They behave as bisphosphonates. These differences influence the biodistribution and pharmacokinetics of the pharmaceutical. Other differences between these agents include the radiation type, the radiation energy and the radionuclide half-life.
One thing that never changed during the last decades and stimulated the search for new agents was the conflict between efficacy and toxicity. The latter consisting of bone marrow suppression in particular. This has even led to a change of indication for the use of ^{32}P-phosphate. It is not used anymore for the palliation of metastatic bone pain but instead for the treatment of myeloproliferative diseases, making use of its bone marrow suppressive potential (Berlin 2000; Cheung and Driedger 1980). Fortunately newer agents have proved to be feasible and relatively safe for the palliative treatment of osseous metastases with acceptable and reversible bone marrow toxicity.

Conclusion	Evidence [a]	Study type [b]
It has been proven that treatment with bone seeking radiopharmaceuticals yields a better pain response than treatment with placebo in patients with painful osseous metastases from diverse cancers including prostate, breast and lung cancer.	Level 1	A1 (Bauman et al. 2005; Finlay, Mason, and Shelley 2005; McQuay et al. 2008; Roque i Figuls et al. 2008) A2 (Han et al. 2002; Lewington et al. 1991; Maxon, III et al. 1991; Sartor et al. 2004; Serafini et al. 1998)
It has been proven that no difference exists with regard to local pain response between treatment with ^{89}Sr-Chloride or external beam radiotherapy in patients with painful osseous metastases from a prostate carcinoma.	Level 1	A2 (Oosterhof et al. 2003; Quilty et al. 1994)
It is likely that no difference exists with regard to pain response between treatment with ^{89}Sr-Chloride and ^{186}Re-HEDP in patients with painful osseous metastases.	Level 2	A2 (Sciuto et al. 2001) B (Piffanelli et al. 2001)

Conclusion	Evidence [a]	Study type [b]
It is likely that the onset of the pain response of ^{186}Re-HEDP is faster than the onset of the pain response of ^{89}Sr-Chloride in patients with painful osseous metastases from a breast carcinoma.	Level 2	A2 (Sciuto et al. 2001)
It is likely that combined treatment with ^{89}Sr-Chloride and chemotherapy (platinum based) yields a better pain response than treatment without chemotherapy in patients with painful osseous metastases from a prostate carcinoma.	Level 2	A2 (Sciuto et al. 2002) C (Sciuto et al. 1996)
It has been suggested that adding ^{89}Sr-Chloride to chemotherapy may lead to improved survival and a longer duration of the pain response compared to treatment with chemotherapy alone.	Level 3	B (Tu et al. 2001)
It has been suggested that no difference exists with regard to the pain response after treatment with chemotherapy or ^{89}Sr-Chloride in patients with painful osseous metastases from a prostate carcinoma.	Level 3	B (Nilsson et al. 2005)
No conclusions can be drawn on the value of adding ^{89}Sr-Chloride to external beam radiotherapy in patients with painful osseous metastases from a prostate carcinoma because of conflicting results.		A2 (Porter et al. 1993; Smeland et al. 2003)

[a] Level of evidence: 1) A1 or at least two independent and consistent A2 studies; 2) One A2 study or at least two independent and consistent B studies; 3) One B or C study; 4) Professional opinion.
[b] Quality and methodology of studies: A1) Systemic review of at least two independent A2 trials; A2) Double-blind randomized trial of sufficient size and quality (comparison with a reference test ('gold standard'), defined endpoints, independent evaluation of both tests, no confounding); B) Comparative trial not meeting A2 criteria;
[c] Non-comparative trial; D) Professional opinion.

Table 1. Evidence based conclusions on treatment with bone seeking radiopharmaceuticals (VIKC 2008).

Radiopharmaceutical	Half-life (days)	β-emission MeV max (mean)	γ-emission keV (%)
^{188}Re-HEDP	0.7	2.12 (0.76)	155 (15%)
^{153}Sm-EDTMP	1.93	0.81 (0.23)	103 (29%)
^{186}Re-HEDP	3.7	1.07 (0.35)	137 (9%)
^{177}Lu-EDTMP	6.7	0.497 (0.15)	208 (11%)
^{223}Ra	11.4	Emits alfa-particles of circa 5.7 MeV	
^{117m}Sn-DTPA	13.6	Emits conversion electrons 127 - 152 keV	
^{32}P-Phosphate	14.3	1.71 (0.70)	None
^{89}Sr	50.5	1.46 (0.58)	910 (0.01%)

Table 2. Bone seeking radiopharmaceuticals categorized by half-life.

All patients with proven osteoblastic (or mixed type) skeletal metastases that accumulate ^{99m}Tc-HDP on skeletal scintigraphy may be candidates for treatment with bone seeking radiopharmaceuticals. They may be cancer patients with advanced disease originating from prostate cancer, breast cancer, lung cancer, medullary thyroid carcinoma, or other tumors (i.e. bronchial carcinoid tumors, medulloblastoma). In routine clinical practice the vast majority of patients are prostate cancer patients. In these patients the incidence of skeletal metastases is very high. They cause high morbidity and mortality (DePuy et al. 2007; Saarto et al. 2002). Metastases originating from prostate cancer are pure osteoblastic with relatively high radionuclide uptake, resulting in high tumor to non-tumor ratio's. And last but not least other treatment options are limited in advanced stages of this disease.

In the growing field of radionuclide therapy many new radiopharmaceuticals are being developed. At the moment $^{89}SrCl_2$ (Metastron®) and ^{153}Sm-EDTMP (Quadramet®) are both FDA approved. Together with ^{186}Re-HEDP (registered in some countries, not in the Netherlands) these bone seeking radiopharmaceuticals are mostly used today.

4. Bone seeking radiopharmaceuticals in clinical practice

4.1 Radiation safety considerations

Patients treated with any kind of radionuclide treatment must be regarded as a potential risk for public health because of a potential radiation hazard. Good understanding of the radionuclide used, its physical characteristics, its biodistribution and its pharmacokinetics, will allow us to draw proper guidelines for this kind of treatment. Does the patient need to be confined after treatment? Are we able to identify the radiation hazard from a qualitative and quantitative perspective? What does that mean for an individual patient in relation to its environment?

Patients treated with 89SrCl2, 186Re-HEDP or 153Sm-EDTMP are a source of radiation, including beta-radiation that has proven to be measurable outside the patient. Beta-particles in superficial tissue (such as in bones, blood vessels) cross the skin and contribute to the ambient equivalent dose. This aspect must be considered when using beta-emitting radiopharmaceuticals in general. The calculated effective doses for bystanders are well below the recommended values and do not lead to unacceptable additional radiation burden to health care workers and patients' families. The mean total effective doses absorbed by bystanders at 30 cm distance from a patient are approximately 0.02 mSv for 89SrCl2, 0.3 mSv for 186Re-HEDP, and 1.6 mSv for 153Sm-EDTMP (Lam et al. 2009b). These observations however should be placed in some perspective. First the

individual variation in effective dose to bystanders and second the potential risk of internal contamination of bystanders.
The total effective dose, as given above, is estimated for bystanders who reside at exactly 30 cm from the patient for an indefinite time. Because this is never the case, these estimations must be corrected for variations in time and distance between bystanders and patients. In a Dutch Ministry of Housing, Spatial Planning and Environment publication accurate calculations were made to cover the various persons who may have contact with patients (VRO92; VROM 2005). These calculations are based on residence times T (in fractions of days) with the patient and distances R (in meters) from the patient. The actual effective doses for bystanders will depend on residence times and distances in relation to the patient. Estimations were made for residence times and distances during a 24-hour period. This was done in the case of an elderly patient in relation to his or her partner and in the case of a patient in relation to his or her child (Tables 3 and 4).

	Without instruction			With instruction		
	Residence time (hrs/24hrs)	Distance (m)	Correction factor [a]	Residence time (hrs/24hrs)	Distance (m)	Correction factor [a]
outdoors activities	3/24	-	0	3/24	-	0
watching TV	5/24	0.5	0.075	5/24	2	0.0047
dinner	2/24	1	0.0075	2/24	1	0.0075
sleeping	8/24	0.7	0.061	8/24	2	0.0075
other	6/24	3	0.0025	6/24	3	0.0025
total			0.15			0.02
	Mean effective dose (mSv)			Mean effective dose (mSv)		
^{153}Sm-EDTMP	0.24			0.03		
^{186}Re-HEDP	0.05			< 0.01		
^{89}Sr-Chloride	< 0.01			< 0.01		

[a] Correction factor applicable for measurements at 30 cm from the patient using the inverse-square law

Table 3. Effective dose (external radiation) of *an elderly partner* with and without instructions.

Assuming that the estimated distances and times are a reflection of reality, corrections were made for these circumstances. Estimations of the effective doses for these persons (partner and child) are given for the three most used radiopharmaceuticals. In the case of a patient and his or her partner, without instructions a correction factor of 0.15 (15%) was applied. This is explained by the fact that bystanders do not stay within 30 cm of patients 24 hours a day. Because of work and other activities a correction factor should be applied. As an example a correction factor of 0.15 may be applied. The effective dose may be further reduced by instructing the patients and their families to keep distance as much as reasonably possible (e.g. watching TV and sleeping apart). With proper instructions to family, residence times may be reduced and distances increased, lowering the correction factor to as low as 0.02 (2%), an almost eight-fold decrease in radiation burden to bystanders (Table 3). In the case of a patient and his or her child an estimated correction factor of about 0.43 (43%) should be applied without instructions and 0.11 (11%) with instructions. In all instances effective doses will be < 1 mSv and with proper instructions they will be < 0.1 mSv or even < 0.01 mSv (Tables 3 and 4). It may be concluded that patients treated with bone seeking radiopharmaceuticals do not pose any threat to others.

	Without instruction			With instruction		
	Residence time (hrs/24hrs)	Distance (m)	Correction factor [a]	Residence time (hrs/24hrs)	Distance (m)	Correction factor [a]
playing	8/24	4	0.0019	8/24	4	0.0019
close contact	1/24	0.1	0.375	0.25/24	0.1	0.094
dinner	2/24	0.5	0.03	2/24	2	0.0019
sleeping	10/24	-	-	10/24	-	-
other	3/24	2	0.0094	3/24	2	0.0094
total			0.43			0.11
	Effective dose (mSv)			Effective dose (mSv)		
^{153}Sm-EDTMP	0.69			0.18		
^{186}Re-HEDP	0.13			0.03		
^{89}Sr-Chloride	< 0.01			< 0.01		

[a] Correction factor applicable for measurements at 30 cm from the patient using the inverse-square law

Table 4. Effective dose (external radiation) of *a young child* with and without instructions.

However, an exception has to be made considering urinary excretion of activity and the possible internal contamination of bystanders. Besides radiation exposure to non-patients from direct emission by the patient, another potential radiation hazard is formed by excreted radioactivity. The calculated mean total urinary excretion percentage of ^{89}Sr during the first 3 days after administration was 16% (Lam et al. 2009b). Using a hypothetical contamination scenario, that is used in radiation protection evaluation (VROM 2005), that 0.01% of the excreted amount of radioactivity will cause internal contamination to non-patients closely related to the patient, an internal dosage of 0.0024 MBq for $^{89}SrCl_2$ therapy (administered dose of 150 MBq) was calculated. For ^{186}Re-HEDP therapy (administered dose of 1295 MBq), the corresponding amount of radioactivity will be 0.064 MBq (49% of the injected dose is excreted (de Klerk et al. 1992)). After treatment with 37 MBq/kg ^{153}Sm-EDTMP 53.1% ± 15.1% of the administered dose was excreted in urine during the first 48 hours (Lam et al. 2007). Potential contamination with 0.01% of the excreted radioactivity will lead to an internal dosage of 0.15 MBq ^{153}Sm-EDTMP. The dose conversion coefficient for ingestion of ^{89}Sr is (e_{ing}) = 2.6 x 10^{-9} Sv/Bq, of ^{186}Re (e_{ing}) = 1.5 10^{-9} Sv/Bq, and of ^{153}Sm (e_{ing}) = 7.4 10^{-10} Sv/Bq. The present data show that the effective radiation absorbed dose, caused by a potential internal contamination (0.01% of the administered dose), is 6.2 microSv for ^{89}Sr, 96 microSv for ^{186}Re and 111 microSv for ^{153}Sm. These numbers are in the same order of magnitude as the numbers given for external exposure (Table 3 and 4).

The total effective dose for non-patients may be caused by both external radiation exposure and internal contamination. In contrast to the mean effective dose caused by external radiation, the effective dose after ingestion of 0.01% of the administered dose is hypothetical and may be much higher or much lower. In the case of ^{131}I it proved to be less. The uptake of ^{131}I in the thyroid of family members was measured (Buchan and Brindle 1970). A maximum uptake of 3.8 Bq per MBq administered was found. So on one hand it must be considered that 0.01% is a hypothetical figure, while the external radiation exposure is a fact. On the other hand, internal contamination poses a real threat to non-patients. Patients that were treated with bone-seeking radiopharmaceuticals are often severely disabled (in contrast to ^{131}I patients). Especially in the case of prostate cancer patients, they often have dysurea. Personal hygiene is not as obvious as it is to others. It is therefore advisable to give the patients simple, easy-to-follow instructions, in order to reduce the risk for non-patients. Using a separate toilet, sitting while urinating and washing hands afterwards, are highly recommended. In the case of incontinence, patients must be catheterized for a certain time depending on urinary excretion of the administered activity. Due to fast renal excretion this may be 12 hours after injection of ^{186}Re-HEDP and ^{153}Sm-EDTMP. $^{89}SrCl_2$ is being administered in relatively low doses and therefore has a relatively low risk for high effective dose due to ingestion of this radiopharmaceutical (6.2 microSv for ^{89}Sr). These patients do not have to be catheterized. The risk for significant internal contamination of non-patients is much lower and acceptable for this radiopharmaceutical.

In general it is advised to hospitalize patients treated with ^{186}Re-HEDP and ^{153}Sm-EDTMP for at least 8 hours. This is mostly based on urinary excretion and the risk for internal contamination, because the radiation exposure to non-patients is < 20 microSv/hour (1 meter from the patients) directly or within a few hours after administration in all cases. In the case of incontinence it is advised to treat patients with either ^{186}Re-HEDP or ^{153}Sm-EDTMP with a urinary catheter for 12 hours after administration. Patients treated with $^{89}SrCl_2$ may return home directly.

After discharge it is advisable to keep distance where possible (Table 3 and 4), following the ALARA ('as low as reasonably achievable') principles. This means, for example, that older patients (> 60 years) may still sleep close to their older partner, while being more stringent towards younger relatives to avoid any unnecessary radiation dose. The ICRP has proposed an effective dose limit of 1 mSv per year for individuals. In special circumstances a higher value may be allowed in a single year provided that the average over 5 years does not exceed 1 mSv per year. In clinical practice, the use of bone-seeking radiopharmaceuticals will give rise to a degree of radiation exposure to all those in contact with patients, albeit in very low doses. The present results further confirm the safety of treatment with bone-seeking radiopharmaceuticals.

4.2 Treatment recommendations

$^{89}SrCl_2$ (Metastron®) and ^{153}Sm-EDTMP (Quadramet®) are both FDA approved and registered in the Netherlands. Together with ^{186}Re-HEDP (registered in some countries, not in the Netherlands) these bone seeking radiopharmaceuticals are mostly used. Most of the randomized double-blind placebo controlled trials have been performed using $^{89}SrCl_2$ or ^{153}Sm-

EDTMP. An evidence based approach would be a choice between these radiopharmaceuticals. One of the differences between these two is the magnitude and rate of renal excretion. Both may be used without confining a patient to the hospital but from a radiation safety perspective it is advised to keep the patient in a controlled setting for at least 8 hours after injection in the case of ^{153}Sm-EDTMP. This could influence the choice on practical grounds in favour of $^{89}SrCl_2$. Not all nuclear medicine departments have such facilities.

Other differences include the longer half-life and higher energy (with higher range in tissue) of $^{89}SrCl_2$ compared to ^{153}Sm-EDTMP. ^{153}Sm-EDTMP and ^{186}Re-HEDP are highly comparable with regard to energy and half-life. Most comparative randomized studies have been performed using $^{89}SrCl_2$ and ^{186}Re-HEDP. It was found that no difference exist with regard to pain response between treatment with ^{89}Sr-Chloride and ^{186}Re-HEDP in patients with painful osseous metastases (Piffanelli et al. 2001; Sciuto et al. 2001). And that the onset of the pain response of ^{186}Re-HEDP is faster than the onset of the pain response of ^{89}Sr-Chloride in patients with painful osseous metastases from a breast carcinoma (Sciuto et al. 2001). So one might argue that when a faster pain response is indicated one should use ^{186}Re-HEDP or ^{153}Sm-EDTMP. Other differences are the longer duration of response of ^{89}Sr-Chloride on one hand, and the prolonged bone marrow toxicity of ^{89}Sr-Chloride on the other hand. These differences were not investigated in direct comparative studies but should be considered nevertheless. In summary: in favour of ^{89}Sr-Chloride are:

- No confinement necessary
- Longer duration of response (suitable in relatively good clinical condition in which a prompt response is not warranted)

In favour of ^{186}Re-HEDP or ^{153}Sm-EDTMP are:

- Fast response (suitable in bad clinical condition in which immediate response is wanted)
- Favourable toxicity profile (suitable in heavily pre-treated patients, in wide spread metastatic disease and possibly in combination with other myelotoxic treatments)

In most cases today a fast response is needed. Besides that most patients, including prostate cancer patients, are heavily pre-treated. They have end stage disease with minimal bone marrow reserve. And last but not least short-living bone seeking radiopharmaceuticals like ^{186}Re-HEDP, ^{153}Sm-EDTMP and others may prove to be more suitable in combination with other treatment modalities, not just because of their toxicity profile but also because of their high dose rate, offering an effective treatment with fast recovery.

5. Enhancement of efficacy

A major concern in the treatment of prostate cancer patients in the more advanced stage of the disease is the delicate balance between efficacy and toxicity. Treatment of metastatic bone pain with analgesics or localized external beam radiotherapy is relatively safe and easy. Treatment with bone seeking radiopharmaceuticals may be more appropriate in selected cases but efficacy is sometimes disappointing and bone marrow toxicity may be high in individual patients. Enhancement of overall efficacy without increasing toxicity could push the clinical decision algorithm in a positive direction with regard to the use of bone seeking radiopharmaceuticals.

One way of improving overall efficacy is combined treatment. Combined treatment regimens may deliver the beneficial effect of two different treatment modalities. These combinations may not only be additive but possibly synergistic to each other, leading to enhancement of overall efficacy with acceptable toxicity.

5.1 Multimodality treatment

The propensity of prostate cancer to metastasize to bone and the prognostic significance of bone metastases suggest that effective treatment of bone metastases may provide clinical benefits (DePuy et al. 2007; Sabbatini et al. 1999). With regard to the 'seed' and 'soil' theory on bone metastases the seed may comprise the so-called cancer stem cells. Whereas the soil may comprise a unique microenvironment, that facilitate the growth and survival of cancer stem cells. Targeting the microenvironment may offer another way to improve treatment of prostate cancer bone metastases. The microenvironment consists of osteoclasts, osteoblasts, endothelium and stroma. In the presence of cancer stem cells they interact leading to a disruption in normal coupling between osteoclasts and osteoblasts. An improved understanding of this process will influence how we select agents to target bone metastases and how we design strategies to treat prostate cancer bone metastases. Treatments may be directed to the cancer stem cells, the osteoblasts, the osteoclasts, the endothelium or the stroma (Tu and Lin 2008).

Osteoblasts may be targeted by several pharmaceuticals including bone seeking radiopharmaceuticals. Other osteoblast directed treatments include endothelin-1-antagonists (atrasentan) (Carducci et al. 2003), vitamin D analogs (1,25-hydroxyvitamin D_3) (Beer et al. 2007), monoclonal IGF-1R (insulin-like growth factor-1-receptor) antibodies (Boyle et al. 2001) and CXRC4 (G-protein-coupled receptor) inhibitors (MSX-122), which inhibit the homing behaviour of cancer stem cells. Osteoclast activity may be inhibited by bisphosphonates (zolendronate) (Saad et al. 2002), RANK ligand inhibitors (denosumab) (Lewiecki 2006), tyrosine kinase inhibitors (dasatinib) or IL-6 antagonists (CNTO328) (Nam et al. 2005). And the endothelium and/or stroma may be targeted by anti-angiogenesis therapies. These include the vascular endothelial growth factor (VEGF) receptor antagonists bevacizumab, thalidomide and lenalidomide (Dahut et al. 2004). They reduce VEGF levels and basic fibroblast growth factor, inhibit growth and survival of tumor cells by modulation of adhesion molecules and mediate various cytokines. Also targeted to the endothelium are platelet-derived growth factor receptor (PDGFR) tyrosine kinase inhibitors (imatinib, sunitinib and tandutinib) (Ko et al. 2001). They may also have anti-angiogenetic potential. Most of these agents are under investigation. Many clinical studies in prostate cancer patients are ongoing (Tu and Lin 2008).

Combining different treatment modalities may be interesting because of additive effects or synergy effects. In the case of bisphosphonates and bone seeking radiopharmaceuticals the combined use has always been contra-indicated because of presumed interaction at the bone matrix level. It was shown that the combined use of ^{153}Sm-EDTMP and bisphosphonates in patients with hormone-refractory prostate carcinoma is feasible. The combined treatment regimen is safe and may prove to be an effective long-term treatment regimen (Lam et al. 2007).

Another combined treatment regimen would be a combination of bone seeking radiopharmaceuticals and chemotherapy. It is likely that combined treatment with ^{89}Sr-Chloride and chemotherapy (platinum based) yields a better pain response than treatment without chemotherapy in patients with painful osseous metastases from a prostate carcinoma (Sciuto et al. 2002), (Sciuto et al. 1996). And it has been suggested that adding

^{89}Sr-Chloride to chemotherapy may lead to improved survival and a longer duration of the pain response compared to treatment with chemotherapy alone (Tu et al. 2001). Studies are yet limited but they are encouraging. Most of them have been performed using ^{89}Sr-Chloride and some using ^{153}Sm-EDTMP (Ricci et al. 2007). Patients may possibly have an improved pain response and longer survival. In prostate cancer patients a most interesting choice would be combining docetaxel and a bone seeking radiopharmaceutical. These studies, using ^{153}Sm-EDTMP or ^{186}Re-HEDP, are underway. Our group investigated the combination of ^{188}Re-HEDP and capecitabine (Xeloda®) (Lam et al. 2009a). This treatment regimen proved to be feasible and safe. Phase II efficacy testing using the maximum tolerable dose of 2500 mg/m^2/day capecitabine is underway. Capecitabine is primarily used as a radiation sensitizer. It offers a convenient therapy with acceptable toxicity, ease of use as oral tablets and low costs. The same is true for ^{188}Re-HEDP. It is homemade on demand and has favourable physical characteristics with a short half-life (16.9 hours) and high beta-energy ($E_{\beta\ max}$ 2.12 MeV; $E_{\beta\ mean}$ 0.76 MeV). In theory, this high dose rate could lead to improved efficacy with rapid recovery. This is ideal for combined treatment regimens and for repeated treatment, which has already shown to be favourable with regard to pain response and survival (Palmedo et al. 2003).

Several other combinations using bone seeking radiopharmaceuticals are under investigation. Currently, a randomized phase III study (MDA-3410/CTSU in M.D. Anderson Cancer Center, Houston, Texas) combining weekly doxorubicin (20 mg/m^2) with ^{89}Sr-Chloride after response to induction chemotherapy is underway, as well as another phase I trial combining docetaxel/prednisone and ^{153}Sm-EDTMP, also at M.D. Anderson (Tu and Lin 2008). It remains to be established whether targeting both the tumor (chemotherapy) and bone compartments will improve therapeutic efficacy. This concept is also being tested in multiple other trials, mostly combining docetaxel/prednisone with bone environment directed treatments, like the agents described above (Tu and Lin 2008). The described studies add to this search for optimized treatment regimens in hormone-refractory prostate cancer patients.

5.2 Predictions of efficacy and toxicity

Most patients with advanced prostate cancer have disease limited to the bone, which is notoriously difficult to assess for response, with a small subset having soft tissue lesions. To limit response evaluation to only patients with bidimensionally measurable disease would eliminate 70% to 80% of patients who would otherwise be evaluable (Figg et al. 1996). With regard to prostate cancer patients efficacy of treatment has been monitored by PSA in a majority of studies. However it is doubtful whether PSA changes correlate with clinical benefit (Bubley et al. 1999). A 50% decrease in PSA level seems a reasonable predictor of a favourable outcome, but this was certainly not the case in all studies (Bauer et al. 1999; Sridhara et al. 1995). It was advised not to use PSA level drops as a surrogate marker for survival (Bubley et al. 1999).

In patients with advanced disease, survival and quality of life, including pain palliation, are the most important criteria of clinical response. Besides survival these parameters are difficult to measure and subject to errors. With an attempt to standardize treatment response monitoring in cancer patients the European Organization for Research and Treatment of Cancer (EORTC) has developed quality of life questionnaires (EORTC QLQ-C30 version 3.0). They were validated in many clinical trials (Aaronson et al. 1993). They include questions on global health status / quality of life, functional scales and symptom scales. The functional scales are subdivided in physical functioning, role functioning, emotional functioning, cognitive functioning and social functioning. The symptom scales are subdivided in fatigue, nausea and vomiting, pain, dyspnoea, insomnia, appetite loss, constipation, diarrhoea and financial difficulties. Each domain was scored on a scale of 0 - 100, according to the EORTC scoring manual (Fayers et al. 2001). The changes in scores may be used to monitor clinical effect.

Other often used clinical monitoring tools include the visual analogue scales (VAS) to monitor pain, changes in analgesic intake and, more basic, the physician's assessment based on anamnesis and physical examination. A matter of debate is the frequency of evaluation. It seems that daily assessment is necessary to appreciate the wide variation in clinical status that patients may experience from day to day (Han et al. 2002). In all cases it is difficult to find a good balance between accuracy and compliance. PSA is therefore still popular to measure an objective level of response (Bubley et al. 1999; Scher et al. 2008).

However, other predictors of response may prove to be much more reliable than PSA. In hormone-refractory prostate cancer patients in advanced stages of their disease the extent of metastatic disease in the skeleton is of high prognostic significance (Sabbatini et al. 1999). Furthermore it was shown that patients with advanced disease who had experienced a so-called Skeletal Related Event (defined as: pathologic fracture, spinal cord compression with vertebral compression fracture, the need for surgery to treat or prevent pathologic fractures or spinal cord compression, or the need for radiation to bone) had a significantly worse survival and poorer quality of life, in comparison with patients who had not experienced a Skeletal Related Event (DePuy et al. 2007). These results further confirm the importance to treat skeletal metastases adequately. Markers of skeletal metabolism were found to be related to outcome and survival. In several clinical studies in prostate cancer patients it was observed that markers of bone metabolism were able to predict outcome, both as absolute levels pre-treatment and as changes after treatment (Jung et al. 2004; Lein et al. 2007). In large series of cancer patients, including a majority of prostate cancer patients, treated with zoledronic acid, it was found that baseline levels of the bone marker urinary N-terminal type I collagen peptide [NTX], as well as changes of NTX after treatment were able to predict improved survival (Coleman et al. 2005; Lipton et al. 2008). Other studies emphasized the importance of the bone marker serum bone specific alkaline phosphatase [BAP] as a predictor of outcome (Cook et al. 2006; Smith et al. 2007). Most of these studies used the same bone markers as we did in the study on the combined treatment of prostate cancer patients with ^{153}Sm-EDTMP and zoledronic acid (i.e. NTX, BAP and serum procollagen type I N propeptide [PINP],). Although this study comprised a small patient population the results are of interest because they confirm the utility of these markers as predictors of clinical outcome, even in small numbers (Lam et al. 2007). Besides, they were first tested in the treatment monitoring of bone seeking radiopharmaceuticals. The bone formation markers BAP and PINP were in agreement with the clinical effect of the combined treatment regimen evaluated by EORTC questionnaires. The bone resorption marker NTX and PSA were not in agreement with the clinical effect. This supports the hypothesis that the extent of osteoblastic metastasis in hormone-refractory prostate cancer patients is an important parameter for clinical outcome. Both treatment itself and treatment monitoring should be directed to these osteoblastic metastases. Bone markers may well prove to be very useful predictors of clinical effect in the treatment with bone seeking radiopharmaceuticals. They should be used in future trials.

Last but not least the importance of imaging modalities should be mentioned with regard to individualized treatment monitoring. Functional rather than anatomical imaging techniques may be used to predict response. Several PET (Positron Emission Tomography) techniques are being developed for this purpose (John et al. 2008; Price et al. 2002). In fact, functional imaging will prove to be one of the major contributions of nuclear medicine to clinical oncology in the future. Does the treatment work? That question needs to be answered for each oncologic treatment on an individual basis. Nuclear imaging and PET in particular may be helpful.

Besides predictors of efficacy, predictors of toxicity are equally important for individualized patient management. Radiopharmaceuticals are important resources in the management of bone pain, but they need to be utilized in a manner that does not prevent other systemic therapy (Rago 1998). Thrombocytopenia is the dose limiting factor in treatment of painful bone metastases with bone seeking radiopharmaceuticals. De Klerk *et al* evaluated thrombocytopenia in patients with hormone refractory prostate carcinoma, treated with ^{186}Re-HEDP (de Klerk et al. 1994). As an index of the extent of bone involvement, the bone scan index (BSI) was determined from the pre-treatment ^{99m}Tc-HDP scintigram. The BSI is a tool to describe the extent of skeletal metastases on a scale from 0 to 100% (Blake et al. 1986). They described a functional relation ($r = 0.78$; $p < 0.001$) of the percentage of platelet decrease after treatment with the extent and distribution of skeletal metastases (BSI) and administered activity, normalized to standard body surface area. Using this relation, it is possible to predict thrombocytopenia by pre-treatment skeletal scintigraphy and to adjust the dosage for each patient to avoid unacceptable toxicity (de Klerk et al. 1994).

However, more sophisticated indices of bone marrow function might also be of paramount importance. Recently, some very interesting reports have been published on 'reticulated platelets' (Briggs et al. 2004; Wang et al. 2002). In systemic radionuclide therapy, the megakaryocyte seems to be most vulnerable to radiation. It is of great interest to gain more knowledge of bone marrow function pre-treatment using 'biological' parameters like 'reticulated platelets'. These newly released platelets are larger and contain RNA. They were suggested to be the platelet analogue of the red cell reticulocyt. Assessment of platelet production using 'reticulated platelets' would distinguish between thrombocytopenia due to bone marrow failure and impending bone marrow recovery after cytotoxic therapy or thrombocytopenia due to increased peripheral platelet destruction and turnover. In both cases platelet levels are low, but in the latter 'reticulated platelet' levels will be high due to increased production (Wang et al. 2002). This non-invasive measurement could further increase our knowledge of platelet production and the influence of radiation on this process.

By adding hematological, chemical and biological parameters, combined with the bone scan index, body surface area, administered activity and retained activity, an extended version of 'De Klerk's formula' may be developed. This is probably best done as a so called nomogram. Smaletz *et al* developed a nomogram to predict survival for patients with hormone refractory prostate carcinoma (Smaletz et al. 2002). A nomogram is a model in which individual parameters lead to a chance (from 0 to 100%) to experience a pre-defined outcome. The outcome may be defined as survival or for example toxicity. Such a model can be made to predict hematological toxicity (thrombocytopenia, leucopenia) after treatment with bone seeking radiopharmaceuticals to improve individualized patient management.

6. Future prospects

Several future implications have already been discussed above. One of the most important developments for bone seeking radiopharmaceuticals will be individualized medicine. The search for an optimized balance between efficacy and toxicity will be found rather in an individualized treatment plan than in new agents. Good predictors of efficacy and toxicity are needed for treatment monitoring. Several potential candidates were described above. They may be found in clinical evaluation, imaging and several laboratory parameters. A combination of these parameters may lead to a prediction model which may be used in daily practice.

Multimodality treatment has also been described above. Many combinations have potential. It has to be investigated which regimen will be most effective. Besides a direct anti-tumor effect which may be reached with chemotherapy (i.e. docetaxel), it is recognized that treatment directed to the bony environment may add to the overall efficacy of the treatment regimen. Bone seeking radiopharmaceuticals are bone-directed and may be of value in combination with other treatment modalities. Besides combinations with chemotherapy or bisphosphonates other interesting combinations may include for example atrasentan, or denosumab.

An important other issue is the timing of treatment with bone seeking radiopharmaceuticals. The frequency and interval of sequential treatment should be considered. Bone seeking radiopharmaceuticals are mostly used as a single shot treatment. When patients respond to the treatment repeated treatment is considered. In most instances this does not happen with a planned interval in mind but rather when symptoms reappear after an initial response. In fact this might be too late. It seems better to treat patients sequentially before symptoms reoccur. This was confirmed in a randomized controlled trial in prostate cancer patients treated with two dosages of 1.1 mCi ^{188}Re-HEDP with an interval of eight weeks compared to single shot treatment. They did not only find an improved pain response with longer duration but surprisingly an improved survival as well (Palmedo et al. 2003). Safety of repeated treatment with bone seeking radiopharmaceuticals was also confirmed (Sartor et al. 2007). This enhancement of efficacy may be attributed to chronic inhibition of osseous metabolism preventing cancer cells to thrive in the bony environment. Most other oncologic compounds are used in a repeated fashion using several cycles to reach sufficient effect. It should be investigated which multiple treatment regimen is most suitable for bone seeking radiopharmaceuticals, and whether it is safe and more effective. It may be suggested that the best result in hormone-refractory will be reached using a multimodality treatment regimen with fractionation of all treatments to be effective over a prolonged period of time.

7. Conclusion

Treatment with bone seeking radiopharmaceuticals in patients with multiple painful skeletal metastases is safe and effective when proper protocols are being used. Important improvements may be found in multimodality treatment in long-term treatment regimens and in individualized patient management. Identification of powerful indicators of toxicity and efficacy may guide patient selection and therapy monitoring to optimize the patient's outcome. This may possibly lead us beyond pain palliation towards improvement of survival.

8. References

Aaronson NK et al (1993) The European Organization for Research and Treatment of Cancer QLQ-C30: a quality-of-life instrument for use in international clinical trials in oncology. *J.Natl.Cancer Inst.* 85 (5):365-376.

Attard G et al (2008) Phase I clinical trial of a selective inhibitor of CYP17, abiraterone acetate, confirms that castration-resistant prostate cancer commonly remains hormone driven. *J.Clin.Oncol.* 26 (28):4563-4571.

Auclerc G et al (2000) Management of advanced prostate cancer. *Oncologist.* 5 (1):36-44.

Bauer KS et al (1999) A pharmacokinetically guided Phase II study of carboxyamido-triazole in androgen-independent prostate cancer. *Clin.Cancer Res.* 5 (9):2324-2329.

Bauman G et al (2005) Radiopharmaceuticals for the palliation of painful bone metastasis-a systemic review. *Radiother.Oncol.* 75 (3):258-270.

Beer TM et al (2007) Double-blinded randomized study of high-dose calcitriol plus docetaxel compared with placebo plus docetaxel in androgen-independent prostate cancer: a report from the ASCENT Investigators. *J.Clin.Oncol.* 25 (6):669-674.

Berlin NI (2000) Treatment of the myeloproliferative disorders with 32P. *Eur.J.Haematol.* 65 (1):1-7.

Berthold DR et al (2008) Docetaxel plus prednisone or mitoxantrone plus prednisone for advanced prostate cancer: updated survival in the TAX 327 study. *J.Clin.Oncol.* 26 (2):242-245.

Berthold DR, Sternberg CN, and Tannock IF (2005) Management of advanced prostate cancer after first-line chemotherapy. *J.Clin.Oncol.* 23 (32):8247-8252.

Blake GM et al (1986) Sr-89 therapy: strontium kinetics in disseminated carcinoma of the prostate. *Eur.J.Nucl.Med.* 12 (9):447-454.

Boyle BJ et al (2001) Insulin-like growth factor binding protein-3 mediates 1 alpha,25-dihydroxyvitamin d(3) growth inhibition in the LNCaP prostate cancer cell line through p21/WAF1. *J.Urol.* 165 (4):1319-1324.

Briggs C et al (2004) Assessment of an immature platelet fraction (IPF) in peripheral thrombocytopenia. *Br.J.Haematol.* 126 (1):93-99.

Bubley GJ et al (1999) Eligibility and response guidelines for phase II clinical trials in androgen-independent prostate cancer: recommendations from the Prostate-Specific Antigen Working Group. *J.Clin.Oncol.* 17 (11):3461-3467.

Buchan RC and Brindle JM (1970) Radioiodine therapy to out-patients - the contamination hazard. *Br.J.Radiol.* 43 (511):479-482.

Carducci MA et al (2003) Effect of endothelin-A receptor blockade with atrasentan on tumor progression in men with hormone-refractory prostate cancer: a randomized, phase II, placebo-controlled trial. *J.Clin.Oncol.* 21 (4):679-689.

Chapman CR and Gavrin J (1999) Suffering: the contributions of persistent pain. *Lancet* 353 (9171):2233-2237.

Cheung A and Driedger AA (1980) Evaluation of radioactive phosphorus in the palliation of metastatic bone lesions from carcinoma of the breast and prostate. *Radiology* 134 (1):209-212.

Coebergh, J. W. W., van de Poll-Franse, L. V., and Alers, J. C. Kanker in Nederland, Trends, prognoses en implicaties voor zorgvraag. Amsterdam. KWF , 65-73. 2004.

Coleman RE et al (2005) Predictive value of bone resorption and formation markers in cancer patients with bone metastases receiving the bisphosphonate zoledronic acid. *J.Clin.Oncol.* 23 (22):4925-4935.

Cook RJ et al (2006) Markers of bone metabolism and survival in men with hormone-refractory metastatic prostate cancer. *Clin.Cancer Res.* 12 (11 Pt 1):3361-3367.

Dahut WL et al (2004) Randomized phase II trial of docetaxel plus thalidomide in androgen-independent prostate cancer. *J.Clin.Oncol.* 22 (13):2532-2539.

de Klerk JM et al (1994) Evaluation of thrombocytopenia in patients treated with rhenium-186-HEDP: guidelines for individual dosage recommendations. *J.Nucl.Med.* 35 (9):1423-1428.

de Klerk JM et al (1992) Pharmacokinetics of rhenium-186 after administration of rhenium-186-HEDP to patients with bone metastases. *J.Nucl.Med.* 33 (5):646-651.

DePuy V et al (2007) Effects of skeletal morbidities on longitudinal patient-reported outcomes and survival in patients with metastatic prostate cancer. *Support.Care Cancer* 15 (7):869-876.

Dijkman GA and Debruyne FM (1996) Epidemiology of prostate cancer. *Eur.Urol.* 30 (3):281-295.

Etches RC (1999) Patient-controlled analgesia. *Surg.Clin.North Am.* 79 (2):297-312.

Fayers, P. M., Aaronson, N. K., Bjordal, K., Groenvold, M., Curran, D., and Bottomley, A. The EORTC QLQ-C30 Scoring Manual. 3rd ed. Brussels: European Organization for Research and Treatment of Cancer . 2001. Brussels. Ref Type: Generic

Figg WD et al (1996) Lack of correlation between prostate-specific antigen and the presence of measurable soft tissue metastases in hormone-refractory prostate cancer. *Cancer Invest* 14 (6):513-517.

Finlay IG, Mason MD, and Shelley M (2005) Radioisotopes for the palliation of metastatic bone cancer: a systematic review. *Lancet Oncol.* 6 (6):392-400.

Han SH et al (2002) The PLACORHEN study: a double-blind, placebo-controlled, randomized radionuclide study with (186)Re-etidronate in hormone-resistant prostate cancer patients with painful bone metastases. Placebo Controlled Rhenium Study. *J.Nucl.Med.* 43 (9):1150-1156.

Hartsell WF et al (2005) Randomized trial of short- versus long-course radiotherapy for palliation of painful bone metastases. *J.Natl.Cancer Inst.* 97 (11):798-804.

James ND et al (2008) Safety and Efficacy of the Specific Endothelin-A Receptor Antagonist ZD4054 in Patients with Hormone-Resistant Prostate Cancer and Bone Metastases Who Were Pain Free or Mildly Symptomatic: A Double-Blind, Placebo-Controlled, Randomised, Phase 2 Trial. *Eur.Urol.*

John SS et al (2008) Newer imaging modalities to assist with target localization in the radiation treatment of prostate cancer and possible lymph node metastases. *Int.J.Radiat.Oncol.Biol.Phys.* 71 (1 Suppl):S43-S47.

Jung K et al (2004) Comparison of 10 serum bone turnover markers in prostate carcinoma patients with bone metastatic spread: diagnostic and prognostic implications. *Int.J.Cancer* 111 (5):783-791.

Kaasa S et al (2006) Prospective randomised multicenter trial on single fraction radiotherapy (8 Gy x 1) versus multiple fractions (3 Gy x 10) in the treatment of painful bone metastases. *Radiother.Oncol.* 79 (3):278-284.

Kelly WK and Scher HI (1993) Prostate specific antigen decline after antiandrogen withdrawal: the flutamide withdrawal syndrome. *J.Urol.* 149 (3):607-609.

Klotz L (2008) Maximal androgen blockade for advanced prostate cancer. *Best.Pract.Res.Clin.Endocrinol.Metab* 22 (2):331-340.

Ko YJ et al (2001) A multi-institutional phase ii study of SU101, a platelet-derived growth factor receptor inhibitor, for patients with hormone-refractory prostate cancer. *Clin.Cancer Res.* 7 (4):800-805.

Krishnamurthy GT and Krishnamurthy S (2000) Radionuclides for metastatic bone pain palliation: a need for rational re-evaluation in the new millennium. *J.Nucl.Med.* 41 (4):688-691.

Lam MG et al (2009a) (188)Re-HEDP combined with capecitabine in hormone-refractory prostate cancer patients with bone metastases: a phase I safety and toxicity study. *Eur.J.Nucl.Med.Mol.Imaging* 36 (9):1425-1433.

Lam MG et al (2007) Combined use of zoledronic acid and 153Sm-EDTMP in hormone-refractory prostate cancer patients with bone metastases. *Eur.J.Nucl.Med.Mol.Imaging.*

Lam MG et al (2009b) Radiation safety considerations for the bone seeking radiopharmaceuticals. 89SrCl2, 186Re-HEDP and 153Sm-EDTMP. *Nuklearmedizin* 48 (1):37-43.

Langley RE et al (2008) Early hormonal data from a multicentre phase II trial using transdermal oestrogen patches as first-line hormonal therapy in patients with locally advanced or metastatic prostate cancer. *BJU.Int.* 102 (4):442-445.

Lein M et al (2007) Serial markers of bone turnover in men with metastatic prostate cancer treated with zoledronic Acid for detection of bone metastases progression. *Eur.Urol.* 52 (5):1381-1387.

Lewiecki EM (2006) RANK ligand inhibition with denosumab for the management of osteoporosis. *Expert.Opin.Biol.Ther.* 6 (10):1041-1050.

Lewington VJ et al (1991) A prospective, randomised double-blind crossover study to examine the efficacy of strontium-89 in pain palliation in patients with advanced prostate cancer metastatic to bone. *Eur.J.Cancer* 27 (8):954-958.

Lipton A et al (2008) Normalization of bone markers is associated with improved survival in patients with bone metastases from solid tumors and elevated bone resorption receiving zoledronic acid. *Cancer* 113 (1):193-201.

Maxon HR, III et al (1991) Rhenium-186(Sn)HEDP for treatment of painful osseous metastases: results of a double-blind crossover comparison with placebo. *J.Nucl.Med.* 32 (10):1877-1881.

McQuay, H. J., Collins, S., Carroll, D., and Moore, R. A. Radiotherapy for the palliation of painful bone metastases. The Cochrane Database of Systemic Reviews Issue 4, 1-22. 2008.

Mithal NP, Needham PR, and Hoskin PJ (1994) Retreatment with radiotherapy for painful bone metastases. *Int.J.Radiat.Oncol.Biol.Phys.* 29 (5):1011-1014.

Nam S et al (2005) Action of the Src family kinase inhibitor, dasatinib (BMS-354825), on human prostate cancer cells. *Cancer Res.* 65 (20):9185-9189.

Nilsson S et al (2005) Palliation of bone pain in prostate cancer using chemotherapy and strontium-89. A randomized phase II study. *J.Pain Symptom.Manage.* 29 (4):352-357.

Oosterhof GO et al (2003) Strontium(89) chloride versus palliative local field radiotherapy in patients with hormonal escaped prostate cancer: a phase III study of the European Organisation for Research and Treatment of Cancer, Genitourinary Group. *Eur.Urol.* 44 (5):519-526.

Palmedo H et al (2003) Repeated bone-targeted therapy for hormone-refractory prostate carcinoma: tandomized phase II trial with the new, high-energy radiopharmaceutical rhenium-188 hydroxyethylidenediphosphonate. *J.Clin.Oncol.* 21 (15):2869-2875.

Piffanelli A et al (2001) Radionuclide therapy for painful bone metastases. An Italian multicentre observational study. Writing Committee of an Ad Hoc Study Group. *Q.J.Nucl.Med.* 45 (1):100-107.

Porter AT et al (1993) Results of a randomized phase-III trial to evaluate the efficacy of strontium-89 adjuvant to local field external beam irradiation in the management of endocrine resistant metastatic prostate cancer. *Int.J.Radiat.Oncol.Biol.Phys.* 25 (5):805-813.

Price DT et al (2002) Comparison of [18 F]fluorocholine and [18 F]fluorodeoxyglucose for positron emission tomography of androgen dependent and androgen independent prostate cancer. *J.Urol.* 168 (1):273-280.

Quilty PM et al (1994) A comparison of the palliative effects of strontium-89 and external beam radiotherapy in metastatic prostate cancer. *Radiother.Oncol.* 31 (1):33-40.

Quirijnen JM et al (1996) Efficacy of rhenium-186-etidronate in prostate cancer patients with metastatic bone pain. *J.Nucl.Med.* 37 (9):1511-1515.

Rago R (1998) Management of Hormone-Sensitive and Hormone-Refractory Metastatic Prostate Cancer. *Cancer Control* 5 (6):513-521.

Ricci S et al (2007) Clinical benefit of bone-targeted radiometabolic therapy with 153Sm-EDTMP combined with chemotherapy in patients with metastatic hormone-refractory prostate cancer. *Eur.J.Nucl.Med.Mol.Imaging* 34 (7):1023-1030.

Roos DE et al (2005) Randomized trial of 8 Gy in 1 versus 20 Gy in 5 fractions of radiotherapy for neuropathic pain due to bone metastases (Trans-Tasman Radiation Oncology Group, TROG 96.05). *Radiother.Oncol.* 75 (1):54-63.

Roque i Figuls, M., Martinez-ZApata, M. J., Alonso-Coello, P., Catala, E., Garcia, J. L., and Ferrandiz, M. Radioisotopes for metastatic bone pain. The Cochrane Database of Systemic Reviews Issue 4, 1-36. 2008.

Saad F et al (2002) A randomized, placebo-controlled trial of zoledronic acid in patients with hormone-refractory metastatic prostate carcinoma. *J.Natl.Cancer Inst.* 94 (19):1458-1468.

Saarto T et al (2002) Palliative radiotherapy in the treatment of skeletal metastases. *Eur.J.Pain* 6 (5):323-330.

Sabbatini P et al (1999) Prognostic significance of extent of disease in bone in patients with androgen-independent prostate cancer. *J.Clin.Oncol.* 17 (3):948-957.

Sartor O et al (2007) Safety and efficacy of repeat administration of samarium Sm-153 lexidronam to patients with metastatic bone pain. *Cancer* 109 (3):637-643.

Sartor O et al (2004) Samarium-153-Lexidronam complex for treatment of painful bone metastases in hormone-refractory prostate cancer. *Urology* 63 (5):940-945.

Scher HI et al (2008) Design and end points of clinical trials for patients with progressive prostate cancer and castrate levels of testosterone: recommendations of the Prostate Cancer Clinical Trials Working Group. *J.Clin.Oncol.* 26 (7):1148-1159.

Sciuto R et al (2001) Metastatic bone pain palliation with 89-Sr and 186-Re-HEDP in breast cancer patients. *Breast Cancer Res.Treat.* 66 (2):101-109.

Sciuto R et al (2002) Effects of low-dose cisplatin on 89Sr therapy for painful bone metastases from prostate cancer: a randomized clinical trial. *J.Nucl.Med.* 43 (1):79-86.

Sciuto R et al (1996) Radiosensitization with low-dose carboplatin enhances pain palliation in radioisotope therapy with strontium-89. *Nucl.Med.Commun.* 17 (9):799-804.

Serafini AN et al (1998) Palliation of pain associated with metastatic bone cancer using samarium-153 lexidronam: a double-blind placebo-controlled clinical trial. *J.Clin.Oncol.* 16 (4):1574-1581.

Smaletz O et al (2002) Nomogram for overall survival of patients with progressive metastatic prostate cancer after castration. *J.Clin.Oncol.* 20 (19):3972-3982.

Small EJ et al (2000) Prospective trial of the herbal supplement PC-SPES in patients with progressive prostate cancer. *J.Clin.Oncol.* 18 (21):3595-3603.

Small EJ et al (2004) Antiandrogen withdrawal alone or in combination with ketoconazole in androgen-independent prostate cancer patients: a phase III trial (CALGB 9583). *J.Clin.Oncol.* 22 (6):1025-1033.

Small EJ and Srinivas S (1995) The antiandrogen withdrawal syndrome. Experience in a large cohort of unselected patients with advanced prostate cancer. *Cancer* 76 (8):1428-1434.

Smeland S et al (2003) Role of strontium-89 as adjuvant to palliative external beam radiotherapy is questionable: results of a double-blind randomized study. *Int.J.Radiat.Oncol.Biol.Phys.* 56 (5):1397-1404.

Smith MR et al (2007) Predictors of skeletal complications in men with hormone-refractory metastatic prostate cancer. *Urology* 70 (2):315-319.

Sridhara R et al (1995) Evaluation of prostate-specific antigen as a surrogate marker for response of hormone-refractory prostate cancer to suramin therapy. *J.Clin.Oncol.* 13 (12):2944-2953.

Tannock I et al (1989) Treatment of metastatic prostatic cancer with low-dose prednisone: evaluation of pain and quality of life as pragmatic indices of response. *J.Clin.Oncol.* 7 (5):590-597.

Tannock IF et al (2004) Docetaxel plus prednisone or mitoxantrone plus prednisone for advanced prostate cancer. *N.Engl.J.Med.* 351 (15):1502-1512.

Tu, S. and Lin, S. Current trials using bone-targeting agents in prostate cancer. Cancer J. 14, 35-39. 2008.

Tu SM et al (2001) Bone-targeted therapy for advanced androgen-independent carcinoma of the prostate: a randomised phase II trial. *Lancet* 357 (9253):336-341.

Van der Linden YM et al (2004) Single fraction radiotherapy is efficacious: a further analysis of the Dutch Bone Metastasis Study controlling for the influence of retreatment. *Int.J.Radiat.Oncol.Biol.Phys.* 59 (2):528-537.

VIKC. Richtlijn 'diagnostiek en behandeling van pijn bij patiënten met kanker' Utrecht. 2008.

Visser, O. and van Noord, K. J. Feiten en fabels over kanker in Nederland. Utrecht. VIKC , 8-9. 2005.

VRO92. Min. VROM, Publicatiereeks Stralenbescherming nr. 1992/55, mei 1992.

VROM. Recommendations: working with therapeutical doses of radionuclides, The Hague. 2005.

Wang C et al (2002) Reticulated platelets predict platelet count recovery following chemotherapy. *Transfusion* 42 (3):368-374.

2

High-Intensity Focused Ultrasound (HIFU) - An Alternative Choice in Prostate Cancer Treatment

Umberto Maestroni and Francesco Ziglioli
Department of Urology, University Hospital of Parma, Parma
Italy

1. Introduction

Prostate cancer is considered one of the most discussed topics in male health with an important social impact on the quality of life.

In Europe, it is the most common solid neoplasm with an incidence rate of 214 cases per 100,000 men[1]. The increasing life expectancy and the more and more widespread use of Prostate Specific Antigen (PSA) are probably the two most important reasons why more patients are diagnosed with prostate cancer. In Europe, 2,6 million new cases of prostate cancer are yearly observed (11% of male cancer diagnosis), responsible for 9% of deaths for male cancer cases.

Radical surgery represents the treatment of choice in clinically localized prostate cancer and in > 10 year life expectancy prostate cancer. Nevertheless, radical surgery itself may be considered a high morbility treatment[2].

Mini-invasive procedure development, such as three-dimensional external radiotherapy, brachytherapy or cryotherapy, especially in elderly or anaesthetically high risk patients, represents a useful treatment in prostate cancer.

HIFU (High-Intensity Focused Ultrasound) is a new and alternative choice in localized and low or intermediate-risk prostate cancer treatment[3-5].

For a variety of reasons, transrectal HIFU appears highly attractive as a minimally invasive treatment for localized prostate cancer. It is a method of delivering ultrasonic energy with resultant heat and tissue destruction to a discrete point without damaging intervening tissue or cells. HIFU has been used for the management of patients diagnosed with various types of cancer, including prostate, breast, liver, pancreas, kidney, bone, and soft tissue.

2. Experimental studies

It has been shown in canines and humans that HIFU is capable of ablating prostatic tissue both contact and irradiation free[6,7].

One of the first investigators who experimented the application of the technique to human beings has been S. Madersbacher[8].

Early studies considered focused ultrasound as a potential technique for neurosurgery (Lynn, 1942; Warwick and Pond, 1968). A significant development was the construction of precision apparatus suitable for human treatment by Fry et al. in 1958.

HIFU has also been used in other clinical fields including ophthalmology (Coleman, 1985), urology (by Foster and Gelet in 1993) and oncology (Chapelon in 1992 and Prat in 1995). To date, focused ultrasound has been used successfully in the management of many tumours, including prostate cancer, in which this technique represents a good treatment option.
HIFU was also used by Madersbacher and colleagues as a treatment for Benign Prostatic Hyperplasia (BPH). To date, this technique is not still used to treat BPH, because of its side effects on bladder neck function.

3. Description of the procedure

HIFU is performed through a computerized surgical device equipped with a treatment table, an ultrasound treatment system connected to an endorectal probe, a safety infrared ray detector, a refrigeration system keeping the rectal mucosa temperature below 14°C and a monitor to set and control the treatment procedure through echographic screening (Fig. 1).
For anatomical reasons, the transrectal approach appears ideally suited to ablate prostatic tissue because the proximity of HIFU transducer and target tissue facilitates HIFU treatment from the technical standpoint.
After introducing the rectal probe, anatomic landmarks must be echographically set (apex, bladder neck, rectal side, prostate capsule), in order to make the computer able to determine the correct subdivision in different prostate portions (generally four).
The probe is equipped with a transducer that gives out a beam of high-focused convergent ultrasounds. The HIFU transducer has an aperture of 37 cm and a focal distance of 25.5 cm.
The focus has a -6 dB beam width of 1.6 mm and axial length of 10 mm. In the ultrasound converging point (focal point), the ultrasound beam absorption generates an immediate growth of temperature (85-100°C), destroying prostate cells in the circumscribed area.

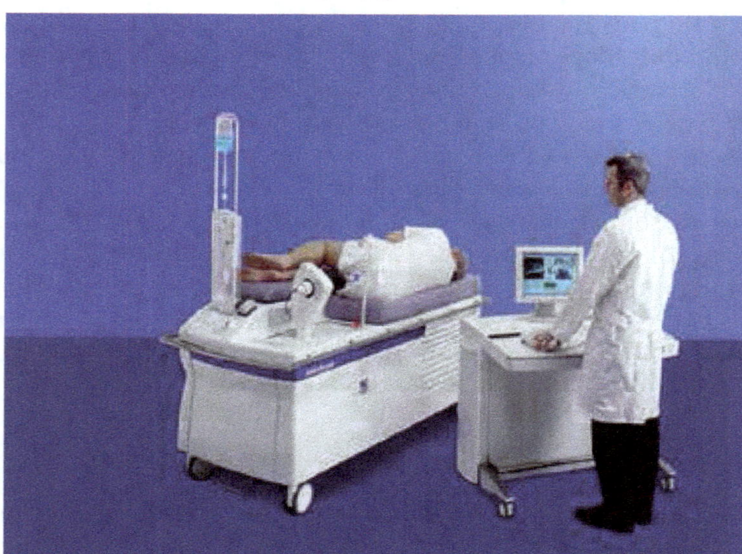

(Ablatherm®-Edap Technomed device).

Fig. 1. Overview of HIFU procedure. The bed with the High-intensity ultrasound probe can be clearly seen. On the right, the ultrasound screen and the screen to set the machine and follow the procedure

Adequately translating the focal point with a robotic and automatic device, the successive ultrasound emissions may destroy all prostate cells (Fig. 2).

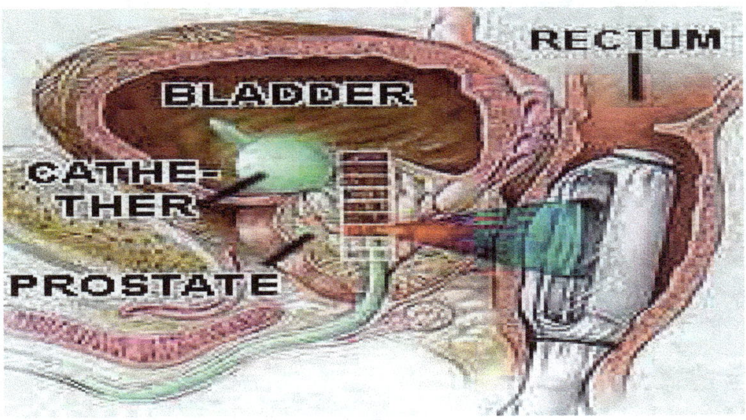

Fig. 2. Anatomical scheme of HIFU endorectal device

These lesions have a predictable size and shape, closely matching the focal region of the ultrasound source. As the lesion width is almost constant along their length, they can be placed side-by-side without leaving gaps (Fig. 3).

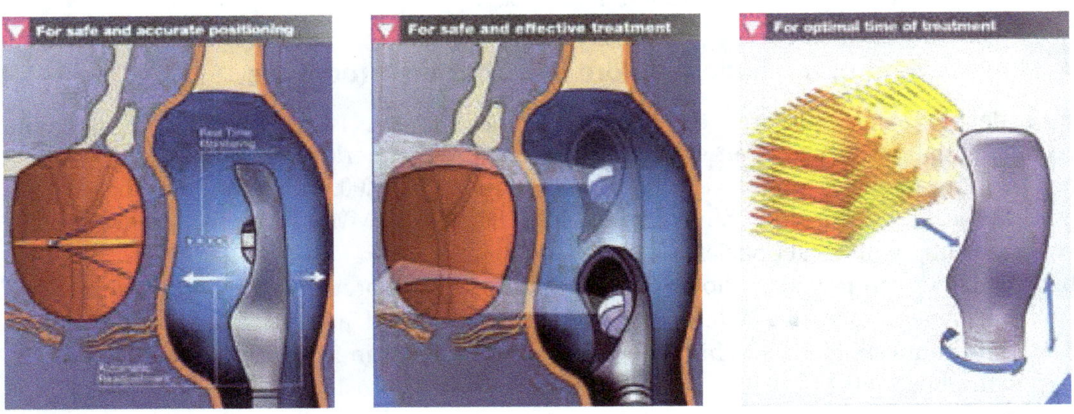

Fig. 3. HIFU mechanism scheme. On the left, ultrasound beam positioning; in the middle, the area to treat; on the right, an overall view of the sections treated by high-intensity ultrasound.

A standard procedure can be personalized in order to obtain ideal treatment settings: ultrasound frequency (standard 3 MHz), shot duration (standard 5 seconds) and waiting-time between shots (standard 5 seconds) may be modified (Fig. 4). Elementary lesion volume measures 19-24 mm and its diameter measures 1.7 mm

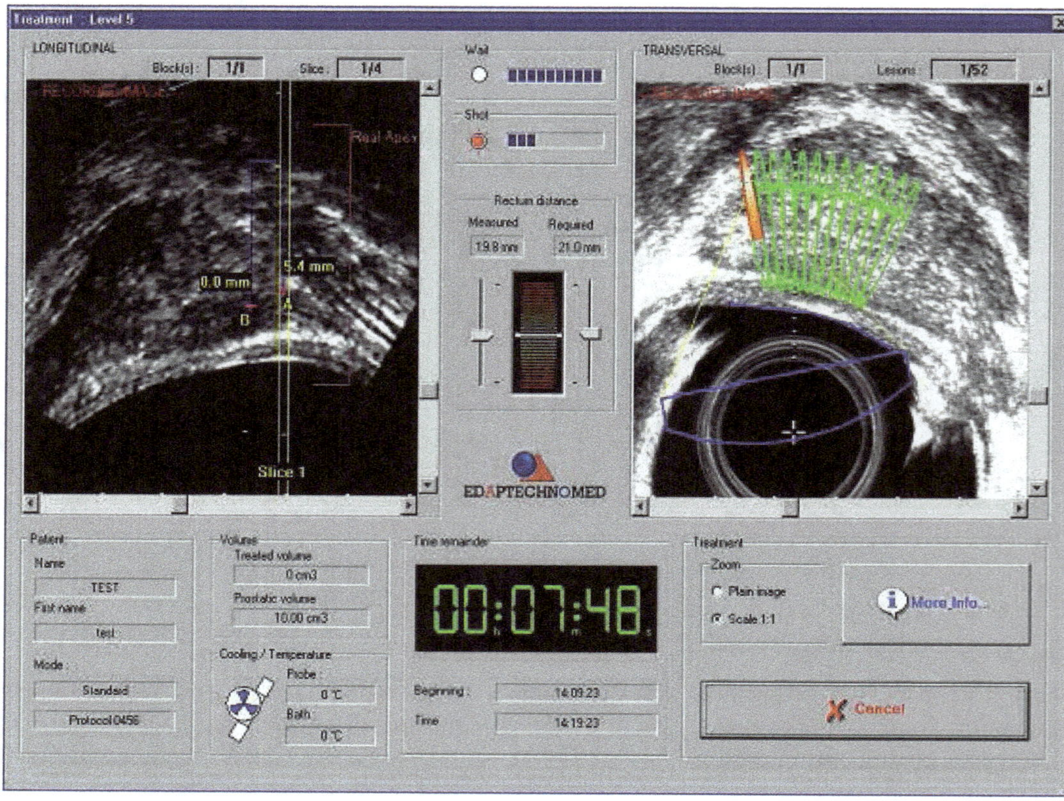

Fig. 4. On the screen, it is possible to follow the procedure and to change settings, such as ultrasound frequency and shot duration. Thus, a safe and optimal treatment can be performed.

4. Management of the patient before and after the procedure

In order to safely perform the treatment, the surgeon is advised to follow some recommendations, in accordance with the European and American guidelines:

a. Anti-trombotic prophylaxis with sodic Dalteparin 5.000 I.U. the day before the procedure. Other low molecular weight heparin (LMWH) can be administrated, according with local policies.
b. Antibiotic prophylaxis should be given in order to prevent infection. A quinolone represents a good choice, but other antibiotic can be used, according with local policies.
c. Careful intestinal toilet. This is an important key point in infection prevention. Also, it is fundamental to obtain a good view of the whole prostate on ultrasound, which is important in order to treat the target area properly. This will also prevent some side effects of the treatment, such as bladder neck irritation, reduces the risk of rectum fistulisation, and improves the erectile function outcome.

All patients undergo intra-spinal block with Chirocaine®.

Marcaine® can be used instead of Chirocaine.

If Marcaine is administrated, it is important to begin the procedure from the left lobe of the prostate, because this lobe is above due to the left decubitus of the patient on the device.

In order to make the procedure more bearable and to obtain the best cooperation from the patient, Midazolam 0,03 mg/kg administration during the procedure is recommended.

Other benzodiazepine can be used, according with their pharmacocynetic and pharmacodynamic features.
Reportedly, patients have no postoperative pain, except in case of complication. Just in the first two hours after the treatment the patient might complain of confusion and dazzling, but these are considered common consequences of the anaesthetic treatment.
The anaesthetist should be involved pre-operatively, intra-operatively and post-operatively, in order to manage the patient properly before and during the treatment and in order to relieve post-operative pain and anaesthetic side-effects and/or complications.

5. Mechanism

Conceptually, a piezoelectric transducer generates a high intensity converging ultrasound beam that destroys local tissues through three mechanisms:

1. Coagulative necrosis;
2. Cavitation;
3. Heat damage.

These three key-points are discussed below.

5.1 Coagulative necrosis

Coagulative necrosis, is due to hyperthermia (85-100°C) generated in the focal point.
Elementary lesion has ellipsoidal shape. The short length of the shot limits heat diffusion around the focal point. Shot by shot, it is possible to generate a plethora of elementary lesions until all prostate tissue is destroyed.
Coagulative necrosis is a non-reversible phenomenon (Fig. 5).

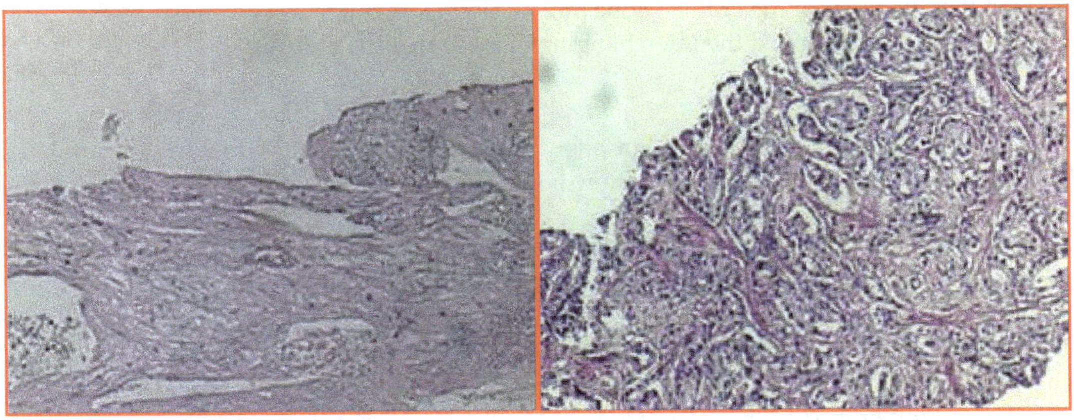

Fig. 5. On the left, pre-HIFU histology aspect; on the right, post-HIFU histology change

This kind of lesion can be clearly seen on optical microscopy. Its effectiveness in cancer treatment is demonstrated by the absence of cell functional structures, such as membranes, active nuclei, and organelles.
After the treatment, glandular structures cannot be seen any longer, thus demonstrating that the HIFU technique provides a lack of function in the treated prostate.
Also liquefactive necrosis and apoptotic necrosis are reported as a common consequence of HIFU treatment (see § 6.1), but these kinds of necrotic lesions do not affect the whole amount of necrotic areas.

5.2 Cavitation

Cavitation is due to the gas microbubble (bubble clouds) vibration dissolved in prostate tissue. Lindau and Lauterborn investigated the collapse and rebound of a cavitation bubble near a flat rigid wall using a high-speed camera[9].

Due to the depression caused by the negative part of the ultrasound wave, intracellular water may enter the gaseous phase.

That would lead to the development of microbubbles.

When they reach the size of resonance, these bubbles suddenly collapse and produce high-pressure shock waves, destroying adjacent tissue.

In a study carried out by Chen H and colleagues[10], the dynamics of cavitation bubble clouds generated at the tissue boundary in continuous HIFU fields has been experimentally investigated by a high-speed photography method.

The experimental results revealed that the cavitation bubble clouds organize into two shapes, which were named ''cone-shape'' bubble cloud structure and ''crown-shape'' bubble cloud structure.

The cavitation bubble cloud is visible at the tissue surface at 200 μs; then a tiny tip becomes obvious at 600 μs. The elongated tip leads to the formation of a cone-shape bubble cloud structure.

After 1.8 ms, the cone-shape bubble cloud attaines a dynamically stable state.

The bubble cluster grows larger and developes a crown-like shape. Meanwhile, it moves forward and finally hits the tissue boundary forming the crown-shape cavitation bubble cloud structure.

Among the 171 image series recorded in the study carried out by Chen H et al, 85% showed the evolution of the cone-shape bubble cloud structure. Another 11% of the image series showed the dynamics of the crown-shape bubble cloud structure.

The remaining 4% exhibited the interchanging of these two structures.

5.3 Heat damage

The tissue ablation induced by high-intensity ultrasound results primarily from bulk heating, with possible contributions from boiling and acoustic cavitation. Bubbles, when present, may enhance local absorption (Fig. 6).

The position and shape of the heated region are determined by the intensity of the field near the focus, the attenuation and the effects of diffusion.

The rate of change of temperature at any point is proportional to the absorbed power density and hence to the incident beam power and attenuation[11].

The irreversible changes in proteins associated with tissue denaturation and coagulation start at low temperature.

When temperatures of approximately 60°C are approached, the rate of denaturation becomes so great that irreversible changes can occur in seconds.

Temperature reached during HIFU treatment is clearly higher, as reported above: When lesioning occurs, the attenuation within the treated volume increases[12], thus altering the absorbed power distribution, depending on the biologic feature of the prostate.

Consequently, the region in which heat is deposited may be expected to change during the heating process.

By a macroscopic point of view, we can say that heat growth is maximal in the middle of the treated volume and minimal in the external area of the treated volume.

This difference allows to surely set the treatment outlines and save the prostate apex, and the striated sphincter and vasculo-nervous bundles.

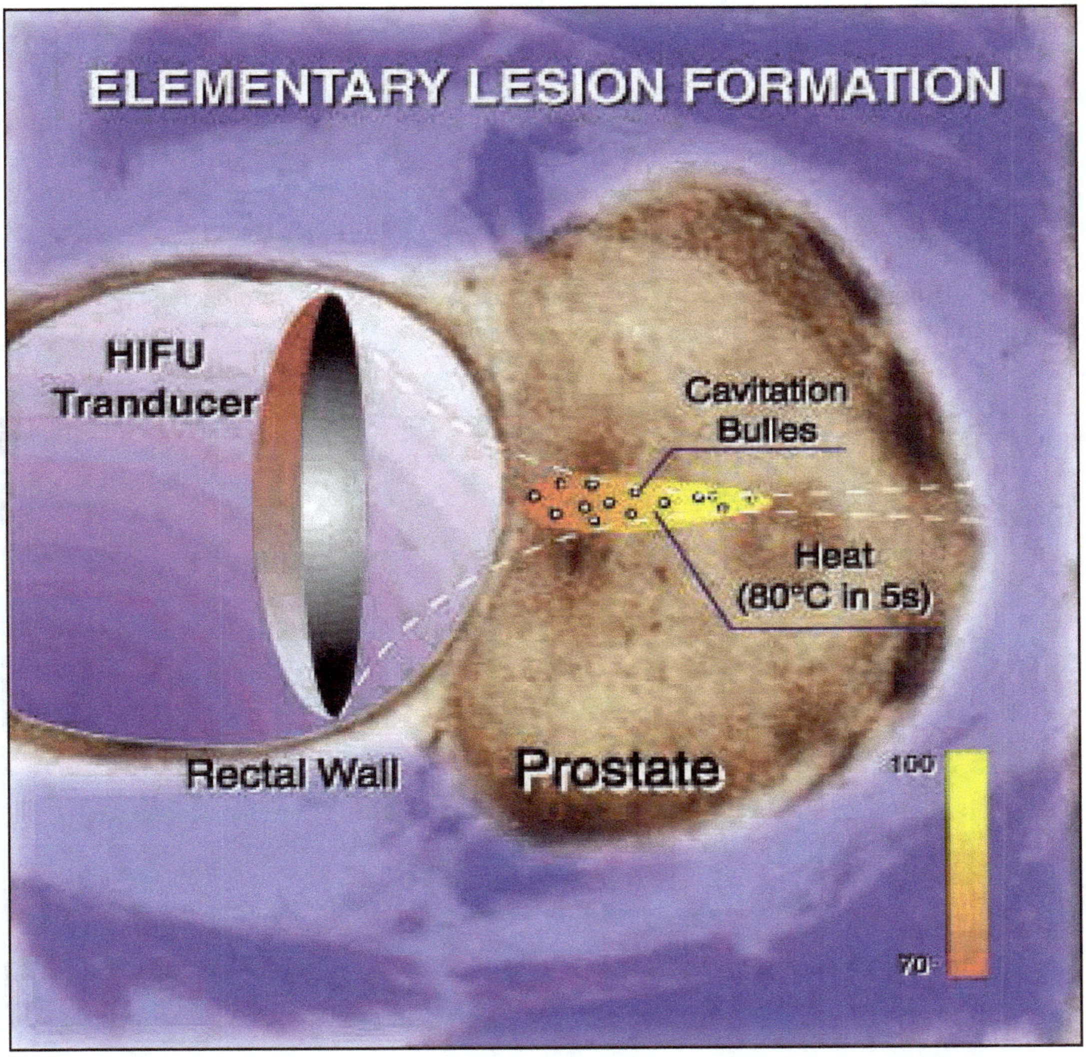

Fig. 6. Elementary lesion formation and its effects on prostate parenchyma, due to heat and mechanical damage.

6. HIFU-induced histopathological changes

HIFU-induced histopathological changes can be studied thanks to light microscopy, immunoistochemistry and electron microscopy.

6.1 Light microscopy

At light microscopy, we can say that the prostatic structure is completely disrupted and hardly recognizable. Three different types of cellular necrosis are generally found:

a. liquefactive necrosis;
b. coagulative necrosis;
c. apoptotic necrosis.

Cell death is generally due to a mixture of the three with liquefactive necrosis being the least common and coagulative necrosis the most common.

Histological findings show consistent coagulative necrosis with precisely defined, sharp margins to normal tissue.

Lesion size and position correlates well with the assumed target zones, thus demonstrating that HIFU permits therapeutic tissue ablation.

Strictly speaking, HIFU treatment induces a spectrum of morphological changes ranging from apparent light microscopic necrosis to more subtle ultrastructural cell damage (see below).

Necrotic tissue in the coagulative necrosis areas consists of homogenously stained eosinophilic fragments (Fig. 7a).

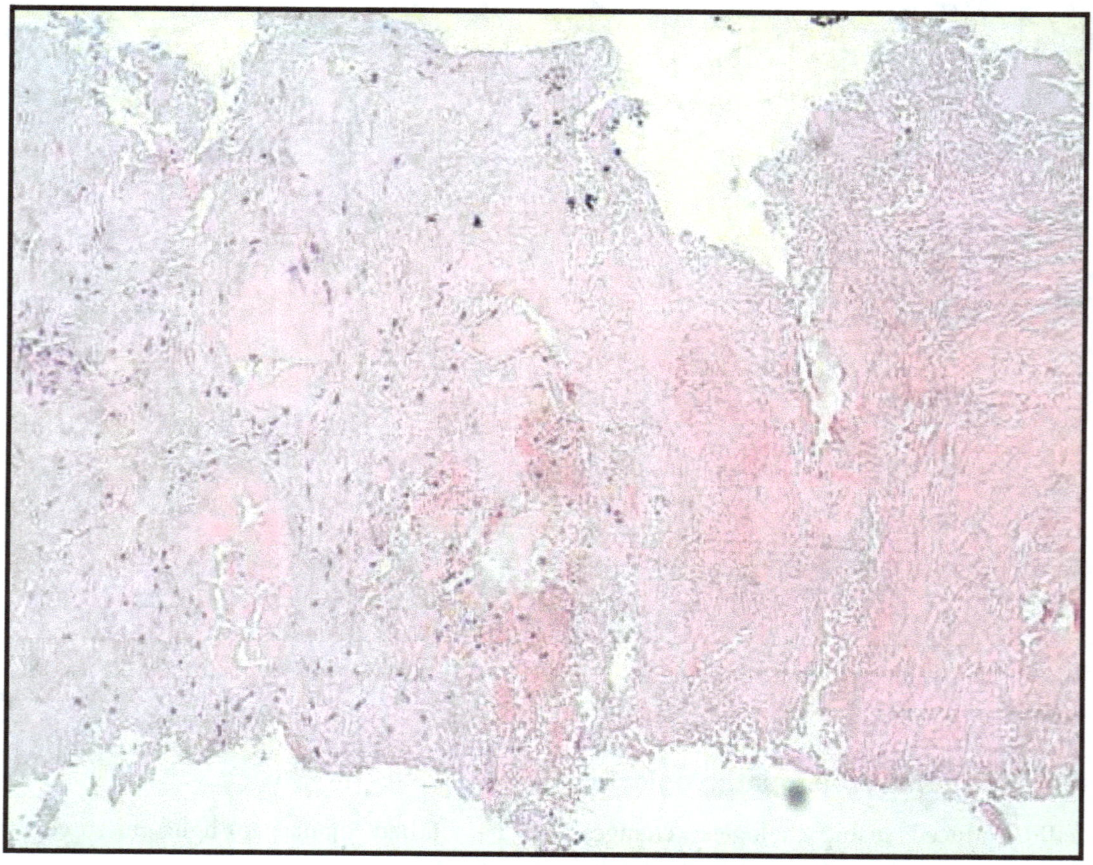

Fig. 7a. Areas of coagulative necrosis can be clearly seen, thus demonstrating the effectiveness of HIFU treatment.

Little structure is apparent aside from some faintly staining collagenous bands and rare indications of the former glandular epithelium. In some cases, necrotic tissue expelled from the coagulative necrosis areas is visible in prostatic ductules of the margin area. Brightly staining blood droplets can be observed on the hematoxylin-eosin slide, of which most are concentrated in the coagulative necrosis area.

The nuclei of epithelial and stromal cells are either pyknotic or totally absent, corresponding to cell necrosis. The nuclei are of normal size with a fine chromatin structure and sporadically small nucleoli.

This epithelial cells also contain pale to eosinophilic cytoplasm, with few vacuoles. Although cell borders are not discernable in most of these cells, they can be identified locally.

Every so often, extended haemorragic areas are found (Fig. 7b).

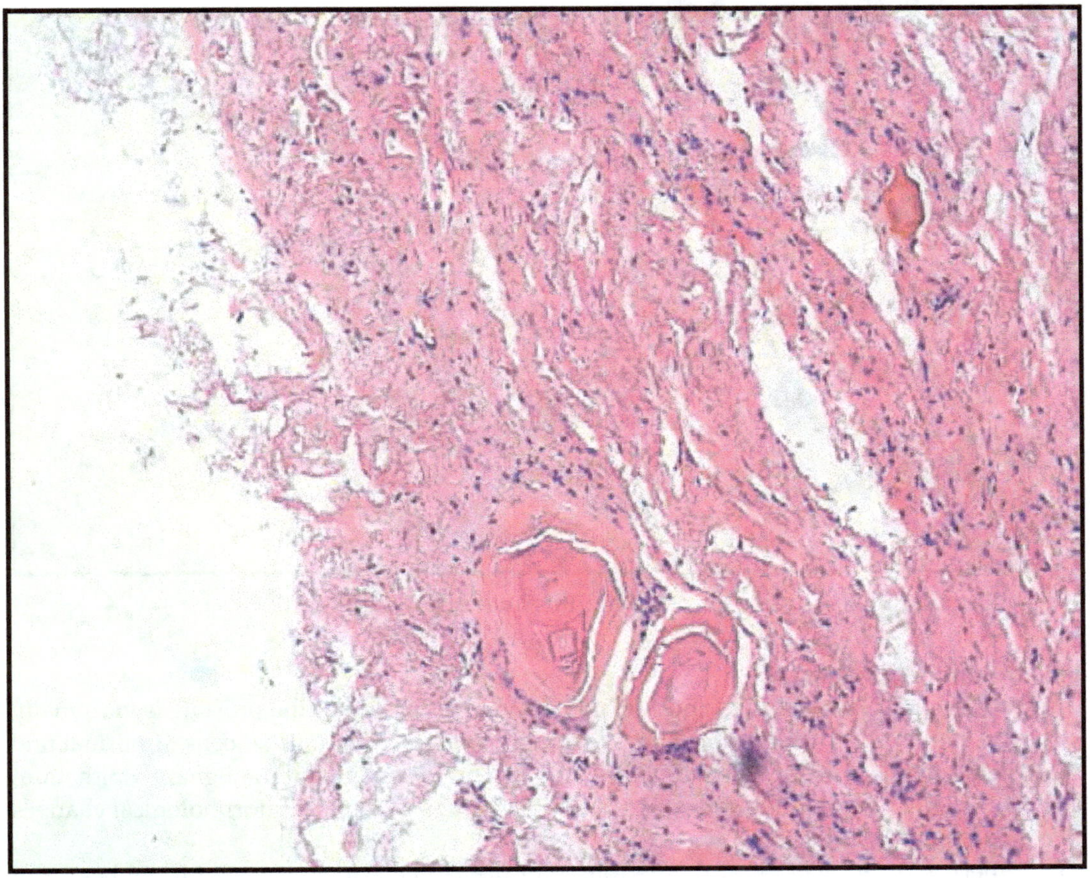

Fig. 7b. Areas of tissue damage, including haemorragic areas

Also, HIFU causes injuries to small vessels, with considerable oedema and swelling of endothelial cells in the margin between the treated and untreated areas. However, in the centre of treated tumor tissue, severely damaged tumor vessels show pyknotic nuclei and debris of nuclei, which indicated endothelial cell death.

Endothelial cells exhibited an irreversible cell death. Almost all of the endothelial cell nuclei disappear, cellular margins were not distinct and junctions between individual cells were disrupted.

The repair of lesions appears to have slow processes of damaged tissue absorption and granulation tissue replacement (Fig. 8).

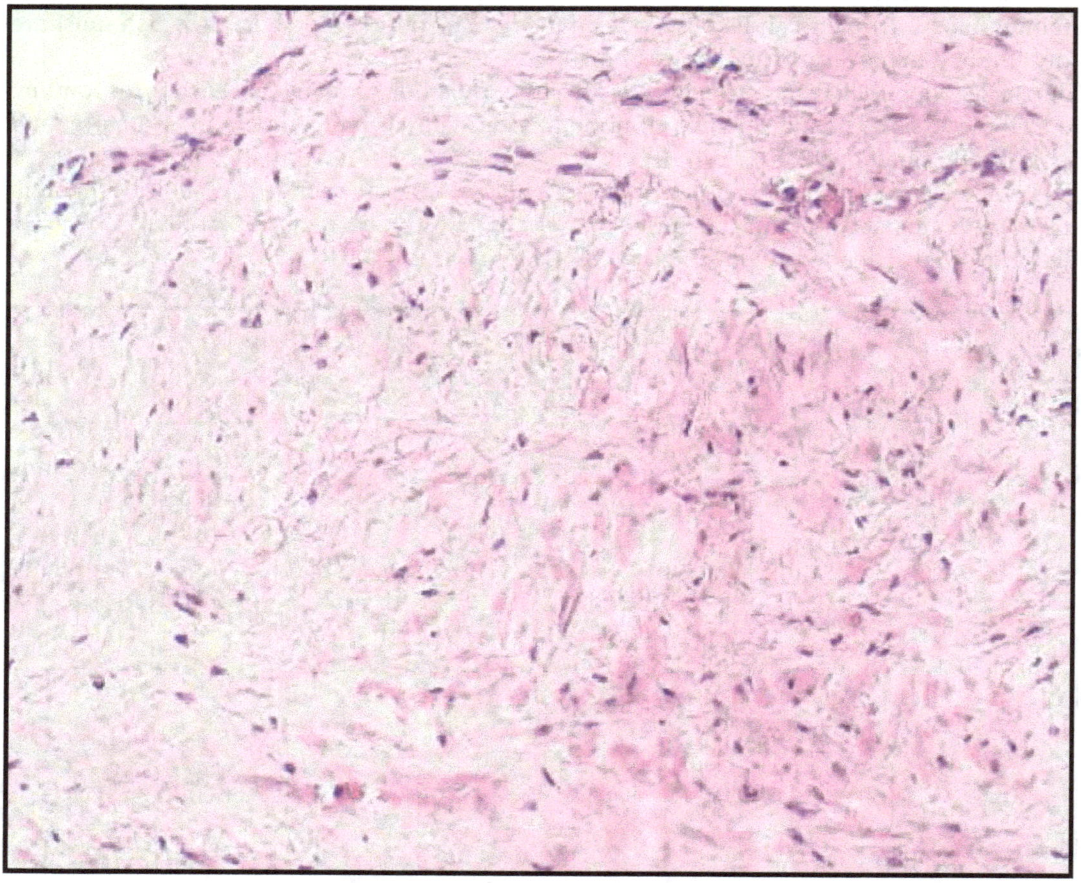

Fig. 8. Granulation tissue and fibrosis 6 months after HIFU treatment.

6.2 Immunoistochemistry

The expression of PSA, panCK, and Ki67 in non-treated regions of the prostate is marginally stronger than in the HIFU region. CK8 is strongly expressed in luminal cells of normal and malignant glands outside the HIFU lesion, but pre-existing and malignant epithelium within the HIFU lesion does not express CK8, regardless of the histomorphological changes in conventional light microscopy.

The hyperplastic epithelium at the periphery of the HIFU lesions reacts with the basal cell antibody 34βE12.

In summary, we can say that prostate glandular epithelium after HIFU treatment reacts with antibodies to pancytokeratin, prostate specific antigen (PSA), and Ki67, but does not express cytokeratin 8, which is indicative of severe cellular damage.

6.3 Electron microscopy

Ultrastructural examination after HIFU reveals disintegration of cellular membranes and cytoplasmic organelles consistent with cell necrosis.

Electron microscopy is not routinely performed. When performed, it confirms submicroscopical cellular damage in the centre of the HIFU lesion.

Electron microscopy is capable to demonstrate cell necrosis also in areas that show no apparent morphological cell necrosis by conventional light microscopy.

Treated areas lack nuclear membranes, but show a fine chromatin pattern that is clumped at the periphery of the nuclei, and conspicuous nucleoli.

The cytoplasm contain some vacuoles, but organelle structures and cell membranes are not generally identified.

7. Immunologic response after HIFU

T-lymphocytes appear in granulation tissue along the ablation margin in all HIFU-treated neoplasms, with no infiltration in those showing typical signs of coagulation necrosis.

The tumor-infiltrating lymphocytes are found mainly in granulation tissue along with immature fibroblasts, new capillaries, and other inflammatory cells.

This observation suggest that their infiltration occurs after HIFU ablation and that these tumor-infiltrating lymphocytes are new lymphocytes moving into the ablated neoplasms from peripheral blood.

As it has been reported by Hartveit and colleagues, this is a typical findings in all tissues treated with HIFU[13].

HIFU treatment may definitively increase the local infiltration of tumor infiltrating lymphocytes in the ablation area, including activated cytotoxic T-Cells and Natural-Killer cells[14].

8. The role of heat-shock proteins (HSP)

Heat shock proteins (HSPs) were first discovered in 1962 as a group of highly conserved proteins that are induced by hyperthermia and other kinds of cellular insults.

There are four principal HSP: HSP-90, HSP-70, HSP-60 and the subgroup of small HSPs including HSP27.

Benign and malignant human prostatic cells respond to heat by increased expression of HSP *in vitro* and *in vivo*.

To obtain a more detailed insight on the effect of heat on prostatic cells, heat shock protein expression of normal and malignant prostatic cells has been studied.

Transrectal HIFU therapy induces intraprostatic necrosis surrounded by a zone characterized by a massive up-regulation of HSP expression.

Recently, several molecular heat shock proteins have been reported to be involved in development and progression of hormone-refractory prostate cancer.

HSP27 and HSP70 are the most strongly induced heat shock proteins during cellular stress (Fig. 9).

HSPs are not all of prognostic value, however some have been demonstrated to have clinical utility as prognostic markers: among this group of heat shock proteins, the most important one is HSP-27, which particularly plays a role in many immunological processes and might stimulate immune defence responses against tumour cells[15].

Accumulating evidence suggests that HSP27 levels correlate with both hormone-refractory prostate cancer and development of resistance to heat. Nevertheless, the functional significance of changes in HSP27 expression associated with heat-resistant prostate cancer remains undefined.

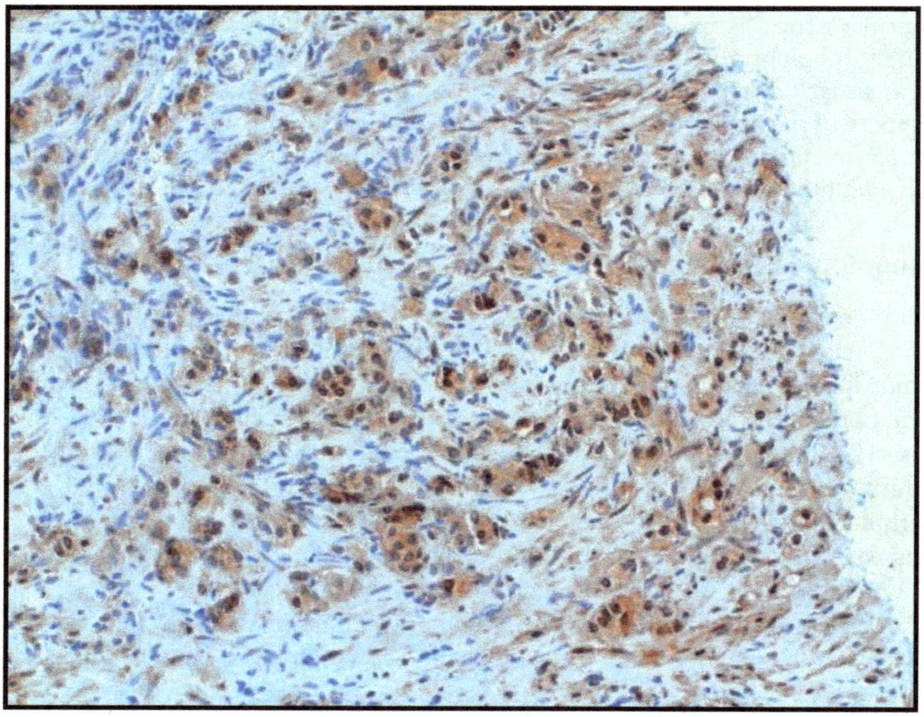

Fig. 9. HSP-70 expression in prostate tissue after HIFU treatment in a case of recurrence

9. Long-term results of HIFU treatment

Many authors have reported their series after HIFU treatment.
One of the most recent is the multicentric study carried out by Crouzet et al[16], who reported a series of 803 patients with a mean follow-up of 43 months. The results of this study are excellent, showing that local control and disease-free survival rate achieved with HIFU were similar to those expected with conformal external-beam radiation therapy (EBRT).
The excellent cancer-specific survival rate reported in this study is also explained by the possibility to repeat HIFU and use salvage EBRT.
The first UK series was reported by Ahmed et al and published on the British Journal of Cancer. 172 men were treated with HIFU with excellent result: 92.4% of patients had no recurrence after a mean follow-up of 346 days[17].
Blana et al published a series of 140 men treated with HIFU, reporting good oncological outcome in long-term follow-up (6.4 years), demonstrating the effective long-term cancer control achieved with HIFU in patients with low- or intermediate-risk localised prostate cancer[18].
Finally, it is correct to cite the negative results reported by Challacombe et al, who interrupted the treatment because of the poor oncological outcome[19].
From all the studies presented, there is clear evidence that the treatment could affect prostate cancer, as shown by both a substantial decrease in serum PSA and negative biopsies after therapy there is clear evidence that the treatment could affect prostate cancer.
The effect has also been demonstrated on radical prostatectomy specimens examined 2 weeks after HIFU.

There are no randomized controlled studies available to compare the outcome of these therapies with each other, other therapies, or watchful waiting.
The combination of a TURP performed just before an HIFU seems to reduce the complications but without affecting the oncologic outcome negatively.
As of today, it is not possible to compare the outcome of HIFU with other treatment modalities for localized prostate cancer.

10. Complications and side effects of HIFU treatment

HIFU is a minimally invasive treatment for prostate cancer, thus resulting in a low complication rate.
Sometimes, minor complications can occour, in the vast majority of cases related to lower urinary tract.
The first one is urinary retention, commonly treated with longer catheterism. The most common is urge incontinence, due to the irritative effect of high-focused ultrasound on the bladder neck. Generally, it disappears in a couple of month, and only in rare cases anticolinergic treatment is required.
Lower urinary tract symptoms, such as frequency, nocturia, weak urinary stream, and so on, are prevented by Trans-Urethral Resection of Prostate (TUR-P), that is recommended to be done 6-8 weeks before HIFU treatment. Anyway, the surgeon is advised to administrate IPSS questionnaire (or equivalent) before the treatment end 3 months after the treatment, in order to assess persistent lower urinary tract symptoms, that should be treated pharmacologically or surgically, if needed.
Infection is another possible complication of this treatment. Antibiotic prophylaxis should prevent this complication, if administrated in accordance with guidelines on infection prevention.
Among the major complications, the most important is recto-vesical or recto-urethral fistula. Only few cases are reported in literature. This complication can be initially treated with longer catheterization, but in some cases surgical repair is required. A common tip to avoid this complication is to safely set the target area on the ultrasound screen, as the slight wall of the rectum can easily lead to fistulization. Also, patients previously diagnosed with ulcerative recto-colitis must not be treated with high-intensity focused ultrasound.
The most important side-effect of HIFU treatment is erectile disfunction and impotency, due to the effect of high intensity ultrasound on the neural bundle. This effect is well known and must be discussed with the patient before the treatment.
Color-doppler-combined technique is reported in literature in order to perform a sort of vessel-sparing procedure, thus resulting in a better outcome by the andrological point of view. However, there is not common agreement among the investigators about the effectiveness and the feasibility of this technique. For this reason, it cannot be recommended at the present time (Fig. 10).
The best management of the patient should include IIEF questionnaire (or equivalent) to be giver before the treatment and 6 months after the treatment in order to assess the sexual outcome.
Patients who are keen on having sexual activity should receive a proper treatment.

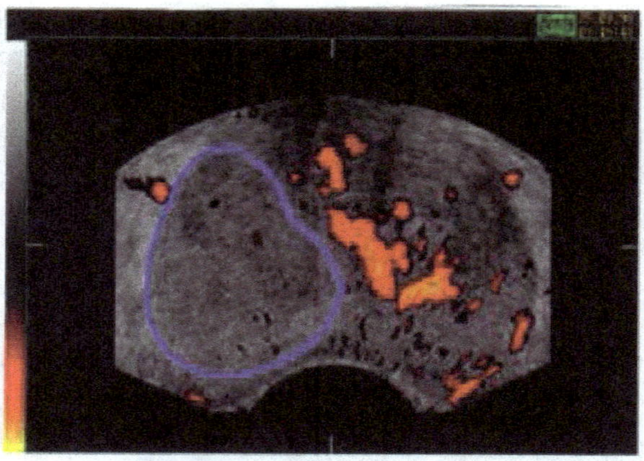

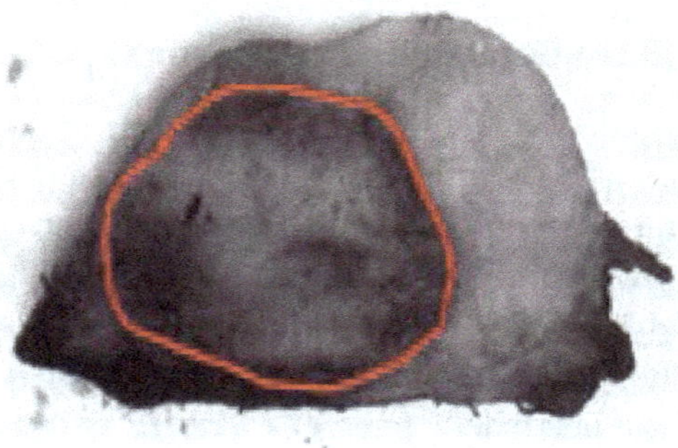

not affected by tumor (red line).

Fig. 10. Color-doppler device for HIFU treatment. Thanks to this additional equipment, it is possible to perform a highly selective treatment (blu line). This can preserve vascular bundle or a portion of prostate

11. Summary

At the time of diagnosis, prostate cancer is organ-confined in 70% of the cases.
The choice of the appropriate treatment for localized prostate cancer is one of the most controversial issues in urologic oncology. Approximately, the most majority of these patients undergo local therapy: surgery or external beam radiation. The rest of the remaining patients do not fit this treatment and are scheduled for Androgen Depriving Therapy (ADT) or watchful waiting.
Besides these treatments, other mini-invasive procedures have emerged in the last few years, such as Brachytherapy, Cryosurgical Ablation, Radiofrequency Interstitial Tumour Ablation and High-Intensity Focused Ultrasound (HIFU).
HIFU represents an alternative choice in mini-invasive treatment of prostate cancer. The treatment is performed under regional anaesthesia and is generally preceeded by limited Trans-Urethral Resection of Prostate (TUR-P).
It is a transrectal procedure: after introducing the rectal probe, anatomic limits must be echographically set (apex, bladder neck, rectal side, prostate capsule), in order to make the computer able to determine the correct subdivision in different prostate portions (generally four).

An absolute contraindication to the procedure is every rectal anatomic or pathologic condition that excludes the transrectal approach.
The technology of the device used to perform the treatment allows to exactly destroy a pre-selected area and to save all the tissues around it.
Conceptually, a piezoelectric trasducer generates a high intensity converging ultrasound beam that destroys local tissues through three mechanisms:

1. *coagulative necrosis*, due to hyperthermia (85-100°C) generated in the focal point. Elementary lesion is ellipsoidal and the short length of the shot limits heat diffusion around the focal point. Shot by shot, it is possible to generate a plethora of elementary lesions until all prostate tissue is destroyed;
2. *cavitation*, due to the gas microbubble vibration dissolved in prostate tissue;
3. *heat growth*, maximal in the middle of the treated volume and minimal in the external area of the treated volume.

This difference allows to surely set the treatment outlines and save the prostate apex (and the striated sphincter) and vasculo-nervous bundles.
HIFU is a minimally invasive ablative technology for managing localized prostate cancer in both the primary and salvage setting. It is a single-session procedure with the possibility of a re-treatment if required.
The advantage of this technique are short hospital stay, reduced convalescence, low morbidity and preservation of continence and erectile function.
As reported in literature, HIFU demonstrated a good oncologic outcome.
The PSA nadir is a major predictive factor for HUFU success and it is generally reached within 6 months after the treatment in all patients.
The most recent results are reported in a study carried out by Crouzet et al. In this multicentric study the mean PSA nadir was 1.0±2.8 ng/mL with a median of 0.25 ng/mL. The 5-year and 7-year Disease Free Survival Rate (DFSR) for low, intermediate-, and high-risk patients (according to D'Amico risk stratification criteria) were, respectively, 83-75%, 72-63% and 68-62%.
As expected by most investigators, the development of more sophisticated technologies should improve these results and lead to a widespread use of this technique. Focal treatment or doppler-combined devices for nerve- or vessel- sparing procedures will be available in the next years.

12. References

Steinberg GD, Carter BS, Beaty TH, et al. Family history and the risk of prostate cancer. Prostate 1990;17:337-47

European Association of Urology. Guidelines 2011 Edition.

Gelet A, Chapelon JY, Bouvier R, Pangaud C, Lasne Y. Local control of prostate cancer by transrectal high intensity focused ultrasound therapy: preliminary results. *J Urol* 1999; 161: 156-62.

Gelet A, Chapelon JY, Bouvier R, Rouviere O, Lyonnet D, Dubernard JM. Transrectal high intensity focused ultrasound of localized prostate cancer: factos influencing the outcome. *Eur Urol* 2001; 40: 124-9

Rebillard X, Gelet A, Davin JL, et al. Transrectal high intensity focused ultrasound in the treatment of localized prostate cancer. *Journal of Endourology* 2005, 19, 6:693-701.

Foster RS, Bihrle R, Sanghvi N, Fry F, Kopecky K, et al. Production of prostatic lesions incanines using transrectally administered high-intensity focused ultrasound. Eur. Urol., 23: 330-336, 1993.

Susani M, Madersbacher S, Kratzik C, Vingcrs L, Marberger M. Morphology of tissue destruction induced by focused ultrasound. Eur. Urol., 23 (Suppl. I): 34-38, 1993.

Madersbacher S, Pedevilla M, Vingers L, et al., Martin Susani, and Michael Marberger. Effect of High-Intensity Focused Ultrasound on human prostate cancer in vivo. Cancer Research 1995; 55: 3346-3351

Lindau O, Lauterborn W., Cinematographic observation of the collapse and rebound of a laser-produced cavitation bubble near a wall, J. Fluid Mech. 479, (2003) 327–348.

Chen H, Li X, Wan M, Wang S. High-speed observation of cavitation bubble clouds near a tissue boundary in high-intensity focused ultrasound fields. Ultrasonics 49 (2009) 289–292.

Clarke RL, Ter Haar GR. Temperature rise recorded during lesion formation by high-intensity focused ultrasound. Ultrasound in Med e Biol 1997;23:299-306.

Bush N. Rivens I, Ter Haar GR, Bamber JC. Acoustic properties of lesions generated with an ultrasound therapy system. Ultrasound Med Biol 1993; 19:789-801.

Hartveit F. Breast cancer: poor short-term prognosis in cases with moderate lymphocyte infiltration at the tumour edge: a preliminary report. Oncol Rep 1998;5:423-6.

Lu P, Zhu XQ, Xu ZL, Zhou Q, Zhang J, Wu F. Increased infiltration of activated tumor-infiltrating lymphocytes after high intensity focused ultrasound ablation of human breast cancer. Surgery 2009; 145: 286-93.

Srivastava, P. Roles of heat-shock proteins in innate and adaptive immunity. *Nat. Rev. Immunol.* 2002, *2*(3): 185-194.

Crouzet S, Rebillard X, Chevallier D, Rischmann P, Pasticer G, Garcia G, et al. Multicentric oncologic outcome of High-Intensity Focused Ultrasound for localized prostate cancer in 803 patients. Eur Urol 2010;58:559-66

Ahmed U, Zacharakis E, Dudderidge T, Armitage JN, Scott R, Calleary J. High-intensity-focused ultrasound in the treatment of primary prostate cancer: the first UK series. Br J Cancer 2009;101:19-26

Blana A, Murat F, Walter B, Thuroff S, Wieland WF, Chaussy C. First analysis of the long-term results with transrectal hifu in patients with localised prostate cancer. Eur Urol 2008;53:1194-203

Challacombe B, Murphy DG, Zakri R, Cahill DJ. High-intensity focused ultrasound for localized prostate cancer: initial experience with a 2-year follow-up. BJU Int 2009;104: 200-4

3

Prostate Specific Membrane Antigen as Biomarker and Therapeutic Target for Prostate Cancer

Philipp Wolf
Department of Urology, University Medical Centre Freiburg
Germany

1. Introduction

The Prostate Specific Membrane Antigen (PSMA) is considered to be the most well established target antigen in prostate cancer, since it is highly and specifically expressed at all tumor stages on the surface of prostate tumor cells. This chapter outlines the structure, function, and expression of PSMA, its relevance as prognostic and diagnostic biomarker, and different therapeutic approaches targeting this antigen.

2. The Prostate Specific Membrane Antigen (PSMA)

2.1 Structure, function and expression

PSMA, also known as Glutamate Carboxypeptidase II (GCPII, EC 3.4.17.21), N-acetyl-α-linked acidic dipeptidase I (NAALADase) or folate hydrolase, is a type II transmembrane protein, which is anchored in the cell membrane of prostate epithelial cells (Carter et al., 1996; Pinto et al., 1996). In 1998, the gene encoding PSMA was mapped to chromosome 11p11-p12, where it encompasses 19 exons spanning about 60 kb of genomic DNA (O'Keefe et al., 1998). The cDNA of PSMA codes for a glycoprotein of 750 amino acids (aa) with a molecular mass of about 100 kDa. The protein is partitioned into a small intracellular domain of 19 aa, a transmembrane domain of 21 amino acids, and a large extracellular domain of 707 aa. Crystallization data revealed that the extracellular domain of PSMA folds into three distinct structural and functional domains: a protease domain (aa 56-116), an apical domain (aa 117-351), and a C-terminal domain (aa 592-750). Furthermore, it was shown that PSMA is expressed as a compact homodimer, which is highly glycosylated with oligosaccharides accounting up to 25% of the molecular weight (Davis et al., 2005; Mesters et al., 2006).

PSMA contains a binuclear zinc site and can act as glutamate carboxypeptidase or folate hydrolase, catalyzing the hydrolytic cleavage of glutamate from poly-γ-glutamated folates (Ghosh & Heston, 2003). Therefore, PSMA is thought to play a role in the folate metabolism of the prostate. This hypothesis is supported by recent studies, where PSMA expression correlated with proliferation and folate uptake of PSMA transfected cells (Yao & Bacich, 2006; Yao et al., 2009).

In contrast to other prostate-related antigens, like prostate specific antigen (PSA), prostate acidic phosphatase (PAP) or prostate secretory protein (PSP), PSMA is not secreted into circulation. Instead of that, PSMA undergoes constitutive internalization, which is about threefold enhanced after antibody binding (Liu et al., 1998). It is therefore suggested that PSMA has transport function and that anti-PSMA antibodies might act as surrogates for a yet unknown ligand. The endocytic pathways of PSMA after antibody binding were specified in a recent study and comprise clathrin-mediated endocytosis, macropinocytosis, and clathrin-, calveolae-independent endocytosis (Liu et al., 2009b).

To examine the PSMA expression in the prostate, immunohistochemical analyses were performed. In a study with prostate tissue specimen from 184 patients with prostate cancer, the percentage of PSMA positive stained cells averaged about 69.5% (range 20%-90%) in the benign epithelium, 77.9% (range 30-100%) in high grade prostatic intraepithelial neoplasia (PIN) and was highest in adenocarcinomas with a mean of 80.2% (range 30-100%). In contrast, tumor stroma, urothelium, normal vasculature and, with rare exceptions, basal cells were PSMA negative (Bostwick et al., 1998). Other immunohistochemical studies demonstrated a heterogeneous, weak to moderate staining of normal prostate epithelial cells, and a homogeneous, extensive staining of prostate adenocarcinomas and metastases (Silver et al., 1997; Wolf et al., 2010a).

PSMA expression is highly organ specific. An extraprostatic expression was only detected in secretory cells of the salivary glands (Israeli et al., 1994; Troyer et al., 1995; Wolf et al., 2010a), in cryptic cells of the duodenal brush border (Chang et al., 1999; Wolf et al., 2010a), and in a subset of proximal renal tubules (Liu et al., 1997; Silver et al., 1997; Chang et al., 1999). In some studies, an additional expression was found in the brain and in the colon, but these results are controversially discussed (Troyer et al., 1995; Silver et al., 1997; Chang et al., 1999; Sacha et al., 2007). Nonetheless, potential side effects of anti-PSMA therapeutics against PSMA expressing normal organs were not described until today.

Interestingly, PSMA is also discussed as an unique anti-angiogenetic target, since it is expressed in the neovascularization of numerous solid tumors (bladder, kidney, breast, pancreas, lung, melanoma), but not in normal blood vessels (Liu et al., 1997; Chang et al., 1999; Chang et al., 2001; Baccala et al., 2007). In this respect, it was found that PSMA regulates cell invasion and tumor angiogenesis by modulating integrin signal transduction in endothelial cells (Conway et al., 2006).

2.2 PSMA as prognostic and diagnostic biomarker

Generally, prostate carcinoma tissues show a higher PSMA expression and an increased enzymatic activity of PSMA compared with normal prostate and benign prostate hyperplasia (BPH) tissues (Lapidus et al., 2000; Burger et al., 2002). Therefore, the question was raised, if PSMA might serve as a valuable biomarker for the management of prostate cancer.

Indeed, in different studies a direct correlation between PSMA expression and the Gleason score, which is used for the staging of prostate cancer, was determined for adenocarcinomas (Su et al., 1995; Kawakami & Nakayama, 1997; Burger et al., 2002). Moreover, an upregulation of PSMA was shown in tumor cells of patients with hormone-refractory prostate cancer (Wright et al., 1996; Kawakami & Nakayama, 1997). In a study with tissue specimen from 136 patients it was demonstrated that PSMA can serve as a prognostic biomarker, because it significantly correlates with adverse prognostic factors, like tumor grade, pathological stage, aneuploidy, and biochemical recurrence, and therefore independently predicts disease outcome (Ross et al., 2003).

Recently, a new splice variant (PSM-E) was described, which is specifically overexpressed in prostate carcinomas and which correlates with the Gleason score (Cao et al., 2007). PSM-E, which is expressed in the cytoplasm, could account for the lack of correlation between histological positive staining of anti-PSMA antibodies with clinical grade (stage) (Mannweiler et al., 2009).

Despite of such controversies, it is apparent that the enhanced expression and enzymatic activity of PSMA in aggressive prostate tumors is indicative of a selective advantage on the part of cells expressing it and that it contributes to prostate carcinogenesis.

PSMA was found to associate with the anaphase-promoting complex and to induce chromosomal instability (Rajasekaran et al., 2008). Moreover, PSMA favoured prostate cancer development in a permissive folate environment (Yao & Bacich, 2006; Yao et al., 2009). One mechanism by which PSMA contributes to prostate tumor growth is its ability to activate IL-6 and CCL5 synthesis. These cytokines acted synergistically to enhance the growth of LNCaP cells by activating the MAPK pathway (Colombatti et al., 2009).

Taken together, assessment of PSMA levels, either alone or in combination with PSA status, might prove useful in future for the diagnosis of metastatic prostate cancer, risk assessment, and the prognosis of disease outcome.

2.3 PSMA as therapeutic target

Specific characteristics of PSMA concerning its structure, function and expression make it an ideal candidate as a target antigen for the treatment of advanced prostate cancer. (1) Its high and specific expression on the prostate cancer cell surface and the fact that it is not shed into the circulation allows an effective systemic delivery of PSMA targeting therapeutics. (2) Its high organ specificity leads to a minimal binding of anti-PSMA drugs to normal organs and therefore to a maximal reduction of potential side effects. (3) Its expression at all tumor stages enables a therapeutic intervention at any time of the disease. (4) Its internalization after ligand binding can be used for the targeted delivery of intracellular acting drugs. (5) Its enzymatic activity allows the cleavage of prodrugs to active molecules on the surface of prostate cancer cells.

Many preclinical and clinical studies were performed in the last years, which used PSMA as target antigen. They include radioimmunotherapy, the use of immunotoxins, targeted virotherapy, retargeting of immune cells, PSMA vaccination, prodrug activation, photodynamic therapy, and PSMA targeting nanoparticles.

2.3.1 Anti-PSMA radioimmunotherapy

Radioimmunoconjugates generally consist of an antibody moiety as target domain coupled to a therapeutic radionuclide (alpha- or beta-particle) with the biologic effect of high linear energy transfer (LET) radiation. Compared to conventional radiotherapy, radioimmunoconjugates allow the targeted delivery of reduced radiation doses to the tumor, which ideally leads to a reduction of side effects. Moreover, the radiation of a radioimmunoconjugate is not restricted to cells presenting the target antigen. It also affects neighboring cells with a heterogeneous antigen expression or insufficient vascularization, which is so called "bystander effect" (Rzeszowska-Wolny et al., 2009).

An initial immunoscintigraphic approach targeting PSMA was done with the ^{111}Indium (^{111}In) labeled anti-PSMA monoclonal antibody 7E11 (Capromab Pendetide (Prosta Scint®), Cytogen, Philadelphia, PA) (Kahn et al., 1994; Sodee et al., 1996; Kahn et al., 1998). With this radioimmunoconjugate a higher sensitivity was reached in the imaging of prostate cancer soft tissue metastases compared to Computed Tomography (CT) or Magnetic Resonance Tomography (MRT) (Murphy et al., 1998). Therefore, Prosta Scint® received approval from the U.S. Food and Drug Administration (FDA) for the detection and imaging of prostate cancer soft tissue metastases (Rosenthal et al., 2001). The reason, why Prosta Scint® is only suitable for the detection of soft tissue metastases, is based on the fact that the 7E11 antibody recognizes an intracellular epitope of PSMA. Therefore, it can not bind to viable tumor cells, but only to PSMA molecules in damaged, dead or dying cells. Lymph node or bone metastatic lesions tend to be relatively small and do not characteristically own a high percentage of apoptotic or necrotic cells. Indeed, in a radioimmunotherapeutic trail with the ^{90}Yttrium-(^{90}Y) labeled 7E11, no objective or biochemical remissions could be measured (Deb et al., 1996; Kahn et al., 1999).

Therefore, monoclonal antibodies, which bind to the extracellular domain of PSMA, were used for the construction of radioimmunoconjugates in subsequent studies. Three anti-PSMA antibodies, called 3/A12, 3/E7, and 3/F11, which recognize different extracellular epitopes, were labeled with ^{64}Copper (^{64}Cu) and used for Positron Emission Tomography (PET) imaging of human prostatic tumors in the SCID mouse xenograft model. Whereas excellent tumor uptakes of all antibodies between 31.6 and 35.1%ID/g were measured in tumors of the PSMA expressing androgen-independent LNCaP subline C4-2, only activities at background levels were detected in PSMA negative DU 145 control xenografts (Elsasser-Beile et al., 2009; Alt et al., 2010). In a first preclinical experiment, the antibody 3/F11 was labeled with the beta particle emitter ^{177}Lutetium (^{177}Lu) and was used for the radioimmunotherapy of mice bearing C4-2 tumors xenografts. Biodistribution studies revealed a tumor to muscle ratio of more than 70 and a tumor to blood ratio of more than 4.5 after 72 h. Treatment of mice with the conjugate resulted in tumor growth inhibition and in a more than 2-fold enhanced survival after application of a single dose of 1 MBq. However, in this study the therapeutic window was small, because mice treated with a dose of 2 MBq apparently died of myelotoxicity (Behe et al., 2011).

Another panel of antibodies binding to extracellular PSMA (J415, J533, and J591) was tested in preclinical and clinical trials for radioimmunotherapy. J591 was labeled with the alpha particle emitter ^{213}Bismuth (^{213}Bi), which is well suited for the radiation of single cell neoplasms and micrometastases in a range between 0.07 and 0.1 mm. [^{213}Bi]J591 caused a high cytotoxicity against LNCaP cells *in vitro. In vivo*, a significant improvement of tumor free survival in nude bearing LNCaP tumors was reached, which was accompanied by a significant reduction of PSA serum levels (McDevitt et al., 2000). In another study, the biodistribution of the ^{131}Iod (^{131}I) labeled antibodies J591, J415, and 7E11 was examined. High tumor uptakes were measured with all antibodies in LNCaP tumor xenografts, which were up to 20-fold higher than in PSMA negative DU 145 or PC-3 tumors. Autoradiographic studies showed that the extracellular binding antibodies J415 and J591 preferentially recognized areas of viable tumor cells, whereas the intracellular binding antibody 7E11 mainly detected necrotic tumor areas (Smith-Jones et al., 2003).

The antibody J591 was chosen for further radioimmunotherapeutic experiments. To reduce a possible immunogenicity of the mouse antibody in prostate cancer patients, J591 was humanized by site directed mutagenesis of putative B- and T-cell epitopes of the variable domains and by exchanging the mouse constant domains into human ones. The humanized antibody J591 (huJ591) was then labeled with ^{131}I and ^{90}Y. Doses of 3.7 to 11.1 MBq ^{131}I-hu591 and of 3.7 to 4.7 MBq ^{90}Y-hu591 led to a reduction of mean tumor volumes between 15 and 90% in nude mice bearing LNCaP tumors. Additionally, both radioimmunoconjugates effected an 2 to 3-fold increase of median survival relative to untreated controls (Vallabhajosula et al., 2004).

In a first phase I clinical trail, prostate cancer patients initially received the ^{111}In-labeled huJ591 for immunoscintigraphy followed by application of ^{90}Y-huJ591 for therapy. With ^{111}In-huJ591 total body images demonstrated a significant metabolism of the radioimmunoconjugate in the liver and to a lesser extend in the kidneys and spleen. Additionally, bone and soft tissue metastases were efficiently targeted. One week later, ^{90}Y-huJ591 was applicated and a maximal tolerated dose (MTD) of 17.5 mCi/m^2 could be determined. PSA stabilisation was noted in 6/29 patients and 2 patients showed a PSA decline of 70 and 85% lasting 8 and 8.6 months, respectively (Milowsky et al., 2004). Another cohort of 35 patients received ^{177}Lu-labeled huJ591 at doses between 10 and 75 mCi/m^2. Blood and urinary pharmacokinetics were similar to those of ^{90}Y-huJ591. But the MTD of 70 mCi/m^2 was about 4-fold higher. Patients treated with 75 mCi/m^2 ^{177}Lu-huJ591 developed grade 3 and 4 thrombocytopenia and grade 4 neutropenia, but retreatment with 30 mCi/m^2 was well tolerated. In 4 patients a PSA decline of more than 50% and in 16 patients a PSA stabilisation was noted (Milowsky et al., 2004). In both clinical trials with radiolabeled huJ591 myelosuppression was dose-limiting. Whereas no clear correlation between myelotoxicity and therapeutic dose was determined for ^{90}Y-huJ591, myelotoxicity and especially thrombocytopenia correlated well with the applicated doses and the bone marrow doses for ^{177}Lu-huJ591 (Vallabhajosula et al., 2005).

To verify PSMA as a target for an anti-angiogenesis therapy, ^{111}In-huJ591 was used for the imaging of known metastases in patients with different solid tumors. Indeed, this radioimmunoconjugate showed a high uptake in metastases of 7/10 kidney cancer patients, 4/4 colon carcinoma patients, 3/3 lung cancer patients, 3/3 pancreatic cancer patients, 1/3 bladder cancer patients, 2/3 breast cancer patients, and 1/1 melanoma patient (Milowsky et al., 2007).

2.3.2 Anti-PSMA immunotoxins

PSMA was also used as a target for the generation of immunotoxins against prostate cancer. Immunotoxins are constructs, where a PSMA binding domain (antibody, antibody fragment, RNA aptamer, peptide) is coupled to a toxin domain. The toxin domain is targeted by the PSMA binding domain to the prostate cancer cell and is cytotoxic after internalization.

Ricin from *Ricinus communis* acts as a very common toxin for the construction of immunotoxins. It consists of the ricin A chain and the ricin B chain held together by a disulfide bond. The ricin A chain is the enzymatically active subunit, which inactivates the protein biosynthesis machinery by irreversible hydrolysis of the N-glycosidic bond of an adenine (A4324) within the 28S rRNA. The ricin B chain binds ubiquitous to cell surface structures and facilitates membrane translocation and intracellular trafficking of the ricin A chain (Sandvig et al., 2002).

The first generation of anti-PSMA immunotoxins was made by chemically coupling of anti-PSMA antibodies to ricin A. An immunotoxin consisting of J591 and ricin A elicited a 50% reduction in cell viability (IC_{50}) of LNCaP cells at a concentration of about 265 pM and showed a more than 5000-fold potentation of cytotoxicity compared to the unconjugated ricin A chain (Fracasso et al., 2002). For another ricin A-based immunotoxin with the rat monoclonal antibody E6 an IC_{50} value of 60 pM was measured. Additionally, a significant inhibition of LNCaP tumor growth in the mouse xenograft model was reached with this molecule (Huang et al., 2004).

In a recent study, the humanized antibody huJ591 was linked to the plant toxin saporin. Saporin is produced is seeds and leaves of the plant *Saponaria officinalis* and belongs to class I ribosome inactivating proteins. With the saporin-based immunotoxin, a percentage of 60.3% apoptotic cells and an IC_{50} value of 140 pM was determined on LNCaP cells after 72 h incubation. Furthermore, a significant inhibition of tumor growth was measured in the LNCaP tumor xenograft model. However, due to its high molecular weight of about 280 kDa, the immunotoxin is thought to have a high immunogenicity and a limited diffusion into tumor tissues. Therefore, further development is focused on saporin-based constructs of smaller size less inherent immunogenicity (Kuroda et al., 2010).

The anti-PSMA antibody J591 was also used for the construction of an immunotoxin containing the melittin-like peptide 101 from honey bee (*Apis mellifera*) venom. This construct successfully inhibited the growth of LNCaP-LN3 tumors and led to a slight improvement of the median survival of treated mice. However, the high affinity of peptide 101 to lipid bilayer membranes also led to a high non-specific cytotoxicity (Russell et al., 2004).

A further immunotoxin was generated by coupling huJ591 to the chemotherapeutic drug maytansinoid 1 (DM1) (Henry et al., 2004), which is a microtubule-depolymerizing analogue of maytansine (Chari et al., 1992). Maytansine is a naturally occurring ansa macrolide and was evaluated as a chemotherapeutic agent in the 1970s and 1980s. Unfortunately, maytansine caused severe, dose-limiting gastrointestinal and central neurological toxicities and was therefore not developed further (Blum et al., 1978). With the DM1-based anti-PSMA immunotoxin, called MLN2704, a growth delay of CWR22Rv1 tumor xenografts of more than 100 days was achieved at an optimized dosage schedule of 60 mg/kg every 14 days (Henry et al., 2004). MLN2704 was also tested in a clinical phase I trial in 9 patients with prostate cancer. Two of these patients, treated with 264 or 343 mg/m^2 immunotoxin respectively, had a more than 50% decrease in their PSA serum level. Additionally, the patient treated with 264 mg/m^2 showed a measurable tumor regression (Galsky et al., 2008).

In another approach, a fully human anti-PSMA antibody was generated in transgenic mice and was conjugated to monomethylauristatin E (MMAE), which is a potent inhibitor of tubulin polymerization. With this construct IC_{50} values of 83 pM on LNCaP cells and of 65 pM on C4-2 cells could be determined. Furthermore, a significant improvement of the median survival of tumor bearing mice 9-fold relative to the controls was reached without any signs of toxicity. Interestingly, 2/5 animals treated with a maximal dose of 6 mg/kg immunotoxin had no detectable tumor or measurable PSA at day 500 and could therefore considered as cure (Ma et al., 2006).

Obstacles of chemically conjugated immunotoxins to be optimal therapeutic agents comprise a high immunogenicity, a possible influence of chemical modifications on antigen binding, and inhomogeneous preparations. This can, at least in part, be overcome by second generation, recombinant immunotoxins.

For the construction of the first recombinant immunotoxin against PSMA, an anti-PSMA single chain antibody fragment (scFv), consisting of one variable domain of the heavy chain (V_H) and one variable domain of the light chain (V_L) connected by a flexible linker, was generated from the monoclonal antibody 3/A12 by phage display. This scFv was called A5.

As toxin domain, the truncated form of *Pseudomonas* exotoxin A (PE40), consisting of the transmembrane domain and the enzymatically active domain of the toxin, was used. The virulence factor *Pseudomonas* Exotoxin A from the human pathogenic bacterium *Pseudomonas aeruginosa* is able to ADP-ribosylate the eukaryotic elongation factor 2 (eEF-2) of a target cell, which leads to the inhibition of protein biosynthesis and finally to apoptosis (Wolf & Elsasser-Beile, 2009). The bacterially expressed anti-PSMA immunotoxin, called A5-PE40, specifically bound to prostate cancer cells with IC_{50} values in the low pM range. Moreover, it induced a significant growth inhibition of C4-2 tumors in the SCID mouse xenograft model (Wolf et al., 2006; Wolf et al., 2008).
A similar immunotoxin was recently generated by using the scFv D7 from the anti-PSMA antibody 3/F11. This immunotoxin, termed D7-PE40, also showed a high binding to C4-2 cells and led to a significant growth inhibition of subcutaneously implanted tumors. In toxicity studies, D7-PE40 was well tolerated in mice at single, but at higher doses the immunotoxin was lethal. Blood analyses indicated that the death of the animals was based on a severe hepatotoxicity, which was marked by increased aspartate transaminase (AST) and alanine transaminase (ALT) serum levels. Histopathological examinations revealed a marked damage of the hepatic parenchyma with disappearance of sinusoidal structures based on apoptosis and vacuolar degeneration of hepatocytes (Wolf et al., 2010b). Hepatotoxicity is a very common side effect of *Pseudomonas* Exotoxin A based immunotoxins and is presumably attributed to a TNF-alpha release of Kupffer cells (Onda et al., 1999). Different strategies are therefore under investigation to reduce the hepatotoxicity, e.g. by PEGylation or lowering of the isoelectric points of the immunotoxins (Onda et al., 2001). Another main research comprises the reduction of the immunogenicity by elimination of immunodominant B-cell epitopes (Onda et al., 2006).
Alternatively to antibodies or antibody fragments, RNA aptamers can be used for the construction of immunotoxins, which are considered to be advantageous with respect to a higher stability, ease of synthesis and lower production costs. One immunotoxin was constructed by coupling of an anti-PSMA RNA aptamer to the plant toxin gelonin from *Gelonium multiflorum*, which has high N-glycosidase activity on the 28S RNA unit of eukaryotic ribosomes. This molecule was found to be toxic against prostate cancer cells with an IC_{50} value of 27 nM (Onda et al., 2006).
Recently, a chemical ligand, termed 2-[3-(1,3-dicarboxypropyl)ureido] pentanedioic acid (DUPA), was synthesized that selectively binds to PSMA (Kularatne et al., 2010). After coupling to different chemotherapeutic drugs, this molecule was capable to mediate the targeted killing of LNCaP cells (Kularatne et al., 2010).

2.3.3 Targeted virotherapy

In a recent study, measles viruses of a live attenuated strain were used for a targeted anti-PSMA virotherapy (Liu et al., 2009a). Measles viruses are very effective against a variety of tumor types, including prostate cancer (Blechacz & Russell, 2008; Msaouel et al., 2009). Generally, measles viruses infect host cells via one of two measles receptors, CD64 or SLAM. CD64 is ubiquitously present on the surface of human cells, whereas SLAM is expressed on immune cells. The viruses take their oncolytic effect by induction of an extensive intracellular fusion between infected cells and neighboring cells to form non-viable multinucleated structures (syncytia). For the construction of the virotherapeutic conjugate, called MVG-αPSMA, the anti-PSMA antibody huJ591 was coupled to a coat protein of measles virus, in which alanine substitutions of specific residues ablated the viral interaction with CD64 and SLAM. After propagation and infection, a MVG-αPSMA mediated cytopathic killing of PSMA expressing LNCaP and PC3/PIP cells was detected. Moreover, a regression or growth inhibition of tumor xenografts could be achieved (Msaouel et al., 2009). A crucial obstacle for a future clinical use of MVG-αPSMA could be pre-existing anti-viral antibodies in patients, who have been vaccinated or infected by wild type measles viruses. These antibodies might quickly neutralize the virus domain after application. Therefore, efforts are undertaken to circumvent the problem, e.g. by intratumoral application of the construct, by hiding the virus in cell carriers, or by the use of immunosuppressive drugs to dampen the patient's immune response (Liu et al., 2009a).

2.3.4 Retargeting of immune cells

The therapeutic concept of immune cell retargeting comprises the activation of T lymphocytes for the targeted cytolysis of tumor cells. For the retargeting of prostate cancer cells via PSMA, two strategies were pursued: the construction of diabodies and the generation of fusion receptors.

Generally, diabodies for T cell retargeting consist of two antibody domains. One domain binds to the tumor antigen and the other one to a T cell activating antigen. The diabody builds a bridge between the tumor cell and the immune effector cell, which then triggers the cytotoxic responses that include perforin and granzyme release.

Anti-PSMA diabodies were constructed by fusing the anti-PSMA scFvs A5 or D7 to a scFv against the CD3 T cell receptor. With these constructs, a retargeting of CD4+ and CD8+ blood lymphocytes with subsequent lysis of C4-2 cells was obtained. Moreover, a significant inhibition of C4-2 tumor growth could be achieved (Buhler et al., 2008; Buhler et al., 2009; Fortmuller et al., 2011).

A fusion receptor targeting PSMA, also referred to as chimeric antigen receptor (CAR), was generated by coupling an anti-PSMA scFv to the zeta-chain of the CD3 T-cell receptor. The CAR can be expressed at the surface of CAR-transfected T cells. Then the CAR can recruit and activate the T cell by binding to PSMA. This mechanism is independent of a human leukocyte antigen expression. Using CAR transfected peripheral blood lymphocytes, a specific killing of PSMA-expressing prostate cancer cells and an elimination of orthotopically or subcutaneously implanted PSMA-positive tumors was reached (Gade et al., 2005). In a subsequent study, the effects of CAR could be optimized by adding combined CD28 and 4-1BBL costimulatory signaling domains. With this strategy, an enhanced cytokine release, a higher *in vivo* T cell survival, and an enhanced anti-tumor activity could be measured in tumor bearing SCID mice (Zhong et al., 2010).

A similar fusion receptor against PSMA, designated as chimeric immunoglobulin T-cell receptor (IgTCR), was also used for the retargeting of immune cells. IgTCR consists of an anti-PSMA scFv from the monoclonal antibody 3D8 and a signaling portion of the CD3 zeta chain. IgTCR transfected T-cells were activated after PSMA binding, which was followed by cytokine release and specific lysis of the prostate cancer cells. Additionally, this molecule showed a high anti-tumor activity in a mouse xenograft model (Ma et al., 2004).

2.3.5 PSMA vaccination

Vaccination with PSMA peptides, which aims for boosting the patient's immune response against PSMA expressing tumor cells, represent another weapon in the battle against prostate cancer. One approach utilizes the patient's dentritic cells (DCs), to present PSMA peptides in association with the MHC class I peptide complex to naïve cytotoxic T lymphocytes (CTL) (Melief, 2008). For DC preparation, patients were leucophoresed and peripheral blood mononuclear cells (PBMCs) were isolated. Adherent cells were differentiated with GM-CSF and IL-4. Then the obtained DCs were pulsed with recombinant PSMA peptides, which were identified in function of their ability to recruit CTLs and to be recognized as CTL targets. In a first phase I/II clinical trial involving 33 prostate cancer patients, 9 partial responders were identified with an average response duration of 225 days (Tjoa et al., 1998). In a phase II study, 2/33 patients with hormone refractory metastatic disease showed a complete response and another 6 patients a partial response (Murphy et al., 1999). In another clinical trial with 37 patients, one complete and 10 partial responses were identified (Salgaller et al., 1998; Tjoa et al., 1999).

Two subsequent protocols used DCs to present a PSMA peptide in combination with peptides from other tumor antigens to treat hormone-refractory patients. In one study, CTL responses and transient decline of serum PSA was observed in 4/8 patients, who received 4 intradermal vaccinations every other week (Fuessel et al., 2006). In the other study, 3 patients were administered with 6 vaccines intradermally at biweekly intervals and showed partial remissions. However, no CTL response against the PSMA peptide could be observed (Waeckerle-Men et al., 2006). The same PSMA peptide was loaded as a single peptide to PBMCs, which were used to treat 12 patients with hormone-resistant tumors. However, no clinical advantages were observed and no immune responses were detected in this trial (Knight et al., 2009).

A further development was the transfection of DCs with plasmids containing the extracellular domain of PSMA to activate autologous lymphocytes in an *in vitro* model. Indeed, PSMA-expressing DCs were able to generate antigen-specific cytotoxic T cell responses (Mincheff et al., 2003).

In a recent study, replication deficient adenoviruses were used to introduce a truncated form of PSMA and the T cell stimulatory molecule 4-1BBL into murine DCs. After infection of the DCs, PSMA-specific proliferative responses and an upregulation of CD80 and CD86 costimulatory molecules were detected. Moreover, vaccination of mice with the transfected DCs induced a potent protective and therapeutic anti-tumor immunity (Kuang et al., 2010).

Other strategies for PSMA vaccination are the application of DNA plasmids or viral immunizations. In a phase I study, prostate cancer patients were intradermally immunized with an expression plasmid or a replication-defective adenoviral vector bearing the PSMA gene according to six different drug regimens. All vaccinations were well tolerated and no immediate- or long-time side effects were reported (Mincheff et al., 2000). Anti-PSMA antibodies were found in 21% of patients at baseline and in 12-50% of patients at longitudinal time points ranging from 3 to 36 months after immunization (Todorova et al., 2005).

In a preclinical study it was shown that immunization of mice with xenogenic PSMA protein followed by a boosting with a vector that encoded autologous PSMA gave the best protection (Mincheff et al., 2006). These data provided the basis for a clinical study with DNA plasmid vaccines, in which 36 patients with recurrent prostate cancer received three vaccinations with mouse or human PSMA. Vaccination was well tolerated and PSA serum levels were maximally reduced at the highest dose level (Gregor et al., 2007).

2.3.6 Prodrug activation

The glutamate carboxy peptidase activity of PSMA can be used for the activation of prodrugs to a fully active compound on the surface of prostate cancer cells. Different methotrexate-based peptide analoges were screened to identify PSMA selective substrates that are stable to unspecific hydrolysis in human and mouse plasma. Analogs containing α-linked or γ-linked glutamic or aspartic acids were most efficiently hydrolyzed by PSMA to release the cytolytic anti-metabolite methotrexate. As a consequence thereof, these analoges showed the highest cytotoxicity against PSMA-expressing prostate cancer cells (Mhaka et al., 2004). In a subsequent study, these peptides were coupled to a cytotoxic analogue of the plant toxin thapsigargin that induces apoptosis by inhibition of the endoplasmatic reticulum Ca-ATPase pump. PSMA hydrolysis of these peptide prodrugs led to a cytotoxicity against PSMA-positive prostate cancer cells that was 10- to 60-fold higher than against PSMA-negative ones. One of these prodrugs was also tested in mice with CWR22H xenografts and elicited tumor growth delay or tumor regressions following a single 3-day or 10-day course of administration (Mhaka et al., 2006).

2.3.7 Photodynamic therapy

The lack of specific delivery of photosensitizers, chemical compounds that can be excited by light of a specific wavelength for the destruction of tumor tissues, represents a significant limitation for photodynamic therapies (PDT). Therefore, a conjugate was generated containing the photosensitizer pyropheophorbide-a and a PSMA inhibitor for the treatment of prostate cancer. This construct demonstrated a high and specific cytotoxicity against LNCaP cells after irradiation, whereas PSMA-negative PC-3 cells remained unaffected. PDT-mediated effects of the photodynamic conjugate were extensively studied and involved cell membrane permeabilization, rapid disruption of microtubules (α-/β-tubulin), microfilaments (actin), and intermediate filaments (cytokeratin 8/18) in the cytoplasm, activation of caspase-3, -8, and -9, Poly [ADP-ribose] Polymerase (PARP)-cleavage, and DNA fragmentation (Liu et al., 2009c; Liu et al., 2010a; Liu et al., 2010b).

2.3.8 Nanoparticles targeting PSMA

Nanotechnology represents a new alternative for the treatment of prostate cancer. The production of nanoparticles enables the targeted delivery and controlled release of thousands of drug molecules per vehicle into the tumor cells and is a promising strategy to overcome the lack of specificity and limited efficacy of conventional chemotherapeutic agents.

One of the first therapeutic nanoparticle against prostate cancer was a docetaxel-encapsulated nanoparticle formulated with biocompatible and biodegradable poly(D,L-lactic acid-co-glycolic acid)-block-poly(ethyleneglycol) copolymer (PLGA-b-PEG), which surface was derivatized with the anti-PSMA RNA-aptamer A10. With this construct, an enhanced cytotoxicity, compared to non-targeted nanoparticles that lack the aptamer, was shown. After a single intratumoral injection, the nanoparticle elicited a complete tumor reduction in 5/7 mice with LNCaP tumor xenografts of about 300 mm^3 in size. The survival rate of these mice in a 109 days study was 100%, compared to 57% of mice treated with the non-targeted nanoparticle and to 14% of mice treated with docetaxel alone (Farokhzad et al., 2006). In a subsequent study, the cisplatin prodrug Pt(IV) was encapsulated in the anti-PSMA nanoparticle. Endocytosis was detected using fluorescence microscopy by colocalization of the encapsulated green fluorescent labeled cholesterol with early endosome marker EEA-1. In a series of *in vitro* cytotoxic assays, the IC_{50} value was determined as 0.03 μM for the nanoparticele compared to 0.13 μM for the non-targeted nanoparticle and to 2.4 μM for free cisplatin on LNCaP cells. However, a high background toxicity of the nanoparticle with an IC_{50} value of 0.11 μM was also detected on PSMA-negative PC-3 cells (Dhar et al., 2008). In a recent study, the anti-PSMA aptamer based nanoparticle was optimized to a self-assembly polymeric nanoparticle carrying cisplatin and docetaxel to prostate cancer cells with synergistic cytotoxicity. The controlled released of both chemotherapeutics was observed over a time period of 48 to 72 h and formation of cisplatin 1,2d(GpG) intrastrand crosslinks could be detected. *In vitro* cytotoxicity of the targeted nanoparticle with an IC_{50} value of 0.09 μM on LNCaP cells was shown to be superior over single drug or non targeted nanoparticles (Kolishetti et al., 2010).

Epigallocatechin 3-gallate (EGCG) is a green tea catechin, which has protective effects against some common types of cancer (Yang et al., 2009). Since it was shown to be chemopreventive against prostate cancer (Bettuzzi et al., 2006; Brausi et al., 2008), an EGCG loaded nanoparticle consisting of PLGA-PEG copolymers was functionalized with an urea-based PSMA inhibitor (Sanna et al., 2011), which is capable of targeting PSMA with a similar affinity and specificity like antibodies and aptamers (Sanna et al., 2011). In *in vitro* experiments LNCaP cells were incubated for 1 or 3 h with the anti-PSMA nanoparticles. In this assay, a significant antiproliferative effect of the nanoparticles to the tumor cells, marked by a growth inhibition up to 60% after 72 h, could be measured (Sanna et al., 2011).

3. Conclusion

In the last years, PSMA arouse increasing interest as a prognostic and diagnostic biomarker as well as an attractive target antigen for new therapeutic approaches against prostate cancer.

Anti-PSMA radioimmunoconjugates demonstrated efficient targeting of soft tissue and bone metastases and led to objective anti-tumor responses in a subset of patients. Moreover, high efficacy and tolerability of anti-PSMA immunotoxins was shown in many preclinical and clinical trials. The future strategy in this field is the recombinant production of immunotoxins, by which different limitations of chemically linked immunotoxins can be overcome.

Retargeting of cytotoxic lymphocytes *in vitro* and *in vivo* led to anti-tumor activities in different preclinical studies. These effects could be enhanced by the evocation of costimulatory signaling. Additionally, early vaccination trials showed that an anti-PSMA immune response can be generated without general toxicity in prostate cancer patients.

The development of PSMA-targeted prodrugs, photosensitizers and nanoparticles is still in an early stage, but such constructs also represent alternative therapeutics in the near future.

It has to be considered that most of the discussed clinical treatments were tested in patients with advanced prostate cancer. However, as shown in preclinical trials, these new therapeutic drugs seem likely to be more effective in patients with minimal residual disease or metastases after primary therapies.

4. References

Alt, K., Wiehr, S., Ehrlichmann, W., Reischl, G., Wolf, P., Pichler, B.J., Elsasser-Beile, U. & Buhler, P. (2010). High-resolution animal PET imaging of prostate cancer xenografts with three different (64)Cu-labeled antibodies against native cell-adherent PSMA. *Prostate*, Vol. 70, No. 13, pp. 1413-1421.

Baccala, A., Sercia, L., Li, J., Heston, W. & Zhou, M. (2007). Expression of prostate-specific membrane antigen in tumor-associated neovasculature of renal neoplasms. *Urology,* Vol. 70, No. 2, pp. 385-390.

Bander, N.H., Milowsky, M.I., Nanus, D.M., Kostakoglu, L., Vallabhajosula, S. & Goldsmith, S.J. (2005). Phase I trial of 177lutetium-labeled J591, a monoclonal antibody to prostate-specific membrane antigen, in patients with androgen-independent prostate cancer. *J Clin Oncol,* Vol. 23, No. 21, pp. 4591-4601.

Behe, M., Alt, K., Deininger, F., Buhler, P., Wetterauer, U., Weber, W.A., Elsasser-Beile, U. & Wolf, P. (2011). In vivo testing of 177Lu-labelled anti-PSMA antibody as a new radioimmunotherapeutic agent against prostate cancer. *In Vivo,* Vol. 25, No. 1, pp. 55-59.

Bettuzzi, S., Brausi, M., Rizzi, F., Castagnetti, G., Peracchia, G. & Corti, A. (2006). Chemoprevention of human prostate cancer by oral administration of green tea catechins in volunteers with high-grade prostate intraepithelial neoplasia: a preliminary report from a one-year proof-of-principle study. *Cancer Res,* Vol. 66, No. 2, pp. 1234-1240.

Blechacz, B. & Russell, S.J. (2008). Measles virus as an oncolytic vector platform. *Curr Gene Ther,* Vol. 8, No. 3, pp. 162-175.

Blum, R.H., Wittenberg, B.K., Canellos, G.P., Mayer, R.J., Skarin, A.T., Henderson, I.C., Parker, L.M. & Frei, E., 3rd. (1978). A therapeutic trial of maytansine. *Cancer Clin Trials,* Vol. 1, No. 2, pp. 113-117.

Bostwick, D.G., Pacelli, A., Blute, M., Roche, P. & Murphy, G.P. (1998). Prostate specific membrane antigen expression in prostatic intraepithelial neoplasia and adenocarcinoma: a study of 184 cases. *Cancer,* Vol. 82, No. 11, pp. 2256-2261.

Brausi, M., Rizzi, F. & Bettuzzi, S. (2008). Chemoprevention of human prostate cancer by green tea catechins: two years later. A follow-up update. *Eur Urol,* Vol. 54, No. 2, pp. 472-473.

Buhler, P., Molnar, E., Dopfer, E.P., Wolf, P., Gierschner, D., Wetterauer, U., Schamel, W.W. & Elsasser-Beile, U. (2009). Target-dependent T-cell activation by coligation with a PSMA x CD3 diabody induces lysis of prostate cancer cells. *J Immunother,* Vol. 32, No. 6, pp. 565-573.

Buhler, P., Wolf, P., Gierschner, D., Schaber, I., Katzenwadel, A., Schultze-Seemann, W., Wetterauer, U., Tacke, M., Swamy, M., Schamel, W.W. & Elsasser-Beile, U. (2008). A bispecific diabody directed against prostate-specific membrane antigen and CD3 induces T-cell mediated lysis of prostate cancer cells. *Cancer Immunol Immunother,* Vol. 57, No. 1, pp. 43-52.

Burger, M.J., Tebay, M.A., Keith, P.A., Samaratunga, H.M., Clements, J., Lavin, M.F. & Gardiner, R.A. (2002). Expression analysis of delta-catenin and prostate-specific membrane antigen: their potential as diagnostic markers for prostate cancer. *Int J Cancer,* Vol. 100, No. 2, pp. 228-237.

Cao, K.Y., Mao, X.P., Wang, D.H., Xu, L., Yuan, G.Q., Dai, S.Q., Zheng, B.J. & Qiu, S.P. (2007). High expression of PSM-E correlated with tumor grade in prostate cancer: a new alternatively spliced variant of prostate-specific membrane antigen. *Prostate,* Vol. 67, No. 16, pp. 1791-1800.

Carter, R.E., Feldman, A.R. & Coyle, J.T. (1996). Prostate-specific membrane antigen is a hydrolase with substrate and pharmacologic characteristics of a neuropeptidase. *Proc Natl Acad Sci U S A,* Vol. 93, No. 2, pp. 749-753.

Chang, S.S., Reuter, V.E., Heston, W.D. & Gaudin, P.B. (2001). Metastatic renal cell carcinoma neovasculature expresses prostate-specific membrane antigen. *Urology,* Vol. 57, No. 4, pp. 801-805.

Chang, S.S., Reuter, V.E., Heston, W.D., Bander, N.H., Grauer, L.S. & Gaudin, P.B. (1999). Five different anti-prostate-specific membrane antigen (PSMA) antibodies confirm PSMA expression in tumor-associated neovasculature. *Cancer Res,* Vol. 59, No. 13, pp. 3192-3198.

Chari, R.V., Martell, B.A., Gross, J.L., Cook, S.B., Shah, S.A., Blattler, W.A., McKenzie, S.J. & Goldmacher, V.S. (1992). Immunoconjugates containing novel maytansinoids: promising anticancer drugs. *Cancer Res,* Vol. 52, No. 1, pp. 127-131.

Chu, T.C., Marks, J.W., 3rd, Lavery, L.A., Faulkner, S., Rosenblum, M.G., Ellington, A.D. & Levy, M. (2006). Aptamer:toxin conjugates that specifically target prostate tumor cells. *Cancer Res,* Vol. 66, No. 12, pp. 5989-5992.

Colombatti, M., Grasso, S., Porzia, A., Fracasso, G., Scupoli, M.T., Cingarlini, S., Poffe, O., Naim, H.Y., Heine, M., Tridente, G., Mainiero, F. & Ramarli, D. (2009). The prostate specific membrane antigen regulates the expression of IL-6 and CCL5 in prostate tumour cells by activating the MAPK pathways. *PLoS One,* Vol. 4, No. 2, pp. e4608.

Conway, R.E., Petrovic, N., Li, Z., Heston, W., Wu, D. & Shapiro, L.H. (2006). Prostate-specific membrane antigen regulates angiogenesis by modulating integrin signal transduction. *Mol Cell Biol,* Vol. 26, No. 14, pp. 5310-5324.

Davis, M.I., Bennett, M.J., Thomas, L.M. & Bjorkman, P.J. (2005). Crystal structure of prostate-specific membrane antigen, a tumor marker and peptidase. *Proc Natl Acad Sci U S A,* Vol. 102, No. 17, pp. 5981-5986.

Deb, N., Goris, M., Trisler, K., Fowler, S., Saal, J., Ning, S., Becker, M., Marquez, C. & Knox, S. (1996). Treatment of hormone-refractory prostate cancer with 90Y-CYT-356 monoclonal antibody. *Clin Cancer Res,* Vol. 2, No. 8, pp. 1289-1297.

Dhar, S., Gu, F.X., Langer, R., Farokhzad, O.C. & Lippard, S.J. (2008). Targeted delivery of cisplatin to prostate cancer cells by aptamer functionalized Pt(IV) prodrug-PLGA-PEG nanoparticles. *Proc Natl Acad Sci U S A,* Vol. 105, No. 45, pp. 17356-17361.

Elsasser-Beile, U., Reischl, G., Wiehr, S., Buhler, P., Wolf, P., Alt, K., Shively, J., Judenhofer, M.S., Machulla, H.J. & Pichler, B.J. (2009). PET Imaging of Prostate Cancer Xenografts with a Highly Specific Antibody against the Prostate-Specific Membrane Antigen. *J Nucl Med,* Vol. 50, No. 4, pp. 606-611.

Farokhzad, O.C., Cheng, J., Teply, B.A., Sherifi, I., Jon, S., Kantoff, P.W., Richie, J.P. & Langer, R. (2006). Targeted nanoparticle-aptamer bioconjugates for cancer chemotherapy in vivo. *Proc Natl Acad Sci U S A,* Vol. 103, No. 16, pp. 6315-6320.

Fortmuller, K., Alt, K., Gierschner, D., Wolf, P., Baum, V., Freudenberg, N., Wetterauer, U., Elsasser-Beile, U. & Buhler, P. (2011). Effective targeting of prostate cancer by lymphocytes redirected by a PSMA x CD3 bispecific single-chain diabody. *Prostate,* Vol. 71, No. 6, pp. 588-596.

Fracasso, G., Bellisola, G., Cingarlini, S., Castelletti, D., Prayer-Galetti, T., Pagano, F., Tridente, G. & Colombatti, M. (2002). Anti-tumor effects of toxins targeted to the prostate specific membrane antigen. *Prostate,* Vol. 53, No. 1, pp. 9-23.

Fuessel, S., Meye, A., Schmitz, M., Zastrow, S., Linne, C., Richter, K., Lobel, B., Hakenberg, O.W., Hoelig, K., Rieber, E.P. & Wirth, M.P. (2006). Vaccination of hormone-refractory prostate cancer patients with peptide cocktail-loaded dendritic cells: results of a phase I clinical trial. *Prostate,* Vol. 66, No. 8, pp. 811-821.

Gade, T.P., Hassen, W., Santos, E., Gunset, G., Saudemont, A., Gong, M.C., Brentjens, R., Zhong, X.S., Stephan, M., Stefanski, J., Lyddane, C., Osborne, J.R., Buchanan, I.M., Hall, S.J., Heston, W.D., Riviere, I., Larson, S.M., Koutcher, J.A. & Sadelain, M. (2005). Targeted elimination of prostate cancer by genetically directed human T lymphocytes. *Cancer Res,* Vol. 65, No. 19, pp. 9080-9088.

Galsky, M.D., Eisenberger, M., Moore-Cooper, S., Kelly, W.K., Slovin, S.F., DeLaCruz, A., Lee, Y., Webb, I.J. & Scher, H.I. (2008). Phase I trial of the prostate-specific membrane antigen-directed immunoconjugate MLN2704 in patients with progressive metastatic castration-resistant prostate cancer. *J Clin Oncol,* Vol. 26, No. 13, pp. 2147-2154.

Ghosh, A. & Heston, W.D. (2003). Effect of carbohydrate moieties on the folate hydrolysis activity of the prostate specific membrane antigen. *Prostate,* Vol. 57, No. 2, pp. 140-151.

Gregor, P., Wolchok, J., Pedraza, A., Orlandi, F., Jefferson, M., Rudolph, J., Curley, T., Houghton, A., Scher, H. & Slovin, S.F., 2007: A xenogeneic PSMA DNA vaccine for patients (pts) with non-castrate metastatic (NCMPC) and castrate metastatic prostate cancer (CMPC): A phase I trial of proof of principle. In 2007 Prostate Cancer Symposium (Orlando).

Henry, M.D., Wen, S., Silva, M.D., Chandra, S., Milton, M. & Worland, P.J. (2004). A prostate-specific membrane antigen-targeted monoclonal antibody-chemotherapeutic conjugate designed for the treatment of prostate cancer. *Cancer Res,* Vol. 64, No. 21, pp. 7995-8001.

Huang, X., Bennett, M. & Thorpe, P.E. (2004). Anti-tumor effects and lack of side effects in mice of an immunotoxin directed against human and mouse prostate-specific membrane antigen. *Prostate,* Vol. 61, No. 1, pp. 1-11.

Israeli, R.S., Powell, C.T., Corr, J.G., Fair, W.R. & Heston, W.D. (1994). Expression of the prostate-specific membrane antigen. *Cancer Res,* Vol. 54, No. 7, pp. 1807-1811.

Kahn, D., Austin, J.C., Maguire, R.T., Miller, S.J., Gerstbrein, J. & Williams, R.D. (1999). A phase II study of [90Y] yttrium-capromab pendetide in the treatment of men with prostate cancer recurrence following radical prostatectomy. *Cancer Biother Radiopharm,* Vol. 14, No. 2, pp. 99-111.

Kahn, D., Williams, R.D., Manyak, M.J., Haseman, M.K., Seldin, D.W., Libertino, J.A. & Maguire, R.T. (1998). 111Indium-capromab pendetide in the evaluation of patients with residual or recurrent prostate cancer after radical prostatectomy. The ProstaScint Study Group. *J Urol,* Vol. 159, No. 6, pp. 2041-2046; discussion 2046-2047.

Kahn, D., Williams, R.D., Seldin, D.W., Libertino, J.A., Hirschhorn, M., Dreicer, R., Weiner, G.J., Bushnell, D. & Gulfo, J. (1994). Radioimmunoscintigraphy with 111indium labeled CYT-356 for the detection of occult prostate cancer recurrence. *J Urol,* Vol. 152, No. 5 Pt 1, pp. 1490-1495.

Kawakami, M. & Nakayama, J. (1997). Enhanced expression of prostate-specific membrane antigen gene in prostate cancer as revealed by in situ hybridization. *Cancer Res,* Vol. 57, No. 12, pp. 2321-2324.

Knight, D., Peterson, A.C., Rini, B.I., Harlin, H., Gajewski, T.F. & Stadler, W.M. (2009). The HLA-A2-restricted PSMA peptide LLHETDSAV is poorly immunogenic in patients with metastatic prostate cancer. *Prostate,* Vol. 69, No. 2, pp. 142-148.

Kolishetti, N., Dhar, S., Valencia, P.M., Lin, L.Q., Karnik, R., Lippard, S.J., Langer, R. & Farokhzad, O.C. (2010). Engineering of self-assembled nanoparticle platform for precisely controlled combination drug therapy. *Proc Natl Acad Sci U S A,* Vol. 107, No. 42, pp. 17939-17944.

Kuang, Y., Weng, X., Liu, X., Zhu, H., Chen, Z., Jiang, B. & Chen, H. (2010). Anti-tumor immune response induced by dendritic cells transduced with truncated PSMA IRES 4-1BBL recombinant adenoviruses. *Cancer Lett,* Vol. 293, No. 2, pp. 254-262.

Kularatne, S.A., Venkatesh, C., Santhapuram, H.K., Wang, K., Vaitilingam, B., Henne, W.A. & Low, P.S. (2010). Synthesis and biological analysis of prostate-specific membrane antigen-targeted anticancer prodrugs. *J Med Chem,* Vol. 53, No. 21, pp. 7767-7777.

Kuroda, K., Liu, H., Kim, S., Guo, M., Navarro, V. & Bander, N.H. (2010). Saporin toxin-conjugated monoclonal antibody targeting prostate-specific membrane antigen has potent anticancer activity. *Prostate,* Vol. 70, No. 12, pp. 1286-1294.

Lapidus, R.G., Tiffany, C.W., Isaacs, J.T. & Slusher, B.S. (2000). Prostate-specific membrane antigen (PSMA) enzyme activity is elevated in prostate cancer cells. *Prostate,* Vol. 45, No. 4, pp. 350-354.

Liu, C., Hasegawa, K., Russell, S.J., Sadelain, M. & Peng, K.W. (2009a). Prostate-specific membrane antigen retargeted measles virotherapy for the treatment of prostate cancer. *Prostate,* Vol. 69, No. 10, pp. 1128-1141.

Liu, H., Moy, P., Kim, S., Xia, Y., Rajasekaran, A., Navarro, V., Knudsen, B. & Bander, N.H. (1997). Monoclonal antibodies to the extracellular domain of prostate-specific membrane antigen also react with tumor vascular endothelium. *Cancer Res,* Vol. 57, No. 17, pp. 3629-3634.

Liu, H., Rajasekaran, A.K., Moy, P., Xia, Y., Kim, S., Navarro, V., Rahmati, R. & Bander, N.H. (1998). Constitutive and antibody-induced internalization of prostate-specific membrane antigen. *Cancer Res,* Vol. 58, No. 18, pp. 4055-4060.

Liu, J., Kopeckova, P., Buhler, P., Wolf, P., Pan, H., Bauer, H., Elsasser-Beile, U. & Kopecek, J. (2009b). Biorecognition and Subcellular Trafficking of HPMA Copolymer-Anti-PSMA Antibody Conjugates by Prostate Cancer Cells. *Mol Pharm,* No. pp.

Liu, T., Wu, L.Y. & Berkman, C.E. (2010a). Prostate-specific membrane antigen-targeted photodynamic therapy induces rapid cytoskeletal disruption. *Cancer Lett,* Vol. 296, No. 1, pp. 106-112.

Liu, T., Wu, L.Y., Choi, J.K. & Berkman, C.E. (2009c). In vitro targeted photodynamic therapy with a pyropheophorbide--a conjugated inhibitor of prostate-specific membrane antigen. *Prostate,* Vol. 69, No. 6, pp. 585-594.

Liu, T., Wu, L.Y., Choi, J.K. & Berkman, C.E. (2010b). Targeted photodynamic therapy for prostate cancer: inducing apoptosis via activation of the caspase-8/-3 cascade pathway. *Int J Oncol,* Vol. 36, No. 4, pp. 777-784.

Ma, D., Hopf, C.E., Malewicz, A.D., Donovan, G.P., Senter, P.D., Goeckeler, W.F., Maddon, P.J. & Olson, W.C. (2006). Potent antitumor activity of an auristatin-conjugated, fully human monoclonal antibody to prostate-specific membrane antigen. *Clin Cancer Res,* Vol. 12, No. 8, pp. 2591-2596.

Ma, Q., Safar, M., Holmes, E., Wang, Y., Boynton, A.L. & Junghans, R.P. (2004). Anti-prostate specific membrane antigen designer T cells for prostate cancer therapy. *Prostate,* Vol. 61, No. 1, pp. 12-25.

Mannweiler, S., Amersdorfer, P., Trajanoski, S., Terrett, J.A., King, D. & Mehes, G. (2009). Heterogeneity of prostate-specific membrane antigen (PSMA) expression in prostate carcinoma with distant metastasis. *Pathol Oncol Res,* Vol. 15, No. 2, pp. 167-172.

McDevitt, M.R., Barendswaard, E., Ma, D., Lai, L., Curcio, M.J., Sgouros, G., Ballangrud, A.M., Yang, W.H., Finn, R.D., Pellegrini, V., Geerlings, M.W., Jr., Lee, M., Brechbiel, M.W., Bander, N.H., Cordon-Cardo, C. & Scheinberg, D.A. (2000). An alpha-particle emitting antibody ([213Bi]J591) for radioimmunotherapy of prostate cancer. *Cancer Res,* Vol. 60, No. 21, pp. 6095-6100.

Melief, C.J. (2008). Cancer immunotherapy by dendritic cells. *Immunity,* Vol. 29, No. 3, pp. 372-383.

Mesters, J.R., Barinka, C., Li, W., Tsukamoto, T., Majer, P., Slusher, B.S., Konvalinka, J. & Hilgenfeld, R. (2006). Structure of glutamate carboxypeptidase II, a drug target in neuronal damage and prostate cancer. *Embo J,* Vol. 25, No. 6, pp. 1375-1384.

Mhaka, A., Gady, A.M., Rosen, D.M., Lo, K.M., Gillies, S.D. & Denmeade, S.R. (2004). Use of methotrexate-based peptide substrates to characterize the substrate specificity of prostate-specific membrane antigen (PSMA). *Cancer Biol Ther,* Vol. 3, No. 6, pp. 551-558.

Mhaka, A., Singh, P., Rosen, M., Dionne, C.A., Christensen, S.B., Isaacs, J.T. & Denmeade, S.R. (2006). Prostate-Specific Membrane Antigen (PSMA) targeted prodrug "smartbombs" as therapy for prostate cancer. *Proc Amer Assoc Cancer Res,* Vol. 47, No. pp. 725.

Milowsky, M.I., Nanus, D.M., Kostakoglu, L., Vallabhajosula, S., Goldsmith, S.J. & Bander, N.H. (2004). Phase I trial of yttrium-90-labeled anti-prostate-specific membrane antigen monoclonal antibody J591 for androgen-independent prostate cancer. *J Clin Oncol,* Vol. 22, No. 13, pp. 2522-2531.

Milowsky, M.I., Nanus, D.M., Kostakoglu, L., Sheehan, C.E., Vallabhajosula, S., Goldsmith, S.J., Ross, J.S. & Bander, N.H. (2007). Vascular targeted therapy with anti-prostate-specific membrane antigen monoclonal antibody J591 in advanced solid tumors. *J Clin Oncol,* Vol. 25, No. 5, pp. 540-547.

Mincheff, M., Zoubak, S. & Makogonenko, Y. (2006). Immune responses against PSMA after gene-based vaccination for immunotherapy-A: results from immunizations in animals. *Cancer Gene Ther,* Vol. 13, No. 4, pp. 436-444.

Mincheff, M., Tchakarov, S., Zoubak, S., Loukinov, D., Botev, C., Altankova, I., Georgiev, G., Petrov, S. & Meryman, H.T. (2000). Naked DNA and adenoviral immunizations for immunotherapy of prostate cancer: a phase I/II clinical trial. *Eur Urol,* Vol. 38, No. 2, pp. 208-217.

Mincheff, M., Zoubak, S., Altankova, I., Tchakarov, S., Makogonenko, Y., Botev, C., Ignatova, I., Dimitrov, R., Madarzhieva, K., Hammett, M., Pomakov, Y., Meryman, H. & Lissitchkov, T. (2003). Human dendritic cells genetically engineered to express cytosolically retained fragment of prostate-specific membrane antigen prime cytotoxic T-cell responses to multiple epitopes. *Cancer Gene Ther,* Vol. 10, No. 12, pp. 907-917.

Msaouel, P., Iankov, I.D., Allen, C., Morris, J.C., von Messling, V., Cattaneo, R., Koutsilieris, M., Russell, S.J. & Galanis, E. (2009). Engineered measles virus as a novel oncolytic therapy against prostate cancer. *Prostate,* Vol. 69, No. 1, pp. 82-91.

Murphy, G.P., Elgamal, A.A., Su, S.L., Bostwick, D.G. & Holmes, E.H. (1998). Current evaluation of the tissue localization and diagnostic utility of prostate specific membrane antigen. *Cancer,* Vol. 83, No. 11, pp. 2259-2269.

Murphy, G.P., Tjoa, B.A., Simmons, S.J., Ragde, H., Rogers, M., Elgamal, A., Kenny, G.M., Troychak, M.J., Salgaller, M.L. & Boynton, A.L. (1999). Phase II prostate cancer vaccine trial: report of a study involving 37 patients with disease recurrence following primary treatment. *Prostate,* Vol. 39, No. 1, pp. 54-59.

O'Keefe, D.S., Su, S.L., Bacich, D.J., Horiguchi, Y., Luo, Y., Powell, C.T., Zandvliet, D., Russell, P.J., Molloy, P.L., Nowak, N.J., Shows, T.B., Mullins, C., Vonder Haar, R.A., Fair, W.R. & Heston, W.D. (1998). Mapping, genomic organization and promoter analysis of the human prostate-specific membrane antigen gene. *Biochim Biophys Acta,* Vol. 1443, No. 1-2, pp. 113-127.

Onda, M., Kreitman, R.J., Vasmatzis, G., Lee, B. & Pastan, I. (1999). Reduction of the nonspecific animal toxicity of anti-Tac(Fv)-PE38 by mutations in the framework regions of the Fv which lower the isoelectric point. *J Immunol,* Vol. 163, No. 11, pp. 6072-6077.

Onda, M., Nagata, S., Tsutsumi, Y., Vincent, J.J., Wang, Q., Kreitman, R.J., Lee, B. & Pastan, I. (2001). Lowering the isoelectric point of the Fv portion of recombinant immunotoxins leads to decreased nonspecific animal toxicity without affecting antitumor activity. *Cancer Res,* Vol. 61, No. 13, pp. 5070-5077.

Onda, M., Nagata, S., FitzGerald, D.J., Beers, R., Fisher, R.J., Vincent, J.J., Lee, B., Nakamura, M., Hwang, J., Kreitman, R.J., Hassan, R. & Pastan, I. (2006). Characterization of the B cell epitopes associated with a truncated form of Pseudomonas exotoxin (PE38) used to make immunotoxins for the treatment of cancer patients. *J Immunol,* Vol. 177, No. 12, pp. 8822-8834.

Pinto, J.T., Suffoletto, B.P., Berzin, T.M., Qiao, C.H., Lin, S., Tong, W.P., May, F., Mukherjee, B. & Heston, W.D. (1996). Prostate-specific membrane antigen: a novel folate hydrolase in human prostatic carcinoma cells. *Clin Cancer Res,* Vol. 2, No. 9, pp. 1445-1451.

Rajasekaran, S.A., Christiansen, J.J., Schmid, I., Oshima, E., Ryazantsev, S., Sakamoto, K., Weinstein, J., Rao, N.P. & Rajasekaran, A.K. (2008). Prostate-specific membrane antigen associates with anaphase-promoting complex and induces chromosomal instability. *Mol Cancer Ther,* Vol. 7, No. 7, pp. 2142-2151.

Rosenthal, S.A., Haseman, M.K. & Polascik, T.J. (2001). Utility of capromab pendetide (ProstaScint) imaging in the management of prostate cancer. *Tech Urol,* Vol. 7, No. 1, pp. 27-37.

Ross, J.S., Sheehan, C.E., Fisher, H.A., Kaufman, R.P., Jr., Kaur, P., Gray, K., Webb, I., Gray, G.S., Mosher, R. & Kallakury, B.V. (2003). Correlation of primary tumor prostate-specific membrane antigen expression with disease recurrence in prostate cancer. *Clin Cancer Res,* Vol. 9, No. 17, pp. 6357-6362.

Russell, P.J., Hewish, D., Carter, T., Sterling-Levis, K., Ow, K., Hattarki, M., Doughty, L., Guthrie, R., Shapira, D., Molloy, P.L., Werkmeister, J.A. & Kortt, A.A. (2004). Cytotoxic properties of immunoconjugates containing melittin-like peptide 101 against prostate cancer: in vitro and in vivo studies. *Cancer Immunol Immunother,* Vol. 53, No. 5, pp. 411-421.

Rzeszowska-Wolny, J., Przybyszewski, W.M. & Widel, M. (2009). Ionizing radiation-induced bystander effects, potential targets for modulation of radiotherapy. *Eur J Pharmacol,* Vol. 625, No. 1-3, pp. 156-164.

Sacha, P., Zamecnik, J., Barinka, C., Hlouchova, K., Vicha, A., Mlcochova, P., Hilgert, I., Eckschlager, T. & Konvalinka, J. (2007). Expression of glutamate carboxypeptidase II in human brain. *Neuroscience,* Vol. 144, No. 4, pp. 1361-1372.

Salgaller, M.L., Lodge, P.A., McLean, J.G., Tjoa, B.A., Loftus, D.J., Ragde, H., Kenny, G.M., Rogers, M., Boynton, A.L. & Murphy, G.P. (1998). Report of immune monitoring of prostate cancer patients undergoing T-cell therapy using dendritic cells pulsed with HLA-A2-specific peptides from prostate-specific membrane antigen (PSMA). *Prostate,* Vol. 35, No. 2, pp. 144-151.

Sandvig, K., Grimmer, S., Lauvrak, S.U., Torgersen, M.L., Skretting, G., van Deurs, B. & Iversen, T.G. (2002). Pathways followed by ricin and Shiga toxin into cells. *Histochem Cell Biol,* Vol. 117, No. 2, pp. 131-141.

Sanna, V., Pintus, G., Roggio, A.M., Punzoni, S., Posadino, A.M., Arca, A., Marceddu, S., Bandiera, P., Uzzau, S. & Sechi, M. (2011). Targeted biocompatible nanoparticles for the delivery of (-)-epigallocatechin 3-gallate to prostate cancer cells. *J Med Chem,* Vol. 54, No. 5, pp. 1321-1332.

Silver, D.A., Pellicer, I., Fair, W.R., Heston, W.D. & Cordon-Cardo, C. (1997). Prostate-specific membrane antigen expression in normal and malignant human tissues. *Clin Cancer Res,* Vol. 3, No. 1, pp. 81-85.

Smith-Jones, P.M., Vallabhajosula, S., Navarro, V., Bastidas, D., Goldsmith, S.J. & Bander, N.H. (2003). Radiolabeled monoclonal antibodies specific to the extracellular domain of prostate-specific membrane antigen: preclinical studies in nude mice bearing LNCaP human prostate tumor. *J Nucl Med,* Vol. 44, No. 4, pp. 610-617.

Sodee, D.B., Conant, R., Chalfant, M., Miron, S., Klein, E., Bahnson, R., Spirnak, J.P., Carlin, B., Bellon, E.M. & Rogers, B. (1996). Preliminary imaging results using In-111 labeled CYT-356 (Prostascint) in the detection of recurrent prostate cancer. *Clin Nucl Med,* Vol. 21, No. 10, pp. 759-767.

Su, S.L., Huang, I.P., Fair, W.R., Powell, C.T. & Heston, W.D. (1995). Alternatively spliced variants of prostate-specific membrane antigen RNA: ratio of expression as a potential measurement of progression. *Cancer Res,* Vol. 55, No. 7, pp. 1441-1443.

Tjoa, B.A., Simmons, S.J., Elgamal, A., Rogers, M., Ragde, H., Kenny, G.M., Troychak, M.J., Boynton, A.L. & Murphy, G.P. (1999). Follow-up evaluation of a phase II prostate cancer vaccine trial. *Prostate,* Vol. 40, No. 2, pp. 125-129.

Tjoa, B.A., Simmons, S.J., Bowes, V.A., Ragde, H., Rogers, M., Elgamal, A., Kenny, G.M., Cobb, O.E., Ireton, R.C., Troychak, M.J., Salgaller, M.L., Boynton, A.L. & Murphy, G.P. (1998). Evaluation of phase I/II clinical trials in prostate cancer with dendritic cells and PSMA peptides. *Prostate,* Vol. 36, No. 1, pp. 39-44.

Todorova, K., Ignatova, I., Tchakarov, S., Altankova, I., Zoubak, S., Kyurkchiev, S. & Mincheff, M. (2005). Humoral immune response in prostate cancer patients after immunization with gene-based vaccines that encode for a protein that is proteasomally degraded. *Cancer Immun,* Vol. 5, No. pp. 1.

Troyer, J.K., Beckett, M.L. & Wright, G.L., Jr. (1995). Detection and characterization of the prostate-specific membrane antigen (PSMA) in tissue extracts and body fluids. *Int J Cancer,* Vol. 62, No. 5, pp. 552-558.

Vallabhajosula, S., Smith-Jones, P.M., Navarro, V., Goldsmith, S.J. & Bander, N.H. (2004). Radioimmunotherapy of prostate cancer in human xenografts using monoclonal antibodies specific to prostate specific membrane antigen (PSMA): studies in nude mice. *Prostate,* Vol. 58, No. 2, pp. 145-155.

Vallabhajosula, S., Goldsmith, S.J., Hamacher, K.A., Kostakoglu, L., Konishi, S., Milowski, M.I., Nanus, D.M. & Bander, N.H. (2005). Prediction of myelotoxicity based on bone marrow radiation-absorbed dose: radioimmunotherapy studies using 90Y- and 177Lu-labeled J591 antibodies specific for prostate-specific membrane antigen. *J Nucl Med,* Vol. 46, No. 5, pp. 850-858.

Waeckerle-Men, Y., Uetz-von Allmen, E., Fopp, M., von Moos, R., Bohme, C., Schmid, H.P., Ackermann, D., Cerny, T., Ludewig, B., Groettrup, M. & Gillessen, S. (2006). Dendritic cell-based multi-epitope immunotherapy of hormone-refractory prostate carcinoma. *Cancer Immunol Immunother,* Vol. 55, No. 12, pp. 1524-1533.

Wolf, P. & Elsasser-Beile, U. (2009). Pseudomonas exotoxin A: from virulence factor to anti-cancer agent. *Int J Med Microbiol,* Vol. 299, No. 3, pp. 161-176.

Wolf, P., Gierschner, D., Buhler, P., Wetterauer, U. & Elsasser-Beile, U. (2006). A recombinant PSMA-specific single-chain immunotoxin has potent and selective toxicity against prostate cancer cells. *Cancer Immunol Immunother,* Vol. 55, No. 11, pp. 1367-1373.

Wolf, P., Alt, K., Buhler, P., Katzenwadel, A., Wetterauer, U., Tacke, M. & Elsasser-Beile, U. (2008). Anti-PSMA immunotoxin as novel treatment for prostate cancer? High and specific antitumor activity on human prostate xenograft tumors in SCID mice. *Prostate,* Vol. 68, No. 2, pp. 129-138.

Wolf, P., Freudenberg, N., Buhler, P., Alt, K., Schultze-Seemann, W., Wetterauer, U. & Elsasser-Beile, U. (2010a). Three conformational antibodies specific for different PSMA epitopes are promising diagnostic and therapeutic tools for prostate cancer. *Prostate,* Vol. 70, No. 5, pp. 562-569.

Wolf, P., Alt, K., Wetterauer, D., Buhler, P., Gierschner, D., Katzenwadel, A., Wetterauer, U. & Elsasser-Beile, U. (2010b). Preclinical evaluation of a recombinant anti-prostate specific membrane antigen single-chain immunotoxin against prostate cancer. *J Immunother,* Vol. 33, No. 3, pp. 262-271.

Wright, G.L., Jr., Grob, B.M., Haley, C., Grossman, K., Newhall, K., Petrylak, D., Troyer, J., Konchuba, A., Schellhammer, P.F. & Moriarty, R. (1996). Upregulation of prostate-specific membrane antigen after androgen- deprivation therapy. *Urology,* Vol. 48, No. 2, pp. 326-334.

Yang, C.S., Wang, X., Lu, G. & Picinich, S.C. (2009). Cancer prevention by tea: animal studies, molecular mechanisms and human relevance. *Nat Rev Cancer,* Vol. 9, No. 6, pp. 429-439.

Yao, V. & Bacich, D.J. (2006). Prostate specific membrane antigen (PSMA) expression gives prostate cancer cells a growth advantage in a physiologically relevant folate environment in vitro. *Prostate,* Vol. 66, No. 8, pp. 867-875.

Yao, V., Berkman, C.E., Choi, J.K., O'Keefe, D.S. & Bacich, D.J. (2009). Expression of prostate-specific membrane antigen (PSMA), increases cell folate uptake and proliferation and suggests a novel role for PSMA in the uptake of the non-polyglutamated folate, folic acid. *Prostate,* Vol. 70, No. 3, pp. 305-316.

Zhong, X.S., Matsushita, M., Plotkin, J., Riviere, I. & Sadelain, M. (2010). Chimeric antigen receptors combining 4-1BB and CD28 signaling domains augment PI3kinase/AKT/Bcl-XL activation and CD8+ T cell-mediated tumor eradication. *Mol Ther,* Vol. 18, No. 2, pp. 413-420.

Zhou, J., Neale, J.H., Pomper, M.G. & Kozikowski, A.P. (2005). NAAG peptidase inhibitors and their potential for diagnosis and therapy. *Nat Rev Drug Discov,* Vol. 4, No. 12, pp. 1015-1026.

4

Combination of Immunotherapy & Radiotherapy for the Treatment of Prostate Cancer

Zsuzsanna Tabi, Lisa K. Spary and John Staffurth
Department of Oncology, School of Medicine, Cardiff University, Cardiff United Kingdom

1. Introduction

There are around 35,000 new cases of prostate carcinoma (PCa) in the UK per annum, making it the most common solid malignancy. Approximately 10,000 men die of PCa each year in the UK (http://infocancerresearchukorg/cancerstats/). Disease incidence is increasing partly due to earlier detection and the increasing age of the population. Environmental causes especially dietary factors have been postulated but this is still an area of research. At presentation ~60% of patients have localised, ~30% locally advanced and 10% metastatic disease.

Radical radiotherapy (RT) can be used as part of curative therapy for both localised and locally advanced disease but has no proven role in the metastatic setting. Recently, radiation has been shown to cause immunogenic tumour cell death and to modify immunosuppression in the tumour environment. Importantly, reduction of tumour burden by RT, in an ablative setting, has been shown to depend largely on T cell responses (Lee et al., 2009). Combination of ionising radiation (IR) and immunological approaches in pre-clinical models of PCa has also proved to be synergistic. Immunotherapy offers a unique co-treatment that enables the patients' own immune cells to contribute to the success of RT. Immunological memory, developing as the result of the combination treatment, may provide long-term protection from tumour recurrence. There are however very few clinical trials addressing how immunotherapy and RT can be best combined for clinical efficiency.

2. Radiotherapy of prostate cancer

There are four major treatment approaches for localised prostate cancer: active surveillance, radical prostatectomy, external beam radiotherapy (EBRT) and low-dose rate (LDR) brachytherapy. RT is conventionally delivered with photons with delivery systems that have developed considerably over the past decade, leading to lower toxicity and allowing safe dose escalation. Higher doses have been demonstrated to improve tumour control outcomes in several large Phase III trials (Viani et al., 2009). Present trials are evaluating the role of intensity modulated radiotherapy (IMRT), hypofractionation (treatment in ~4 weeks) and improved imaging during treatment with image-guided radiotherapy (IGRT) (Khoo & Dearnaley, 2008). Further developments in EBRT delivery systems allow highly targeted treatment in 5-7 fractions, called stereotactic body radiotherapy (SBRT), although tumour control outcomes are not yet known (King et al., 2011; Madsen et al., 2007).

Proton therapy is the delivery of EBRT using protons instead of photons. Protons have a different pattern of dose delivery within tissue, with energy deposited in a very tightly defined area as the protons slow. This results in less radiation being delivered beyond the target, and has become the radiotherapeutic modality of choice for childhood cancers and several other tumors. The evidence base for proton therapy for prostate cancer is less established, but its use in some countries has become widespread partly due to the results of a dose escalation trial using protons (Coen & Zietman, 2009). Proton therapy has not been compared to dose-equivalent photon-RT. LDR brachytherapy, which uses multiple permanently planted radioactive seeds, can be used to deliver a very high radiation dose to a highly targeted volume in a single treatment with equivalent outcomes to EBRT and surgery.

Locally advanced disease is usually treated with a combination of EBRT and androgen deprivation therapy (ADT) (Shelley et al., 2009; Shelley et al., 2009; Warde et al., 2010). However, the outcome is still relatively poor. Recent and ongoing UK-based trials are currently exploring the potential advantage of dose escalation in either systemic therapies (James et al., 2009; Guerrero Urbano et al., 2010). High dose rate (HDR) brachytherapy, which uses a single high-intensity radiation source that is temporarily inserted into multiple positions in the prostate, may also have a role in locally advanced disease as a single agent or in combination with ADT and/or RT (Hoskin, 2008). EBRT has a proven role as adjuvant or salvage therapy after radical prostatectomy. In the adjuvant setting, it has been shown to reduce the rate of relapse in high risk patients by approximately 50% in three randomised trials (Bolla et al., 2007; Thompson et al., 2006; Wiegel et al., 2009).

The commonest site of metastases in castrate refractory metastatic PCa is bone, with 80% of patients dying with prostate cancer dying with bone metastases. They can cause one of several skeletal-related events, but pain is the predominant problem. Palliative EBRT is highly efficacious for single sites of disease. An alternative approach is the use of therapeutic bone-targeted radioisotopes. The interim results of a trial with a novel alpha-emitting isotope, Radium-223, have reported a 3-month overall survival advantage, (http://www.algeta.com) suggesting that these drugs will be used more widely in the future. Radioimmunotherapy (RIT) refers to the use of antibody labelled with a therapeutic radionuclide, with the aim of delivering a cytotoxic radiation dose specifically to the tumour. The concept is equivalent to bone-targeted radioisotopes, but with the targeting of tumour-associated antigens (TAA) rather than osteoblastic metastases. The same principle can be used for imaging of micrometastatic disease if radionuclides of different properties (radiation type and energy) are used. There is much research in this field over recent years (Bouchelouche et al., 2011), partly due to the increasing number of PCa-specific TAA, as discussed later in this chapter.

3. Immunological aspects of PCa

PCa is an immunogenic cancer, as evidenced by a positive correlation between the frequency of $CD8^{+}$ tumour-infiltrating T cells and prostate-specific antigen (PSA) recurrence-free survival (Kärjä et al., 2005). Immune cell behaviour towards tumour cells has been described by three stages: (1) elimination of tumour cells, (2) equilibrium between tumour, and immune cells - maintained by active immunological control of the tumour - and (3) escape of tumour cells from immunological control. Apart from evidence from animal models underpinning this theory (Teng et al., 2008), clinical observations of donor-derived melanoma developing in immunosuppressed organ transplant recipients provide indirect evidence about the immune system's role in tumour-control (Strauss & Thomas, 2010). Overcoming anti-tumour immune responses is described as an emerging hallmark of cancer (Hanahan & Weinberg, 2011). Further observations and experiments are accumulating in order to provide firm evidence about the role of anti-tumour immune responses in the control of cancer.

3.1 Tumour-associated antigens in PCa

The specificity of tumour-infiltrating T cells reflects engagement with TAA. The presence of TAA-specific T cells in the TIL pool results in longer median survival compared to those patients whose TIL did not contain tumour-specific T cells, as observed in melanoma (22.5 months vs. 4.5 months) (Haanen et al., 2005). There is no such prognostic correlation for the frequency of TAA-specific T cells in the peripheral blood of patients. TAA-specific T cell infiltration is likely to be important in PCa too.

PCa-associated antigens include prostate-specific differentiation antigens, expressed both on healthy and malignant prostate epithelial cells, such as kallikrein-4, PAP (prostatic acid phosphatase) and PSA. Tumour antigens that are overexpressed on malignant cells (not all specific for PCa) compared to healthy epithelial cells are: PSMA (prostate specific membrane antigen), PSCA (prostate stem cell antigen), Her-2, MUC-1, survivin, STEAP (six transmembrane epithelial antigen of the prostate) and telomerase. Cancer-germline or cancer-testis oncofoetal antigens observed in PCa are not expressed on normal cells, but may be expressed by placental trophoblasts and testicular germ cells, such as NY-ESO, MAGE-C1, MAGE-C2 and 5T4 (Chen et al., 1997; Hudolin et al., 2006; Southall et al., 1990).

More recent additions to the list of potential TAAs in PCa are; AMACR (Honma et al., 2009), WT-1 (Nakatsuka et al., 2006), ADAM-17 (Sinnathamby et al., 2011), RHAMM (CD168) (Gust et al., 2009), SIM2 (Arredouani et al., 2009), TARP (Epel et al., 2008), SH3GLB2 (Fassò et al., 2008) and the androgen receptor (Olson & McNeel, 2011). T cells specific for some of these antigens have been identified in PCa patients and T cell clones or lines killed PCa cells, confirming the suitability of most of these TAA-antigens for targeted therapies.

3.2 Tumour-infiltrating immune cells in PCa

Prostate cancer has a complex microenvironment which develops during the course of tumour development. Tumour cells are surrounded by endothelial cells of blood vessels, stromal fibroblasts, bone marrow-derived cells and lymphocytes. These cells produce growth factors and enzymes that enhance tumour growth and survival, aid stroma-remodelling and recruit further immune cells into the tumour. The two main immune cell types infiltrating the tumour are lymphocytes and myeloid cells.

3.2.1 Lymphocytes

The presence of activated T and/or natural killer (NK) cells in the tumour tissue is a positive prognostic factor in several solid cancers, including PCa (Kärjä et al., 2005; Gannon et al., 2009). $CD8^+$ T cells are responsible for direct killing of target cells which express appropriate peptides on MHC Class I molecules, while NK cells play a role in killing tumour cells which downregulate MHC Class I molecules as an evasion mechanism from T cell recognition. Target cell killing occurs via delivering perforin and apoptosis-inducing granzyme complexes into the target cell (Thiery et al., 2011). $CD4^+$ T cells, depending on their subtype: Th1, Th2, Th17 or T regulatory cells (Treg) produce cytokines which support pro- or anti-inflammatory responses, respectively. CD4+, CD8+ and regulatory T cells are all present in PCa tumour tissue, with CD8+ T cells being predominant, unlike in the peripheral blood where CD4+ T cell frequencies are higher (Bronte et al., 2005). The majority of tumour-infiltrating CD8+ T cells are memory or terminally differentiated cells but their ability to upregulate activation markers is impaired (Bronte et al., 2005; Drake, 2010). In radical prostatectomy specimens of PCa, IFN-γ and perforin expression is lower than in T cells in healthy prostate tissue (Ebelt et al., 2008). Lymphocytes can mainly be observed in clusters in peritumoural areas while only a few infiltrate the tumour areas (Fig. 1).

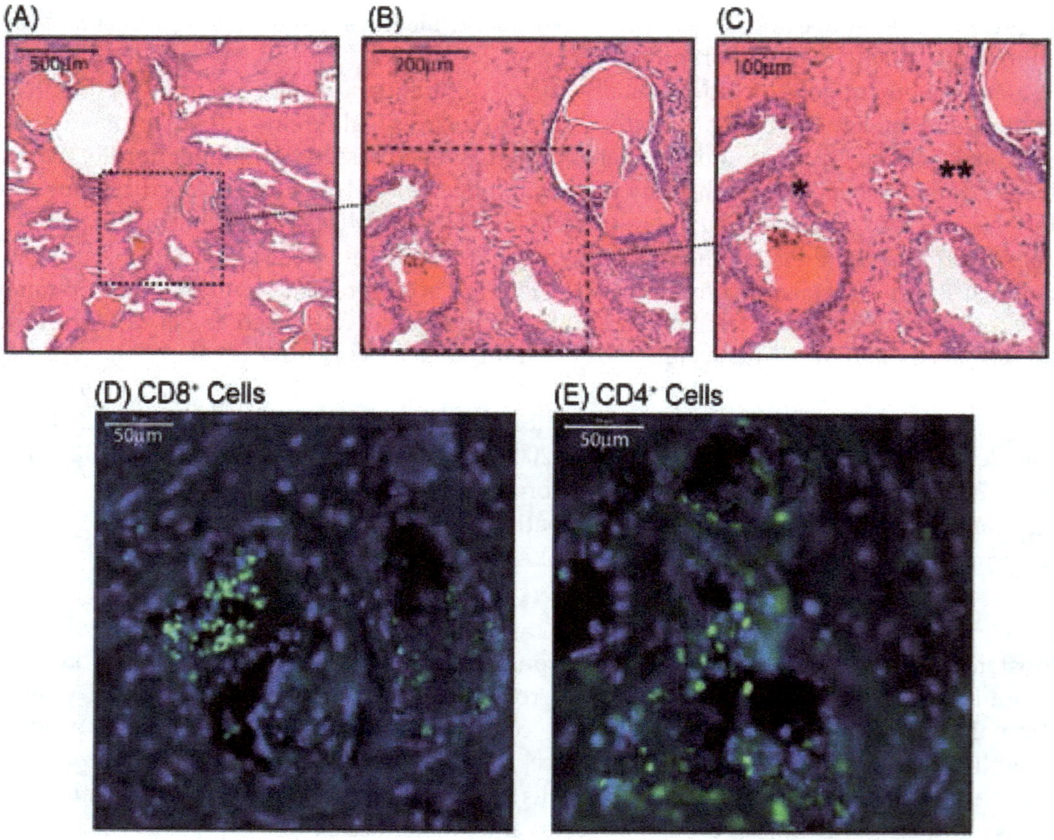

Fig. 1. (A-C) PCa prostatectomy sections stained with haematoxylin and eosin shown at increasing magnifications; (C) a region with glandular (★) and stromal areas (★★). (D) peritumoural CD8+ T lymphocyte cluster, identified by fluorescence microscopy. (E) CD4+ cells are also present in this region.

T cells with regulatory function (CD4+CD25+Foxp3+) are present at higher frequencies in PCa than in healthy tissue. They can be found mainly in T cell clusters surrounding prostate cancer lesions or in the stroma (Ebelt et al., 2009; Miller et al., 2006; Sfanos et al., 2008). Some of these Treg cells express the glucocorticoid-induced TNF-receptor (GITR) and ICOS (a CD28-superfamily costimulatory molecule) at higher levels than in blood, indicating recent activation. They also express CCL22 which mediates Treg cell trafficking into the tumour (Miller et al., 2006). T cell clusters infiltrated by Treg cells often express high levels of PD-1 and B7-H1 markers (Ebelt et al., 2008) which indicates T cell exhaustion and functional impairment.

3.2.2 Myeloid cells

$CD68^+$ monocytes and macrophages have been observed at higher frequencies in PCa compared to benign prostate tissues in a Gleason-score and disease stage-associated manner (Lindholm et al., 2010). $CD68^+$ monocytes and less differentiated $CD11b^+CD33^+$ myeloid cells have been shown by immunohistochemistry to be present in PCa stroma (Sorrentino et al., 2011). There is no information available as to whether these cells function as tumour-associated macrophages (TAM) or myeloid-derived suppressor cells (MDSC). Monocytic MDSC have been characterised as $CD11b^+$, $CD14^+$, $CD15^{+/-}$, $CD16^-$, $CD33^+$, $CD66b^+$, $CD124^+$, $VEGFR1^-$ and $HLA\text{-}DR^{low}$ cells (Gabrilovich & Nagaraj, 2009; Marigo et al., 2008). More work is needed to establish if immunosuppressive MDSC are present in the microenvironment in PCa. Myeloid-derived dendritic cells (DC) have also been documented in PCa tissues although at relatively low frequencies and in a minimally activated state (Troy et al., 1998).

3.3 Immune evasion in PCa

The most common immunosuppressive factors in the tumour tissue include vascular endothelial growth factor (VEGF), transforming growth factor beta (TGF-β), interleukin (IL)-10 and adenosine which inhibit proliferation, differentiation and activation of T lymphocytes and DC.

VEGF supports tumour growth and metastasis by initiating endothelial cell proliferation and the formation of new blood vessels, thus providing a continuous blood supply to the tumour (Carmeliet & Jain, 2000). Increased angiogenesis has been observed in PCa tissue compared to benign prostatic hyperplasia (BPH) (Jackson et al., 1997). VEGF production by PCa cells in vitro is enhanced by addition of IL-1 and tumour necrosis factor alpha (TNF-α), both of which are found in the tumour microenvironment in PCa (Ferrer et al., 1997). VEGF is also important in immune suppression not only by inhibiting DC maturation and T cell development but also by acting as a chemoattractant for MDSC (Gabrilovich et al., 1996; Ohm et al., 2003; Oyama et al., 1998).

TGF-β is a pleiotropic cytokine. During PCa development it first acts as a tumour suppressor and later switches roles to become a tumour promoter and immunosuppressor in the tumour environment. TGF-β regulates immune cells by inhibiting cytotoxic T cell function, supporting the development of Treg cells and interfering with DC differentiation (Wan & Flavell, 2007; Wrzesinski et al., 2007). PCa-derived TGF-β has been shown to convert $CD4^+CD25^-$ T cells into $CD4^+$ $CD25^+$ $Foxp3^+$ Treg cells (Liu et al., 2007).

The anti-inflammatory cytokine IL-10 secreted by tumour and stromal cells can inhibit proliferation, differentiation and activation of T lymphocytes via impaired DC (Sato et al., 2002). In the presence of IL-10, alternatively activated DC maintain an immature phenotype in the tumour microenvironment and induce tolerance rather than immune activation and support Treg cell development (H Huang et al., 2010).

Extracellular adenosine is generated from ATP or ADP via the combined action of CD39 and CD73. These are ecto-nucleoside triphosphate diphosphohydrolases which, in the tumour tissue, are predominantly expressed on Treg cells while CD73 is also expressed on CD8+ T cells and tumour cells (CD73) (Stagg & Smyth, 2010). CD39 and CD73 are also expressed on tumour-derived exosomes, thus potentially extending the immunosuppressive tumour microenvironment (Clayton et al., 2010). Adenosine, generated by CD39 (ATP to ADP) and CD73 (ADP and AMP to adenosine) engage androgen receptors on effector T cells, monocytes and DC. As a consequence, pro-inflammatory cytokine production (IL-2, IL-4, IFNγ, TNFα, IL-12) and co-stimulatory molecule expression (e.g. CD86) decreases and cyclic AMP (cAMP) accumulates in these cells. cAMP further amplifies anti-inflammatory responses (Ernst et al., 2010).

Cytokines, such as monocyte chemotactic protein-1 (MCP-1) and stromal-derived factor-1 alpha (SDF-1α) secreted by tumour cells and tumour-associated stromal cells have been associated with enhanced prostate epithelial cell proliferation and migration (Begley et al., 2005; Lu et al., 2006). They also induce the recruitment of myeloid cells at the tumour site and suppress immune responses (Allavena et al., 2008; Loberg et al., 2007). TAM also produce MCP-1 resulting in an amplification loop for further monocyte recruitment (Allavena et al., 2008).

4. Immunological aspects of radiation therapy

The effects of IR on human tissue have been studied for decades. The key therapeutic effect is thought to be via direct killing of tumour cells by initiating irreparable double-stranded DNA breaks. However, the consequences of RT are much more complex than that, as radiation also affects tumour stroma, including tumour-resident immune cells, and results in the re-modelling of the tumour microenvironment. One of the consequences is the reduction of immunosuppression in the tumour tissue.

4.1 IR-mediated release of cellular tumour antigens

The details of the multiple cellular events downstream of radiation-induced DNA damage are beyond the scope of this chapter. The damage results in activation of damage recognition pathways and proliferative arrest, which can ultimately be repaired (fully or partially), or lead to cell death. RT-induced apoptotic and necrotic tumour cell death provide a cellular source of tumour antigens. The tissue damage attracts phagocytic cells to the site of radiation. Monocytes, macrophages and dendritic cells (DC) phagocytose and process dead tumour cells and carry TAA into draining lymph nodes where antigen presentation and T cell stimulation occur. Contrary to natural cell death which occurs without generating an inflammatory response, IR-treated tumour cells express heat shock proteins, translocate antigens such as calreticulin (CR) from the endoplasmic reticulum to the cell surface and passively release high mobility group protein B1 (HMGB1). DNA, RNA and ATP release are also observed at the site of radiation damage. Phagocytosis and simultaneous signalling in DC by HMGB1 via Toll-like receptors (TLR) such as TLR4 and TLR2, or via RAGE (receptor for advanced glycan end products) trigger DC to release IL-1β and present TAA in an immunogenic manner to T cells and B cells (Ma et al., 2011). ATP, released by damaged cells, also contributes to DC maturation via stimulating purinergic P2RX7 receptors and driving IL-1β secretion (Aymeric et al., 2010). Local radiation of mouse B16 tumour has generated DC efficiently cross-present tumour antigens in a Type I interferon (IFN)-dependent manner (Burnette et al., 2011). Single nucleotide polymorphisms (SNP) of TLR4 (Asp299Gly and Thr399Ilr) or P2RX7 (Glu496Ala) (Sluyter et al., 2004; Arbour et al., 2000), which affect the function of these molecules, may be associated with worse prognosis, as shown in breast cancer patients undergoing chemotherapy (Apetoh et al., 2007).

4.2 Chemokine and cytokine induction by IR

Tumour cells, not killed by IR, respond to radiation by increasing the production of pro-inflammatory cytokines that include TNFα, IL-1α/β, IL-6 and IL-8 (Shiao & Coussens, 2010; Formenti & Demaria, 2009; Van Der Meeren et al., 1999; Matsumura & Demaria, 2010). The main effect of these cytokines is an inflammatory response and the recruitment of activated T cells and macrophages to irradiated tumours (Formenti & Demaria, 2009). The widely used PCa cell line, LNCaP, is extremely sensitive to TNFα (Chopra et al., 2004). TNFα-treatment results in growth-arrest and apoptosis of LNCaP cells but not of normal prostate epithelial cells, suggesting that IR-induced TNFα expression may selectively induce apoptosis of tumour cells without affecting normal prostate epithelial cells. Immune cell recruitment is further enhanced by the production of the chemokine CXCL16 which is induced by IL-1β and TNFα, both upregulated by IR (Lu et al., 2008). PCa cell lines (LNCaP, DU145, C4-2B and PC3) produce CXCL16 in culture without IR treatment (Lu et al., 2008).

4.3 Irradiated tumour cells become sensitive to immune cell attack

In tumour cells, not killed by IR, surface molecules such as MHC, the death receptor Fas and heat-shock proteins become upregulated (Shiao & Coussens, 2010; Garnett et al., 2004; Lugade et al., 2008). IR-induced upregulation of MHC Class I molecules, on both tumour cells and APC, improves antigen presentation and may enhance tumour cell recognition by activated $CD8^+$ cells that infiltrate the tumour at an enhanced rate following radiation (Reits et al., 2006; Lugade et al., 2005).

Adhesion molecules, such as intracellular adhesion molecule (ICAM)-1, vascular cell adhesion molecule (VCAM)-1 and platelet endothelial cell adhesion molecule (PECAM)-1, along with integrins, selectins and cadherins are also upregulated in the tumour tissue by IR (Baluna et al., 2006; Lugade et al., 2008). ICAM-1 is known to be upregulated by inflammatory cytokines such as TNFα, IL-1α/β and IL-6 thus resulting in lymphocyte and macrophage accumulation in inflamed tissues. As previously discussed, these cytokines are upregulated in the tumour tissue as a response to IR. ICAM-1 has an important role in enhancing T cell killing via cell-cell adhesion to lymphocyte function-associated antigen (LFA)-1 and by directly co-stimulating activated T cells (Garnett et al., 2004; Baluna et al., 2006). PCa cells express ICAM-1 and VCAM-1 and in tissue areas of high lymphocyte and neutrophil accumulation the expression of ICAM-1 is significantly elevated (Fujita et al., 2008; Rokhlin & Cohen, 1995). These data suggest that ICAM-1 upregulation by IR may facilitate immune responses by recruiting lymphocytes and macrophages to the tumour site. Increased adhesion between tumour cells with upregulated ICAM-1 and activated $CD8^+$ T cells expressing LFA-1^+ may result in more powerful cytotoxic T cell activity.

4.4 Direct effect of IR on immune cells

Immune cells are highly susceptible to IR-induced damage and readily undergo apoptosis. Therapeutic doses of RT often result in lymphopenia. One of the potential immunologically positive effects of direct IR on tumour-infiltrating immune cells is the depletion of Treg cells. However, there is some controversy regarding this question. Cao et al. observed that the proportion of $Foxp3^+$ cells within purified $CD4^+CD25^+$ T cell population decreased significantly (48.2% to 23.3%) following irradiation with 1.8 Gy in vitro and was abolished (1.2%) by 30 Gy. The suppressive function of these Treg cells was also impaired by IR probably due to loss of membrane-bound TGF-β (Cao et al., 2009). Tregs were especially sensitive to low-dose radiation compared to effector T cells (Cao et al., 2011). Another study, in TRAMP mice, had the opposite findings: Treg cell numbers increased in immune organs after local or whole body irradiation without changes to their functional activity (Kachikwu et al., 2010), indicating relative resistance to 0-20 Gy radiation. It remains to be seen what happens to Tregs in situ during RT of PCa.

We showed recently that lymphopenia following prostate and pelvic RT causes preferential death of naïve or unstimulated T-cells (Tabi et al., 2010). Elevated frequencies of Treg cells were observed in the circulation following 44 Gy radiation in 20 fractions to the pelvic nodes and 55 Gy to the prostate (Fig.2). T cell proliferative function was also impaired (Tabi et al., 2010) but it was restored in vitro with exogenous IL-2 without increasing Treg frequencies (Fig. 2). This indicates that IL-2 maybe used to support T cell function after patients completed standard RT.

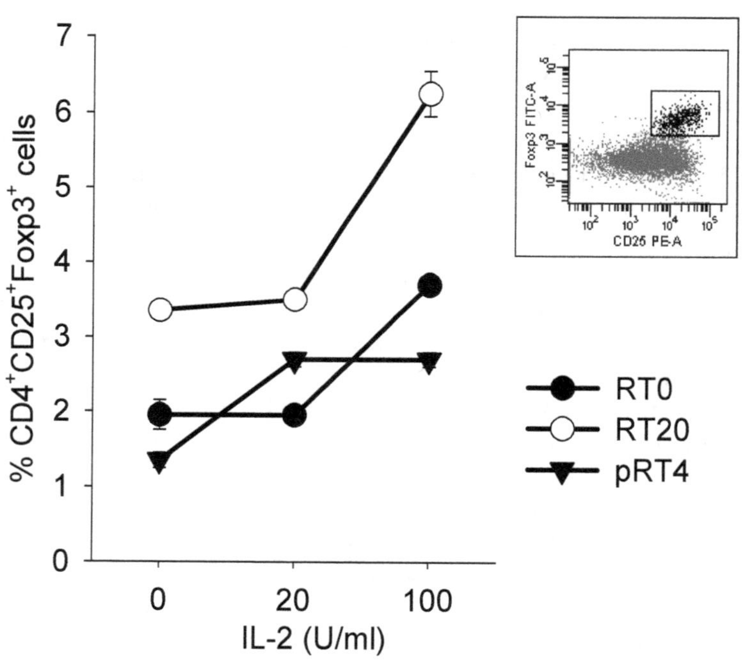

Fig. 2. IL-2 response of Treg cells from the peripheral blood of PCa patients undergoing standard RT. Frequencies of CD4+CD25+Foxp3+ T cells (see gate in insert) were measured before (RT0), immediately after radical radiation in 20 fractions (RT20) and 4 weeks after the last fraction (pRT4). Means and SD of triplicates are shown from a representative patient. Frequencies of Tregs were elevated at RT20, but returned to pre-radiation (RT0) level at pRT4. Unlike at RT0 or RT20, exogenous IL-2, added to the cells in vitro, did not increase Treg frequencies at pRT4.

Most importantly, we identified novel TAA-specific T-cell responses post-RT (Tabi et al., 2010), which were not present before RT. Similar findings were observed by others (Nesslinger et al., 2007; Schaue et al., 2008), indicating the ability of radiation to shift the balance between tumour-specific regulatory and effector immune mechanisms.

5. RT and immunotherapy combination modalities

5.1 Pre-clinical models

The use of IL-2 as a monotherapy in cancer has been extensively researched but due to issues with toxicity its clinical use has been limited. In the murine renal adenocarcinoma model, IR was found to augment the response of pulmonary metastases to IL-2 therapy (Younes et al., 1995). Following IR to one lung, plus systemic IL-2 treatment, a reduction in tumour size was observed in both lungs. The effect is dose-dependent and immunohistological studies show significant infiltration of T cells and macrophages at the tumour site. IL-2 is capable of rescuing T cells from IR-induced apoptosis and restores T cell proliferation after RT (Tabi et al., 2010). Its use in combination with RT may minimise the immunosuppressive effects of RT and enhance tumour cell killing via T cells (Mor & Cohen, 1996). In PCa, the combination of IL-2 and radiation in a mouse bone metastases model demonstrated a ~50% inhibition of tumour growth (Hillman et al., 2003). There was a greater degree of tumour destruction in IL-2-treated irradiated tumours than in irradiated tumours alone and the histology revealed increased fibrosis and elevated numbers of infiltrating inflammatory immune cells.

Antitumour effects were also observed in a model utilising IL-12 and RT. IL-12 is secreted by mature DC and macrophages and required for IFNγ and TNFα production from T cells and mediates a Th1-type immune response. Adenovirus-derived IL-12 plus RT significantly increased local antitumour and systemic antimetastatic effects in a preclinical model of metastatic PCa when compared to either treatment alone (Fujita et al., 2008). This antimetastatic activity is due to the antitumoural activities of natural killer (NK) cells. These results were also observed in the 4T1 mammary carcinoma. The combination of RT and an adenoviral vector encoding IL-12 and the co-stimulatory molecule CD80 resulted in a significant reduction in tumour growth (Lohr et al., 2000). The antitumour effect observed in the combination therapy group was far superior if the IL-12 and CD80-expressing adenovirus was administered after the final fraction of radiation.

Further cytokine studies have evaluated the combined effect of IL-3 and RT. IL-3 differentiates haematopoietic stem cells into myeloid progenitor cells and stimulates the proliferation of myeloid-derived cells such as DC and monocytes. In mouse models of fibrosarcoma and PCa, IL-3 was found to increase the tumour response to radiation. Combining adenoviral-IL-3 and radiation in the TRAMP-C1 mouse prostate model caused significant delays in tumour growth. Further reports indicated that adenoviral-IL-3 plus radiation enhanced IFNγ-producing $CD4^+$ and $CD8^+$ T cell responses in the spleen (Oh et al., 2004). This shifted the immune response to a Th1-type response from a suppressive Th2-type response (Tsai et al., 2006).

The combination of the pro-inflammatory cytokine TNFα and RT in mouse mammary carcinoma delayed tumour growth at a greater extent than either treatment alone (Nishiguchi et al., 1990). Similar synergistic effects have also been observed in mouse melanoma, lung adenocarinoma and brain tumours. The combined effects were attributed to increased recruitment and enhanced activation of lymphocytes and neutrophils (Gridley et al., 1996; Gridley et al., 2002; Gridley et al., 2000; Jin et al., 2005; Li et al., 1998).

Adoptive-cell-transfer (ACT) therapy is the passive transfer of tumour-specific T cells that have been expanded ex vivo. Local tumour irradiation can enhance the therapeutic efficacy of ACT therapy (Teitz-Tennenbaum et al., 2009). Combination of RT with ACT of carcinoembryonic antigen (CEA)-specific $CD8^+$ T cells in a mouse colon carcinoma demonstrated increased tumour rejection, that could be attributed to the upregulation of the death receptor Fas on the surface of irradiated tumour cells (Chakraborty et al., 2003).

The anti-tumour effect can be further enhanced by intratumoural administration of DC. In a murine metastatic melanoma model reduction in the size of tumour and extent of spontaneous metastasis and prolonged survival were observed after irradiation and intratumoural DC administration. This was associated with an increase in proliferation, accumulation and cytokine production of $CD4^{+}$ cells. Similar results were observed in DC plus irraditation in melanoma and sarcoma models (J. Huang et al., 2007). Kjaergaard et al. (2005) reported a method of fusing DC with tumour cells via an electric field resulting in a TAA-DC primed vaccine. These DC/tumour cell fusions induce a potent immune response in combination with local cranial RT in mouse glioma. Both $CD4^{+}$ and $CD8^{+}$ T cells infiltrate the tumours, leading to complete tumour regression. Tumour rejection was also observed after subsequent tumour challenge, indicating the presence of immunological memory.

Vaccines containing either modified tumour cells that are more immunogenic than the "native" tumour cells or TAA-vaccines have been tested extensively in preclinical models. Combination of cytokine-producing vaccines with local RT in mouse glioma demonstrated that IL-4 and GM-CSF vaccines alone were capable of curing 20-40% of mice but in combination with local RT 80-100% of the mice were cured. The brain tumours were heavily infiltrated with $CD4^{+}$ T cells (Lumniczky et al., 2002). The increased anti-tumour effect of GM-CSF and RT was also demonstrated in mouse glioma using a vaccine which contained GM-CSF-secreting tumour cells (Newcomb et al., 2006).

Strategies using RT in combination with monoclonal antibodies that are specific for TAA are now commonly used in clinical oncology (reviewed by Drake, 2010). In a mouse lung cancer model, monoclonal antibody to OX40 (a secondary co-stimulatory molecule expressed on activated $CD4^{+}$ and $CD8^{+}$ T cells) and RT resulted in a synergistic effect on survival compared to either treatment alone (Yokouchi et al., 2008). The effect was $CD8^{+}$ T cell dependent. Antibody-based immunotherapy strategies aiming to neutralise molecules implied in immune tolerance have also been examined. Antibodies for the cytotoxic T lymphocyte antigen (CTLA)-4 (a CD28-superfamily molecule causing T cell functional inhibition) have been shown to induce effective anti-tumour responses via lowering the threshold of tumour-specific T cell activation (reviewed by Drake, 2010). Based on the preclinical findings, CTLA-4 inhibition by the antibody Ipilimumab is now an FDA approved treatment of metastatic melanoma (Chambers et al., 2001). Its combination with RT is being tested in animal models (Dewan et al., 2009) and in clinical trials (see next section).

5.2 Clinical trials

There is huge potential for augmentation of the radiation response with the use of immunotherapy but as yet there are only a few clinical trials published. These were carried out in PCa patients at the National Cancer Institute, using a recombinant viral vaccine consisting of recombinant vaccinia virus (rV) encoding PSA, admixed with rV encoding the co-stimulatory molecule B7.1, followed by booster vaccinations with recombinant fowlpox (rFP) vector expressing PSA prior to RT. The product has been further developed and is presently marketed as Prostvac® which encodes ICAM-1 and LFA-3 in addition to B7.1 (PSA-TRICOM). This agent has been shown to improve median overall survival from 16.6 months to 25.1 months in a phase II multi-centre randomized controlled trial in 125 men with asymptomatic or minimally symptomatic metastatic castrate refractory prostate cancer (Kantoff et al., 2010). There was similar progression-free survival in the two arms of the trial, but the hazard ratio for death was 0.56 (95% CI 0.37 to 0.85) in the PSA-TRICOM arm and the treatment was generally well tolerated.

The initial results of the phase II trial in combination with radiation were highly encouraging. Thirty patients were randomised in a 2:1 ratio to receive vaccine plus EBRT or EBRT alone. In this trial the vaccine consisted of a priming vaccine with rV-PSA plus rV-B7.1 followed by monthly booster vaccines with rFP-PSA. The immunological adjuvants used were GMCSF and high dose IL-2. PSA-specific T cell responses generated prior to RT were not adversely affected by RT, confirming our observation (Tabi et al., 2010). In total, 13 of the 17 patients in the combination arm had increases in PSA-specific T cells and epitope spreading to 4 other prostate cancer TAA (PSMA, PAP, PSCA and MUC-1) was noted (Gulley et al., 2005), possibly due to cross-presentation of a mix of TAA from dying tumour cells by DC (Obeid et al., 2007). There was some IL-2 toxicity, which was reduced in a single-arm follow-up study using lower doses but longer durations of IL-2, immunological effects were equivalent (Gulley et al., 2005; Lechleider et al., 2008).

There is one other reported ongoing work of immunotherapy-radiotherapy combination with intraprostatic injections of autologous DC. The first report confirms the safety of this approach in 5 HLA-A2+ patients with high risk, localised disease, also treated with ADT, EBRT to 45 Gy and LDR brachytherapy. Autologous intraprostatic DC injections were given at four timepoints during EBRT. Measurable, induced increases in TAA-specific T cell frequencies in peripheral blood using ELISPOT were observed in some patients. The pattern of distribution of $CD8^+$ cells in tissue was consistent with PCa TAA-targeting, rather than non-specific organ infiltration (Finkelstein et al., 2011).

There are no other published studies in PCa patients of EBRT in combination with cytokines, antibodies, immune modulators or immunologically relevant gene therapy. However, there are a few prostate cancer clinical trials combining RT and immunotherapy currently recruiting according to the ClinicalTrials.gov website, such as anti-CTLA-4 (Ipilimumab) antibody therapy in castration-resistant prostate cancer following RT (Phase III trial, Bristol-Myers Squibb; NCT00861614) and treatment with anti-OX40 and cyclophosphamide in combination with RT in metastatic prostate cancer (Providence Health & Services, Oregon USA, Phase I/II trial; NCT01303705).

5.3 Designs of combination clinical trials

Clinical trial design, investigating the benefit of immunotherapy in addition to EBRT is challenging in PCa, as long-term tumour control outcome is already good in both localised (assuming dose escalated image-guided IMRT) and locally advanced disease (assuming combination of long term ADT and EBRT). Phase III trials, adequately powered to show a clinically relevant improvement, would need to address biochemical relapse-free survival or overall survival, both of which require prolonged follow-up of many hundreds and perhaps thousands of patients. Before such trials were undertaken, it is important to optimise the immunotherapy-RT schedules. Reliable biomarkers of treatment-efficacy are needed and this is difficult, especially if neoadjuvant or adjuvant ADT is used, as changes in PSA-kinetics become redundant in these patients. Therefore, development of reliable immunological biomarkers is crucial. We believe that the presence of systemic TAA-specific T cell responses is likely to be the most reliable and easily detectable indicator of a sustainable immunological effect. It may also assist patient selection for optimised treatment of those patients who are most likely to benefit from combination therapies.

The successful result of the IMPACT trial showing the survival advantage with Sipuleucel-T is expected to lead to a dramatic increase in the use of systemic immunotherapy for prostate cancer (Sonpavde et al., 2011). Presently there are only production facilities within the USA and the cost is likely to remain prohibitive for many healthcare systems. Radiation has great potential to augment the effect of systemic immunotherapy and we can expect many combination trials in the future. Clinical trial design in this setting will remain challenging as immunotherapy appears to improve overall survival but demonstrable tumour or biochemical responses are often delayed. Augmenting immunotherapy with radiation may improve overall advantage further.

6. Conclusions

PCa has become a huge burden on the health and wealth of Western societies. It is now the commonest solid malignancy and in spite of an excellent general outcome it is expected to become the main cause of cancer-related death in men. There is therefore an urgent need for improved therapies. Sipuleucel-T for PCa was the first immunotherapy to show a survival advantage in cancer, and it has been quickly followed by ipilimumab in melanoma. Radiotherapy has many applications for PCa and it is clear that there are many interactions between immunotherapy and radiation. In general these are positive such that immunotherapy may improve outcomes for those being irradiated and vice versa. The challenge is to move the science into the clinical setting, optimising combinations and sequences, identification of appropriate biomarkers and designing appropriate trials.

7. Acknowledgements

Experimental work presented in this chapter was supported by Cancer Research Wales (Cardiff UK) to ZT, LKS and JS and by Velindre NHS Trust R&D (Cardiff, UK) to JS.

8. References

Allavena, P., Sica, A., Solinas, G., Porta, C. & Mantovani, A. (2008). The inflammatory micro-environment in tumor progression: the role of tumor-associated macrophages. *Critical Reviews in Oncology/Hematology* 66, 1, (Apr), 1-9.

Apetoh, L., Ghiringhelli, F., Tesniere, A., Criollo, A., Ortiz, C., Lidereau, R., Mariette, C., Chaput, N., Mira, J.P., Delaloge, S., Andre, F., Tursz, T., Kroemer, G. & Zitvogel, L. (2007). The interaction between HMGB1 and TLR4 dictates the outcome of anticancer chemotherapy and radiotherapy. *Immunol Rev* 220, (Dec), 47-59.

Arbour, N., Lorenz, E., Schutte, B., Zabner, J., Kline, J., Jones, M., Frees, K., Watt, J. & Schwartz, D. (2000). TLR4 mutations are associated with endotoxin hyporesponsiveness in humans. *Nat Genet* 25, 2, 187-191.

Arredouani, M., Lu, B., Bhasin, M., Eljanne, M., Yue, W., Mosquera, J., Bubley, G., Li, V., Rubin, M., Libermann, T. & Sanda, M. (2009). Identification of the transcription factor single-minded homologue 2 as a potential biomarker and immunotherapy target in prostate cancer. *Clin Cancer Res* 15, 18, 5794-5802.

Aymeric, L., Apetoh, L., Ghiringhelli, F., Tesniere, A., Martins, I., Kroemer, G., Smyth, M. & Zitvogel, L. (2010). Tumor cell death and ATP release prime dendritic cells and efficient anticancer immunity. *Cancer Res* 70, 3, 855-858.

Baluna, R.G., Eng, T.Y. & Thomas, C.R. (2006). Adhesion molecules in radiotherapy. *Radiat Res* 166, 6, (Dec), 819-831.

Begley, L., Monteleon, C., Shah, R.B., Macdonald, J.W. & Macoska, J.A. (2005). CXCL12 overexpression and secretion by aging fibroblasts enhance human prostate epithelial proliferation in vitro. *Aging Cell* 4, 6, (Dec), 291-298.

Bolla, M., Van Poppel, H. & Collette, L. (2007). [Preliminary results for EORTC trial 22911: radical prostatectomy followed by postoperative radiotherapy in prostate cancers with a high risk of progression]. *Cancer Radiother* 11, 6-7, (Nov), 363-369.

Bouchelouche, K., Tagawa, S.T., Goldsmith, S.J., Turkbey, B., Capala, J. & Choyke, P. (2011). PET/CT imaging and radioimmunotherapy of prostate cancer. *Semin Nucl Med* 41, 1, (Jan), 29-44.

Bronte, V., Kasic, T., Gri, G., Gallana, K., Borsellino, G., Marigo, I., Battistini, L., Iafrate, M., Prayer-Galetti, T., Pagano, F. & Viola, A. (2005). Boosting antitumor responses of T lymphocytes infiltrating human prostate cancers. *J Exp Med* 201, 8, 1257-1268.

Burnette, B.C., Liang, H., Lee, Y., Chlewicki, L., Khodarev, N.N., Weichselbaum, R.R., Fu, Y.X. & Auh, S.L. (2011). The efficacy of radiotherapy relies upon induction of type I interferon -dependent innate and adaptive immunity. *Cancer Res* 71, 7, (Apr 1), 2488-2496.

Cao, M., Cabrera, R., Xu, Y., Liu, C. & Nelson, D. (2009). Gamma irradiation alters the phenotype and function of CD4+CD25+ regulatory T cells. *Cell Biol Int* 33, 5, (May), 565-571.

Cao, M., Cabrera, R., Xu, Y., Liu, C. & Nelson, D. (2011). Different radiosensitivity of CD4+CD25+ regulatory T cells and effector T cells to low dose gamma irradiation in vitro. *Int J Rad Biol* 87, 1, 71-80.

Carmeliet, P. & Jain, R.K. (2000). Angiogenesis in cancer and other diseases. *Nature* 407, 6801, (Sep 14), 249-257.

Chakraborty, M., Abrams, S.I., Camphausen, K., Liu, K., Scott, T., Coleman, C.N. & Hodge, J.W. (2003). Irradiation of tumor cells up-regulates Fas and enhances CTL lytic activity and CTL adoptive immunotherapy. *J Immunol* 170, 12, (Jun 15), 6338-6347.

Chambers, C., Kuhns, M., Egen, J. & Allison, J. (2001). CTLA-4-mediated inhibition in regulation of T cell responses: mechanisms and manipulation in tumor immunotherapy. *Ann Rev Immunol* 19, 565-594.

Chen, Y., Scanlan, M., Sahin, U., Türeci, O., Gure, A., Tsang, S., Williamson, B., Stockert, E., Pfreundschuh, M. & Old, L. (1997). A testicular antigen aberrantly expressed in human cancers detected by autologous antibody screening. *Proc Natl Acad Sci USA* 94,5,1914-1918.

Chopra, D.P., Menard, R.E., Januszewski, J. & Mattingly, R.R. (2004). TNF-alpha-mediated apoptosis in normal human prostate epithelial cells and tumor cell lines. *Cancer Lett* 203, 2, (Jan 20), 145-154.

Clayton, A., Al-Taei, S., Webber, J., Mason, M.D. & Tabi, Z. (2011). Cancer exosomes express CD39 and CD73, which suppress T cells through adenosine production. *J Immunol* 187, 2, (July 15) 676-683.

Coen, J. & Zietman, A. (2009). Proton radiation for localized prostate cancer. *Nat Rev Urol* 6, 6, 324-330.

Dewan, M., Galloway, A., Kawashima, N., Dewyngaert, J., Babb, J., Formenti, S. & Demaria, S. (2009). Fractionated but not single-dose radiotherapy induces an immune-mediated abscopal effect when combined with anti-CTLA-4 antibody. *Clin Cancer Res* 15, 17, 5379-5388.

Drake, C.G. (2010). Prostate cancer as a model for tumour immunotherapy. *Nat Rev Immunol* 10, 8, (Aug), 580-593.

Ebelt, K., Babaryka, G., Figel, A., Pohla, H., Buchner, A., Stief, C., Eisenmenger, W., Kirchner, T., Schendel, D. & Noessner, E. (2008). Dominance of CD4+ lymphocytic infiltrates with disturbed effector cell characteristics in the tumor microenvironment of prostate carcinoma. *Prostate* 68, 1, 1-10.

Ebelt, K., Babaryka, G., Frankenberger, B., Stief, C., Eisenmenger, W., Kirchner, T., Schendel, D. & Noessner, E. (2009). Prostate cancer lesions are surrounded by FOXP3+, PD-1+ and B7-H1+ lymphocyte clusters. *Eur J Cancer* 45, 9, 1664-1672.

Epel, M., Carmi, I., Soueid-Baumgarten, S., Oh, S., Bera, T., Pastan, I., Berzofsky, J. & Reiter, Y. (2008). Targeting TARP, a novel breast and prostate tumor-associated antigen, with T cell receptor-like human recombinant antibodies. *Eur J Immunol* 38, 6, 1706-1720.

Ernst, P.B., Garrison, J.C. & Thompson, L.F. (2010). Much ado about adenosine: adenosine synthesis and function in regulatory T cell biology. *J Immunol* 185, 4, (Aug 15) 1993-1998.

Fassò, M., Waitz, R., Hou, Y., Rim, T., Greenberg, N., Shastri, N., Fong, L. & Allison, J. (2008). SPAS-1 (stimulator of prostatic adenocarcinoma-specific T cells)/SH3GLB2: A prostate tumor antigen identified by CTLA-4 blockade. *Proc Natl Acad Sci USA* 105, 9, 3509-3514.

Ferrer, F.A., Miller, L.J., Andrawis, R.I., Kurtzman, S.H., Albertsen, P.C., Laudone, V.P. & Kreutzer, D.L. (1997). Vascular endothelial growth factor (VEGF) expression in human prostate cancer: in situ and in vitro expression of VEGF by human prostate cancer cells. *J Urol* 157, 6, (Jun), 2329-2333.

Finkelstein, S.E., Gabrilovich, D., Rodriguez, F.A., Chuang, T., Kang, L., Torres-Roca, J., Heysek, R., Pow-Sang, J.M., Antonia, S., Fishman, M.N. & Immunotherapy Research Group. (2011). Know when to say when: Serial assessment of apoptosis and lymphocyte infiltrates with combined intraprostatic autologous dendritic cell immunotherapy radiation therapy in high-risk prostate cancer. *ASCO Meeting Abstracts* 29, 7S, 149.

Formenti, S.C. & Demaria, S. (2009). Systemic effects of local radiotherapy. *Lancet Oncol* 10, 7, (Jul), 718-726.

Fujita, K., Ewing, C.M., Sokoll, L.J., Elliott, D.J., Cunningham, M., De Marzo, A.M., Isaacs, W.B. & Pavlovich, C.P. (2008). Cytokine profiling of prostatic fluid from cancerous prostate glands identifies cytokines associated with extent of tumor and inflammation. *Prostate* 68, 8, (Jun 1), 872-882.

Gabrilovich, D.I., Chen, H.L., Girgis, K.R., Cunningham, H.T., Meny, G.M., Nadaf, S., Kavanaugh, D. & Carbone, D.P. (1996). Production of vascular endothelial growth factor by human tumors inhibits the functional maturation of dendritic cells. *Nat Med* 2, 10, (Oct), 1096-1103.

Gabrilovich, D.I. & Nagaraj, S. (2009). Myeloid-derived suppressor cells as regulators of the immune system. *Nat Rev Immunol* 9, 3, (Mar), 162-174.

Gannon, P., Poisson, A., Delvoye, N., Lapointe, R., Mes-Masson, A. & Saad, F. (2009). Characterization of the intra-prostatic immune cell infiltration in androgen-deprived prostate cancer patients. *J Immunol Methods* 348, 1-2, 9-17.

Garnett, C.T., Palena, C., Chakraborty, M., Tsang, K.Y., Schlom, J. & Hodge, J.W. (2004). Sublethal irradiation of human tumor cells modulates phenotype resulting in enhanced killing by cytotoxic T lymphocytes. *Cancer Res* 64, 21, (Nov 1), 7985-7994.

Gridley, D.S., Andres, M.L., Garner, C., Mao, X.W. & Slater, J.M. (1996). Evaluation of TNF-alpha effects on radiation efficacy in a human lung adenocarcinoma model. *Oncol Res* 8, 12, 485-495.

Gridley, D.S., Li, J., Kajioka, E.H., Andres, M.L., Moyers, M.F. & Slater, J.M. (2000). Combination of pGL1-TNF-alpha gene and radiation (proton and gamma-ray) therapy against brain tumor. *Anticancer Res* 20, 6B, (Nov-Dec), 4195-4203.

Gridley, D.S., Baer, J.R., Cao, J.D., Miller, G.M., Kim, D.W., Timiryasova, T.M., Fodor, I. & Slater, J.M. (2002). TNF-alpha gene and proton radiotherapy in an orthotopic brain tumor model. *Int J Oncol* 21, 2, (Aug), 251-259.

Guerrero Urbano, T., Khoo, V., Staffurth, J., Norman, A., Buffa, F., Jackson, A., Adams, E., Hansen, V., Clark, C., Miles, E., McNair, H., Nutting, C., Parker, C., Eeles, R., Huddart, R., Horwich, A. & Dearnaley, D.P. (2010). Intensity-modulated Radiotherapy Allows Escalation of the Radiation Dose to the Pelvic Lymph Nodes in Patients with Locally Advanced Prostate Cancer: Preliminary Results of a Phase I Dose Escalation Study. *Clin Oncol* 22, 3, 236-244.

Gulley, J.L., Arlen, P.M., Bastian, A., Morin, S., Marte, J., Beetham, P., Tsang, K.Y., Yokokawa, J., Hodge, J.W., Menard, C., Camphausen, K., Coleman, C.N., Sullivan, F., Steinberg, S.M., Schlom, J. & Dahut, W. (2005). Combining a recombinant cancer vaccine with standard definitive radiotherapy in patients with localized prostate cancer. *Clin Cancer Res* 11, 9, (May 1), 3353-3362.

Gust, K., Hofer, M., Perner, S., Kim, R., Chinnaiyan, A., Varambally, S., Moller, P., Rinnab, L., Rubin, M., Greiner, J., Schmitt, M., Kuefer, R. & Ringhoffer, M. (2009). RHAMM (CD168) is overexpressed at the protein level and may constitute an immunogenic antigen in advanced prostate cancer disease. *Neoplasia* 11, 9, 956-963.

Haanen, J., Baars, A., Gomez, R., Weder, P., Smits, M., de Gruijl, T., von Blomberg, B., Bloemena, E., Scheper, R., van Ham, S., Pinedo, H. & van den Eertwegh, A. (2005). Melanoma-specific tumor-infiltrating lymphocytes but not circulating melanoma-specific T cells may predict survival in resected advanced-stage melanoma patients. *Cancer Immunol Immunother* 1-8.

Hanahan, D. & Weinberg, R. (2011). Hallmarks of cancer: the next generation. *Cell* 144, 5, 646-674.

Hillman, G.G., Maughan, R.L., Grignon, D.J., Yudelev, M., Che, M., Abrams, J., Wang, Y., Layer, A., Wright, J.L., Rubio, J. & Forman, J.D. (2003). Responsiveness of experimental prostate carcinoma bone tumors to neutron or photon radiation combined with cytokine therapy. *Int J Radiat Oncol Biol Phys* 56, 5, (Aug 1), 1426-1437.

Honma, I., Torigoe, T., Hirohashi, Y., Kitamura, H., Sato, E., Masumori, N., Tamura, Y., Tsukamoto, T. & Sato, N. (2009). Aberrant expression and potency as a cancer immunotherapy target of alpha-methylacyl-coenzyme A racemase in prostate cancer. *J Transl Med* 7, 103.

Hoskin, P. (2008). High dose rate brachytherapy for prostate cancer. *Cancer Radiother* 12, 6-7, (Nov), 512-514.

Huang, H., Dawicki, W., Zhang, X., Town, J. & Gordon, J. (2010). Tolerogenic dendritic cells induce CD4+CD25hiFoxp3+ regulatory T cell differentiation from CD4+CD25-/loFoxp3- effector T cells. *J Immunol* 185, 9, 5003-5010.

Huang, J., Wang, Y., Guo, J., Lu, H., Lin, X., Ma, L., Teitz-Tennenbaum, S., Chang, A.E. & Li, Q. (2007). Radiation-induced apoptosis along with local and systemic cytokine elaboration is associated with DC plus radiotherapy-mediated renal cell tumor regression. *Clin Immunol* 123, 3, (Jun), 298-310.

Hudolin, T., Juretic, A., Spagnoli, G., Pasini, J., Bandic, D., Heberer, M., Kosicek, M. & Cacic, M. (2006). Immunohistochemical expression of tumor antigens MAGE-A1, MAGE-A3/4, and NY-ESO-1 in cancerous and benign prostatic tissue. *Prostate* 66, 1, 13 - 18.

Jackson, M.W., Bentel, J.M. & Tilley, W.D. (1997). Vascular endothelial growth factor (VEGF) expression in prostate cancer and benign prostatic hyperplasia. *J Urol* 157, 6, (Jun), 2323-2328.

James, N.D., Sydes, M.R., Clarke, N.W., Mason, M.D., Dearnaley, D.P., Anderson, J., Popert, R.J., Sanders, K., Morgan, R.C., Stansfeld, J., Dwyer, J., Masters, J. & Parmar, M.K.B. (2009). Systemic therapy for advancing or metastatic prostate cancer (STAMPEDE): a multi-arm, multistage randomized controlled trial. *BJU Internatl* 103, 4, 464-469.

Jin, G.H., Jin, S.Z., Liu, Y., Xu, R.M., Yang, J.Z., Pan, X.N. & Liu, S.Z. (2005). Therapeutic effect of gene-therapy in combination with local X-irradiation in a mouse malignant melanoma model. *Biochem Biophys Res Commun* 330, 3, (May 13), 975-981.

Kachikwu, E., Iwamoto, K., Liao, Y., Demarco, J., Agazaryan, N., Economou, J., McBride, W. & Schaue, D. (2010). Radiation enhances regulatory T Cell representation. *Int J Radiat Oncol Biol Phys* Epub ahead of print Nov 17.

Kantoff, P.W., Higano, C.S., Shore, N.D., Berger, E.R., Small, E.J., Penson, D.F., Redfern, C.H., Ferrari, A.C., Dreicer, R., Sims, R.B., Xu, Y., Frohlich, M.W. & Schellhammer, P.F. (2010). Sipuleucel-T Immunotherapy for castration-resistant prostate cancer. *N Engl J Med* 363, 5, 411-422.

Kärjä, V., Aaltomaa, S., Lipponen, P., Isotalo, T., Talja, M. & Mokka, R. (2005). Tumour-infiltrating lymphocytes: A prognostic factor of PSA-free survival in patients with local prostate carcinoma treated by radical prostatectomy. *Anticancer Res* 25, 6C, 4435-4438.

Khoo, V.S. & Dearnaley, D.P. (2008). Question of dose, fractionation and technique: ingredients for testing hypofractionation in prostate cancer--the CHHiP trial. *Clin Oncol* 20, 1, (Feb), 12-14.

King, C.R., Brooks, J.D., Gill, H. & Presti, J.C., Jr. (2011). Long-Term Outcomes from a Prospective Trial of Stereotactic Body Radiotherapy for Low-Risk Prostate Cancer. *Int J Radiat Oncol Biol Phys*, (Feb 5).

Kjaergaard, J., Wang, L.X., Kuriyama, H., Shu, S. & Plautz, G.E. (2005). Active immunotherapy for advanced intracranial murine tumors by using dendritic cell-tumor cell fusion vaccines. *J Neurosurg* 103, 1, (Jul), 156-164.

Lechleider, R., Arlen, P., Tsang, K., Steinberg, S., Yokokawa, J., Cereda, V., Camphausen, K., Schlom, J., Dahut, W. & Gulley, J. (2008). Safety and immunologic response of a viral vaccine to prostate-specific antigen in combination with radiation therapy when metronomic-dose interleukin 2 is used as an adjuvant. *Clin Cancer Res* 14, 16, 5284-5291.

Lee, Y., Auh, S.L., Wang, Y., Burnette, B., Wang, Y., Meng, Y., Beckett, M., Sharma, R., Chin, R., Tu, T., Weichselbaum, R.R. & Fu, Y.-X. (2009). Therapeutic effects of ablative radiation on local tumor require CD8+ T cells: changing strategies for cancer treatment. *Blood* 114, 3, (July 16), 589-595.

Li, J., Andres, M.L., Fodor, I., Nelson, G.A. & Gridley, D.S. (1998). Evaluation of pGL1-TNF-alpha therapy in combination with radiation. *Oncol Res* 10, 7, 379-387.

Lindholm, P., Lu, Y., Adley, B., Vladislav, T., Jovanovic, B., Sivapurapu, N., Yang, X. & Kajdacsy-Balla, A. (2010). Role of monocyte-lineage cells in prostate cancer cell invasion and tissue factor expression. *Prostate* 70, 15, 1672-1682.

Liu, V.C., Wong, L.Y., Jang, T., Shah, A.H., Park, I., Yang, X., Zhang, Q., Lonning, S., Teicher, B.A. & Lee, C. (2007). Tumor evasion of the immune system by converting CD4+CD25- T cells into CD4+CD25+ T regulatory cells: role of tumor-derived TGF-beta. *J Immunol* 178, 5, (Mar 1), 2883-2892.

Loberg, R.D., Ying, C., Craig, M., Yan, L., Snyder, L.A. & Pienta, K.J. (2007). CCL2 as an important mediator of prostate cancer growth in vivo through the regulation of macrophage infiltration. *Neoplasia* 9, 7, (Jul), 556-562.

Lohr, F., Hu, K., Haroon, Z., Samulski, T.V., Huang, Q., Beaty, J., Dewhirst, M.W. & Li, C.Y. (2000). Combination treatment of murine tumors by adenovirus-mediated local B7/IL12 immunotherapy and radiotherapy. *Mol Ther* 2, 3, (Sep), 195-203.

Lu, Y., Cai, Z., Galson, D.L., Xiao, G., Liu, Y., George, D.E., Melhem, M.F., Yao, Z. & Zhang, J. (2006). Monocyte chemotactic protein-1 (MCP-1) acts as a paracrine and autocrine factor for prostate cancer growth and invasion. *Prostate* 66, 12, (Sep 1), 1311-1318.

Lu, Y., Wang, J., Xu, Y., Koch, A.E., Cai, Z., Chen, X., Galson, D.L., Taichman, R.S. & Zhang, J. (2008). CXCL16 functions as a novel chemotactic factor for prostate cancer cells in vitro. *Mol Cancer Res* 6, 4, (Apr), 546-554.

Lugade, A., Moran, J., Gerber, S., Rose, R., Frelinger, J. & Lord, E. (2005). Local radiation therapy of B16 melanoma tumors increases the generation of tumor antigen-specific effector cells that traffic to the tumor. *J Immunol* 174, 12, 7516-7523.

Lugade, A., Sorensen, E., Gerber, S., Moran, J., Frelinger, J. & Lord, E. (2008). Radiation-induced IFN-gamma production within the tumor microenvironment influences antitumor immunity. *J Immunol* 180, 5, 3132-3139.

Lumniczky, K., Desaknai, S., Mangel, L., Szende, B., Hamada, H., Hidvegi, E.J. & Safrany, G. (2002). Local tumor irradiation augments the antitumor effect of cytokine-producing autologous cancer cell vaccines in a murine glioma model. *Cancer Gene Therapy* 9, 1, (Jan), 44-52.

Ma, Y., Aymeric, L., Locher, C., Kroemer, G. & Zitvogel, L. (2011). The dendritic cell-tumor cross-talk in cancer. *Current Op Immunol* 23, 1, 146 - 152.

Madsen, B.L., Hsi, R.A., Pham, H.T., Fowler, J.F., Esagui, L. & Corman, J. (2007). Stereotactic hypofractionated accurate radiotherapy of the prostate (SHARP), 33.5 Gy in five fractions for localized disease: first clinical trial results. *Int J Radiat Oncol Biol Phys* 67, 4, (Mar 15), 1099-1105.

Marigo, I., Dolcetti, L., Serafini, P., Zanovello, P. & Bronte, V. (2008). Tumor-induced tolerance and immune suppression by myeloid derived suppressor cells. *Immunol Rev* 222, (Apr), 162-179.

Matsumura, S. & Demaria, S. (2010). Up-regulation of the pro-inflammatory chemokine CXCL16 is a common response of tumor cells to ionizing radiation. *Radiat Res* 173, 4, (Apr), 418-425.

Miller, A., Lundberg, K., Ozenci, V., Banham, A., Hellström, M., Egevad, L. & Pisa, P. (2006). CD4+CD25high T cells are enriched in the tumor and peripheral blood of prostate cancer patients. *J Immunol* 177, 10, 7398-7405.

Mor, F. & Cohen, I.R. (1996). IL-2 rescues antigen-specific T cells from radiation or dexamethasone-induced apoptosis. Correlation with induction of Bcl-2. *J Immunol* 156, 2, (Jan 15), 515-522.

Nakatsuka, S., Oji, Y., Horiuchi, T., Kanda, T., Kitagawa, M., Takeuchi, T., Kawano, K., Kuwae, Y., Yamauchi, A., Okumura, M., Kitamura, Y., Oka, Y., Kawase, I., Sugiyama, H. & Aozasa, K. (2006). Immunohistochemical detection of WT1 protein in a variety of cancer cells. *Mod Pathol* 19, 6, 804-814.

Nesslinger, N.J., Sahota, R.A., Stone, B., Johnson, K., Chima, N., King, C., Rasmussen, D., Bishop, D., Rennie, P.S., Gleave, M., Blood, P., Pai, H., Ludgate, C. & Nelson, B.H. (2007). Standard treatments induce antigen-specific immune responses in prostate cancer. *Clin Cancer Res* 13, 5, (March 1, 2007), 1493-1502.

Newcomb, E.W., Demaria, S., Lukyanov, Y., Shao, Y., Schnee, T., Kawashima, N., Lan, L., Dewyngaert, J.K., Zagzag, D., McBride, W.H. & Formenti, S.C. (2006). The combination of ionizing radiation and peripheral vaccination produces long-term survival of mice bearing established invasive GL261 gliomas. *Clin Cancer Res* 12, 15, (Aug 1), 4730-4737.

Nishiguchi, I., Willingham, V. & Milas, L. (1990). Tumor necrosis factor as an adjunct to fractionated radiotherapy in the treatment of murine tumors. *Int J Radiat Oncol Biol Phys* 18, 3, (Mar), 555-558.

Obeid, M., Tesniere, A., Ghiringhelli, F., Fimia, G.M., Apetoh, L., Perfettini, J.L., Castedo, M., Mignot, G., Panaretakis, T., Casares, N., Métivier, D., Larochette, N., van Endert, P., Ciccosanti, F., Piacentini, M., Zitvogel, L. & Kroemer, G. (2007). Calreticulin exposure dictates the immunogenicity of cancer cell death. *Nat Med* 13, 1, 54-61.

Oh, Y.T., Chen, D.W., Dougherty, G.J. & McBride, W.H. (2004). Adenoviral interleukin-3 gene-radiation therapy for prostate cancer in mouse model. *Int J Radiat Oncol Biol Phys* 59, 2, (Jun 1), 579-583.

Ohm, J.E., Gabrilovich, D.I., Sempowski, G.D., Kisseleva, E., Parman, K.S., Nadaf, S. & Carbone, D.P. (2003). VEGF inhibits T-cell development and may contribute to tumor-induced immune suppression. *Blood* 101, 12, (Jun 15), 4878-4886.

Olson, B. & McNeel, D. (2011). CD8+ T cells specific for the androgen receptor are common in patients with prostate cancer and are able to lyse prostate tumor cells. *Cancer Immunol Immunother* 60, 6, 781-792.

Oyama, T., Ran, S., Ishida, T., Nadaf, S., Kerr, L., Carbone, D.P. & Gabrilovich, D.I. (1998). Vascular endothelial growth factor affects dendritic cell maturation through the inhibition of nuclear factor-kappa B activation in hemopoietic progenitor cells. *J Immunol* 160, 3, (Feb 1), 1224-1232.

Reits, E., Hodge, J., Herberts, C., Groothuis, T., Chakraborty, M., Wansley, E., Camphausen, K., Luiten, R., de Ru, A., Neijssen, J., Griekspoor, A., Mesman, E., Verreck, F., Spits, H., Schlom, J., van Veelen, P. & Neefjes, J. (2006). Radiation modulates the peptide repertoire, enhances MHC class I expression, and induces successful antitumor immunotherapy. *J Exp Med* 203, 5, 1259-1271.

Rokhlin, O.W. & Cohen, M.B. (1995). Expression of cellular adhesion molecules on human prostate tumor cell lines. *Prostate* 26, 4, (Apr), 205-212.

Sato, K., Yamashita, N. & Matsuyama, T. (2002). Human peripheral blood monocyte-derived interleukin-10-induced semi-mature dendritic cells induce anergic CD4(+) and CD8(+) T cells via presentation of the internalized soluble antigen and cross-presentation of the phagocytosed necrotic cellular fragments. *Cell Immunol* 215, 2, (Feb), 186-194.

Schaue, D., Comin-Anduix, B., Ribas, A., Zhang, L., Goodglick, L., Sayre, J., Debucquoy, A., Haustermans, K. & McBride, W. (2008). T-cell responses to survivin in cancer patients undergoing radiation therapy. *Clin Cancer Res* 14, 15, 4883-4890.

Sfanos, K., Bruno, T., Maris, C., Xu, L., Thoburn, C., DeMarzo, A., Meeker, A., Isaacs, W. & Drake, C. (2008). Phenotypic analysis of prostate-infiltrating lymphocytes reveals TH17 and Treg skewing. *Clin Cancer Res* 14, 11, 3254-3261.

Shelley, M.D., Kumar, S., Coles, B., Wilt, T., Staffurth, J. & Mason, M.D. (2009). Adjuvant hormone therapy for localised and locally advanced prostate carcinoma: A systematic review and meta-analysis of randomised trials. *Cancer Treatment Reviews* 35, 7, 540-546.

Shelley, M.D., Kumar, S., Wilt, T., Staffurth, J., Coles, B. & Mason, M.D. (2009). A systematic review and meta-analysis of randomised trials of neo-adjuvant hormone therapy for localised and locally advanced prostate carcinoma. *Cancer Treatment Reviews* 35, 1, 9-17.

Shiao, S.L. & Coussens, L.M. (2010). The tumor-immune microenvironment and response to radiation therapy. *J Mammary Gland Biol Neoplasia* 15, 4, (Dec), 411-421.

Sinnathamby, G., Zerfass, J., Hafner, J., Block, P., Nickens, Z., Hobeika, A., Secord, A., Lyerly, H., Morse, M. & Philip, R. (2011). ADAM metallopeptidase domain 17 (ADAM17) is naturally processed through major histocompatibility complex (MHC) class I molecules and is a potential immunotherapeutic target in breast, ovarian and prostate cancers. *Clin Exp Immunol* 163, 3, 324-332.

Sluyter, R., Shemon, A. & Wiley, J. (2004). Glu496 to Ala polymorphism in the P2X7 receptor impairs ATP-induced IL-1 beta release from human monocytes. *J Immunol* 172, 6, 3399-3405.

Sonpavde, G., Agarwal, N., Choueiri, T. & Kantoff, P. (2011). Recent advances in immunotherapy for the treatment of prostate cancer. *Expert Opin Biol Ther* 11, 8, 997-1009.

Sorrentino, C., Musiani, P., Pompa, P., Cipollone, G. & Di Carlo, E. (2011). Androgen deprivation boosts prostatic infiltration of cytotoxic and regulatory T lymphocytes and has no effect on disease-free survival in prostate cancer patients. *Clin Cancer Res* 17, 6, 1571-1581.

Southall, P., Boxer, G., Bagshawe, K., Hole, N., Bromley, M. & Stern, P. (1990). Immunohistological distribution of 5T4 antigen in normal and malignant tissues. *Br J Cancer* 61, 1, 89-95.

Stagg, J. & Smyth, M.J. (2010). Extracellular adenosine triphosphate and adenosine an cancer. *Oncogene* 29, (Sept 30), 5346-5358.

Strauss, D. & Thomas, J. (2010). Transmission of donor melanoma by organ transplantation. *Lancet Oncol* 11, 8, 790-796.

Tabi, Z., Spary, L., Coleman, S., Clayton, A., Mason, M.D. & Staffurth, J. (2010). Resistance of CD45RA- T cells to apoptosis and functional impairment, and generation of tumor-antigen specific T cell responses during radiation therapy of prostate cancer. *J Immunol* 185, 2, (Jul 15), 1330-1339.

Teitz-Tennenbaum, S., Li, Q., Davis, M.A., Wilder-Romans, K., Hoff, J., Li, M. & Chang, A.E. (2009). Radiotherapy combined with intratumoral dendritic cell vaccination enhances the therapeutic efficacy of adoptive T-cell transfer. *J Immunother* 32, 6, (Jul), 602-612.

Teng, M., Swann, J., Koebel, C., Schreiber, R. & Smyth, M. (2008). Immune-mediated dormancy: an equilibrium with cancer. *J Leukocyte Biol* 84, 4, 988-993.

Thiery, J., Keefe, D., Boulant, S., Boucrot, E., Walch, M., Martinvalet, D., Goping, I., Bleackley, R., Kirchhausen, T. & Lieberman, J. (2011). Perforin pores in the endosomal membrane trigger the release of endocytosed granzyme B into the cytosol of target cells. *Nat Immunol*, 19 Jun, Epub ahead of print.

Thompson, I.M., Jr., Tangen, C.M., Paradelo, J., Lucia, M.S., Miller, G., Troyer, D., Messing, E., Forman, J., Chin, J., Swanson, G., Canby-Hagino, E. & Crawford, E.D. (2006).

Adjuvant radiotherapy for pathologically advanced prostate cancer: a randomized clinical trial. *Jama* 296, 19, (Nov 15), 2329-2335.

Troy, A., Davidson, P., Atkinson, C. & Hart, D. (1998). Phenotypic characterisation of the dendritic cell infiltrate in prostate cancer. *J Urol* 160, 1, (Jul), 214-219.

Tsai, C.H., Hong, J.H., Hsieh, K.F., Hsiao, H.W., Chuang, W.L., Lee, C.C., McBride, W.H. & Chiang, C.S. (2006). Tetracycline-regulated intratumoral expression of interleukin-3 enhances the efficacy of radiation therapy for murine prostate cancer. *Cancer Gene Therapy* 13, 12, (Dec), 1082-1092.

Van Der Meeren, A., Squiban, C., Gourmelon, P., Lafont, H. & Gaugler, M.H. (1999). Differential regulation by IL-4 and IL-10 of radiation-induced IL-6 and IL-8 production and ICAM-1 expression by human endothelial cells. *Cytokine* 11, 11, (Nov), 831-838.

Viani, G., Stefano, E. & Afonso, S. (2009). Higher-than-conventional radiation doses in localized prostate cancer treatment: a meta-analysis of randomized, controlled trials. *Int J Radiat Oncol Biol Phys* 74, 5, 1405-1418.

Wan, Y. & Flavell, R. (2007). 'Yin-Yang' functions of transforming growth factor-beta and T regulatory cells in immune regulation. *Immunol Rev* 220, 199-213.

Warde, P., Mason, M., Sydes, M., Gospodarowicz, M., Swanson, G., Kirkbride, P., Kostashuk, E. & al., e. (2010). Intergroup randomised phase III study of androgen deprivation therapy (ADT) plus radiation therapy (RT) in locally advanced prostate cancer (CaP) (NCIC-CTG, SWOG, MRC-UK, INY: T94-0110; NCT00002633). *J Clin Oncol* 28, 18s, CRA 4504.

Wiegel, T., Bottke, D., Steiner, U., Siegmann, A., Golz, R., Storkel, S., Willich, N., Semjonow, A., Souchon, R., Stockle, M., Rube, C., Weissbach, L., Althaus, P., Rebmann, U., Kalble, T., Feldmann, H.J., Wirth, M., Hinke, A., Hinkelbein, W. & Miller, K. (2009). Phase III postoperative adjuvant radiotherapy after radical prostatectomy compared with radical prostatectomy alone in pT3 prostate cancer with postoperative undetectable prostate-specific antigen: ARO 96-02/AUO AP 09/95. *J Clin Oncol* 27, 18, (Jun 20), 2924-2930.

Wrzesinski, S., Wan, Y. & Flavell, R. (2007). Transforming growth factor-beta and the immune response: implications for anticancer therapy. *Clin Cancer Res* 13, 18 Pt 1, 5262-5270.

Yokouchi, H., Yamazaki, K., Chamoto, K., Kikuchi, E., Shinagawa, N., Oizumi, S., Hommura, F., Nishimura, T. & Nishimura, M. (2008). Anti-OX40 monoclonal antibody therapy in combination with radiotherapy results in therapeutic antitumor immunity to murine lung cancer. *Cancer Sci* 99, 2, (Feb), 361-367.

Younes, E., Haas, G.P., Dezso, B., Ali, E., Maughan, R.L., Kukuruga, M.A., Montecillo, E., Pontes, J.E. & Hillman, G.G. (1995). Local tumor irradiation augments the response to IL-2 therapy in a murine renal adenocarcinoma. *Cell Immunol* 165, 2, (Oct 15), 243-251.

5

Radical Prostatectomy in High Risk Prostate Cancer

Jorge Rioja, Carlos Blanco and Jorge Aranda
Dept Urology, University Hospital Miguel Servet, Zaragoza
Spain

1. Introduction

Prostate cancer is the leading cancer diagnosis in men, and the second cuase, after lung cancer, of cancer death in men in the U.S. Worldwide is the fourth most common cancer in men with variable incidence and mortality rates, based on geographic regions (1). In Europe is the most common solid tumor, with an incidence of 214 cases per 1000 men, outnumbering the lung and colorectal cancers, and is the second most common cause of cancer death in men.

In recent years, the incidence of prostate cancer is increasing in most countries due to the improvement and widespread use of PSA, aging and probably a real increase in incidence. In men after 40 years there is a progressively incidence increase, with a peak at age 80. The countries with the highest mortality rate for prostate cancer are: Switzerland, Scandinavia and the USA-adjusted death rates by age group between 15-20/100.000 inhabitants. By contrast, the Asian countries with Japan and China leading the way, have the lowest mortality rate (less than 5 per 100,000 population) (1).

The geographic incidence variations of prostate Cancer are multiple and complex, but there are genetic and environmental factors, which seem to be more involved in its genesis. African Americans are those who have higher rates of prostate ca. As mentioned above, China and Japan have lower rates in the incidence of prostate ca and USA one of the highest in the world, well, it is noteworthy that Asian Americans have lower incidence rate of prostate cancer than white Americans, the indicating that the genetic factor is crucial in the development of the disease.

The overall increase in the incidence of prostate cancer worldwide in recent decades, is justified with the development of PSA screening protocols of prostate Cancer. The diagnosis of prostate cancer is based on the determination of serum PSA. The risk of prostate cancer is depending on Serum PSA (2):

PSA 0-2 ng / ml: 15-25%.
PSA 2-4 ng / ml: 17-32%
PSA 4-10 ng / ml: 17-32%
PSA> 10 ng / ml: 43-65%.

There is still much controversy among health professionals about what is the best protocol for the screening of prostate cancer. The long awaited results of two prospective, randomised trials were published in 2009. The Prostate, Lung, Colorectal, and Ovarian

(PLCO) Cancer Screening Trial randomly assigned 76,693 men at 10 US centres to receive either annual screening with PSA and DRE or standard care as the control. After 7 years' follow-up, the incidence of prostate cancer per 10,000 person-years was 116 (2,820 cancers) in the screening group and 95 (2,322cancers) in the control group (rate ratio, 1.22) (3). The incidence of death per 10,000 person-years was 2.0 (50 deaths) in the screened group and 1.7 (44 deaths) in the control group (rate ratio, 1.13). The data at 10 years were 67% complete and consistent with these overall findings. The PLCO project team concluded that prostate cancer related mortality was very low and not significantly different between the two study groups. The European Randomized Study of Screening for Prostate Cancer (ERSPC) included a total of 162,243 men from seven countries aged between 55 and 69 years. The men were randomly assigned to a group offered PSA screening at an average of once every 4 years or to an unscreened control group. During a median follow-up of 9 years, the cumulative incidence of prostate cancer was 8.2% in the screened group and 4.8% in the control group (4). The rate ratio for death from prostate cancer was 0.80 in the screened group compared with the control group. The absolute risk difference was 0.71 deaths per 1,000 men. This means that 1410 men would need to be screened and 48 additional cases of prostate cancer would need to be treated to prevent one death from prostate cancer. The ERSPC investigators concluded that PSA-based screening reduced the rate of death from prostate cancer by 20%, but was associated with a high risk of over-diagnosis.

Both trials have received considerable attention and comments. In the PLCO trial, the rate of compliance in the screening arm was 85% for PSA testing and 86% for DRE. However, the rate of contamination in the control arm was as high as 40% in the first year and increased to 52% in the sixth year for PSA testing and ranged from 41% to 46% for DRE. Furthermore, biopsy compliance was only 40-52% versus 86% in the ERSPC. Thus, the PLCO trial will probably never be able to answer whether or not screening can influence prostate cancer mortality. In the ERSCP trial, the real benefit will only be evident after 10-15 years of follow-up, especially because the 41% reduction of metastasis in the screening arm will have an impact.

Recent sub-analysis, with longer follow up have shown a potential benefit of screening, lowering the number of men needed to screen, and the number of patients needed to treat to safe one life.

Two key items remain open and empirical:

- at what age should early detection start
- what is the interval for PSA and DRE.

A baseline PSA determination at age 40 years has been suggested upon which the subsequent screening interval may then be based (5) (GR: B). A screening interval of 8 years might be enough in men with initial PSA levels < 1 ng/mL (6) . Further PSA testing is not necessary in men older than 75 years and a baseline PSA < 3 ng/mL because of their very low risk of dying from prostate cancer (7).

D'Amico in 1998 proposed a classification according to risk group for prostate cancer based on T stage, PSA value and Gleason. This has allowed to simplify the classification of patients with prostate cancer as well as trying to unify its treatment. (Table 1)

The widespread use of PSA testing has led to a significant migration in stage and grade of prostate cancer, with > 90% of men in the current era diagnosed with clinically localised disease (8). Despite the trends towards lower-risk prostate cancer, 20-35% of patients with newly diagnosed prostate cancer are still classified as high risk, based on either PSA > 20 ng/mL, Gleason score > 8, or an advanced clinical stage (9). Patients classified with high-risk prostate cancer are at an increased risk of PSA failure, the need for secondary therapy, metastatic progression and death from prostate cancer. Nevertheless, not all high-risk patients have a uniformly poor prognosis after RP (10). There is no consensus regarding the optimal treatment of men with high-risk prostate cancer. Decisions on whether to elect surgery as local therapy should be based on the best available clinical evidence.

Low risk	Intermediate risk	High risk
T1-T2a & PSA<10 y Gleason ≤6	T2b or PSA 10-20 or Glesason 7	T2c-T3-T4 or PSA > 20 or Gleason ≥8

Table 1. D'Amico classification of patients according to risk group

As expected, survival and success of the treatment applied in prostate cancer is closely linked to the stadium and the risk presented by the patient.
In this chapter we will focus on Prostate Cancer at high risk as well as the different therapeutic options, focusing on the radical prostatectomy as an effective treatment of the disease.

2. Defining high risk prostate cancer

The factors that best define the high risk prostate cancer are those described by D'Amico (11) approved by the American Urological Association in 2007 are:

Gleason ≥ 8 points and / or PSA ≥ 20 and / or clinical stage ≥ T2c

These high-risk tumors are at high risk for recurrence, either local or remote, so they are also traditionally called "locally advanced" (12) or "poorly differentiated" (13). If the patient has the 3 items they are considered "very high risk" and have a high probability to die from prostate cancer (14).
Another factor that has been added as a fourth factor is pretreatment *PSA velocity* which if greater 2ng/ml/year is included as criteria for high-risk disease (15,16).
The simplification of the term "risk" has led many doctors to select patients and improperly included in high-risk groups. Also, following the analysis of these high-risk criteria, we can not quantify the individual risk to a patient, for example, with stage T2c and Gleason 8 would have the same risk that a patient with a PSA 70 and stage T3a (17). That is why this classification system is inadequate and we must use another tool to individualize the risk of each patient; this tool are *Nomograms* which individually allow to analyze and quantify the risk presented by each patient in response to multiple risk factors or variables, integrated in a complex mathematical formula (18). There are plenty of nomograms (19) that have been designed for use in prostate cancer in recent years and could be classified into 3 groups:
Diagnostic nomograms: those who pretend to estimate the probability of a patient developing prostate cancer. For example, the Vienna nomogram (20) that analyzes the number of cylinders to take a biopsy of the prostate.
Staging nomograms: such as the Partin tables (21), which indicates the likelihood of organ-confined disease. Or A. Borque neural network for predicting pathological stage in men undergoing radical prostatectomy. (22)

Prognostic nomograms: are tools that estimate the probability of success in applying a certain treatment to analyze different variables. The most famous and globally applied is Kattan nomogram (23). It analyzes a combination of three factors to determine the probability of PSA relapse after local therapy. These factors are: PSA, Gleason score and clinical stage. They apply both to radical prostatectomy, radiotherapy and brachytherapy. Nomograms derived from the results of treating thousands of patients. The statistical probability of relapse depends on the presence of pre-existing micro metastases at the time of local therapy (23). Hence the likelihood of relapse determined by the Kattan nomograms can be taken as an indication of the presence of micro metastases at the time of local therapy, resulting in an estimate to calculate the probability of success / failure when applying a certain treatment.

In summary, nomograms are useful modern tools that exist today, which may help us making treatment decisions in patients with prostate cancer, especially those with high-risk prostate cancer. As well as providing more information to the patient.

2.1 Locally advanced prostate cancer cT3a

When the disease has overpassed the prostate capsule, it is a T3a stage. Typically, when a patient is at this stage we are advise against radical prostatectomy (24) as primary treatment based on the high rate of positive surgical margins and lymph node metastases (25,26). Numerous studies have shown that the risk/benefit of a radical prostatectomy is even more clear in the treatment of high risk prostate cancer (27-32), but unfortunately, there are not studies comparing combination therapy (radiotherapy plus hormones) with RP.

Between 13% and 27% of patients diagnosed with stage T3 are overstimated (31,32).

The development of CT imaging or MRI, as well as directed needle biopsies of lymph nodes or seminal vesicles (32), help identify patients who have less probability to benefit from a surgical treatment (33) as well as to plan surgery upon results.

Due to an increased sophistication and experience of the different surgical techniques, there has been a decreased in operative morbidity and better functional outcomes after RP in stage T3 cancer than before (31,33). Urinary incontinence and erectile dysfunction remain the two major consequences of the surgery, but due to surgical expertise and experience, as well as a proper surgical planning, an improvement in functional results has been shown (35).

2.2 High grade prostate cancer: Gleason score 8-10

Patients with high Gleason score 8-10 tumors, which are confined to the prostate on histopathological examination, they still have a good prognosis after RP (36). The differences between the Gleason score biopsy and the Gleason score regarding the surgical specimen are between 36 and 60% of cases, although a study by Dr. Grossfeld (37) shows that 39% of patients had Gleason 8-10 in the biopsy specimen, showed a Gleason score of 7 or less in the prostatectomy speciem.

In a recent publication (38) in which the outcome of 781 patients undergoing RP clinically localized stages T1-T2 was analysed, they divided into 2 groups according to Gleason: Gleason patients 2-7 and another group with Gleason 8-10. Over all, they showed a worse prognostic features and higher PSA relapse. (Table 2)

Patients with Gleason score 8-10 prostate cancer have a higher likelihood of recurrence, but due to the PSA era, many of these patients are diagnosed with an early stage and therefore a potential local curative treatment is applicable successful (38).

Various studies such as those of Mian et al (39), Lau et al (40) and Soloway et al (41) analyze and study the survival in these patients concluded similarly.
The clinical Gleason 8-10 is an independent prognostic factor for biochemical progression-free survival. The radical prostatectomy remains one of the most valid treatments for these short of patients and providing good oncological and functional outcomes.

	Group Gleason 2-7	Group Gleason 8-10	P value
N° of patients	673	108	
PSA (ng/ml)	Av 13,48 Median 9,8	Av. 16,89 Median 12	<0,01
T1c	55%	50%	<0,0001
>T1c	45%	50%	
<pT3b	69%	44%	<0,0001
pT3b	30%	56%	
Surgical Margin-	67%	48%	<0,0001
Surgical Margin +	33%	53%	
Biochemical Progression -	74,3%	52,5%	<0,0001
Biochemical Progression +	25,7%	47,5%	

Table 2.

2.3 Prostate cancer with PSA > 20

Different studies show that the RP in patients with a PSA> 20 is associated with a high recurrence rate, D'Amico and colleagues found that males with a PSA level higher than 20 ng/ml had risk recurrence of 50% at 5 years after RP (42). Similarly, Yossepowitch published the results of their series of patients with PSA> 20ng/ml who underwent radical prostatectomy, showing a PSA recurrence rate of 44 and 53% at 4 and 20 years respectively (10). It is perhaps the high preoperative PSA, the factor that best relates to a worse prognosis preoperatively.
On the other hand, Inman and colleagues, in their series of patients with PSA> 50ng/ml who underwent RP with multimodal adjuvant therapy, had biochemical progression-free survival at 10 years of 83% with a cancer-specific survival 87% (43). These highlights the potential benefit of surgery with in a multimodal approach.

3. Therapeutic options in "high risk" prostate cancer

3.1 Introduction

Localized prostate cancer

The lack of evidence regarding the effectiveness of treatment options for clinically localised prostate cancer continues to impact on clinical decision-making. The two such options are radical prostatectomy (RP) and active surveillance (AS). (44)
For the majority of men with favorable-risk localized disease, older than 65, surveillance will be an attractive option that avoids adverse effects of treatment(45). But the existing trials,

provide insufficient evidence to allow confident statements to be made about the relative beneficial and harmful effects of RP and AS for patients with localised prostate cancer.(44)
Klotz L et al. assure that active surveillance with treatment reserved for evidence of rapid PSA progression or increase in tumor volume or grade is associated with about a 3% risk of prostate cancer death at 10 years. (46)

Advanced prostate cancer

In the other hand, patients with prostate cancer continue to present with metastatic disease or to relapse following initial hormone therapy; for these men, the optimal combination and sequencing of new medical treatments must be defined. (45)

High risk prostate cancer

For these patients, (T2c-T3-T4 or PSA >20 or Gleason score ≥8) it is very important to give information about the different treatment options, and trying to adequate them to their live expectancy and quality of live.
Urologist, traditionally recommended radiotherapy or androgen deprivation therapy over RP, not because oncologic outcomes were better with radiotherapy, but because incontinence and impotence rates with RP were higher, and cure rates was discouraging. (47)
Actually, RP and radiotherapy have potential benefits and cumulative toxicities that must be matched to disease characteristics and patient expectations in selecting a treatment course. (48)

3.2 Pre-treatment management in high risk prostate cancer

A critical assessment of the location, size, and extent of the primary tumor provides prognostic information, is essential for treatment planning.
D'Amico and colleagues have defined high-risk prostate cancer as that associated with any 1 of 3 risk factors: biopsy Gleason score ≥8, PSA ≥20 ng/mL, or clinical stage ≥T2c. (11)
More recently, D'Amico and colleagues refined their high-risk definition to incorporate an absolute number of high-risk features (stage ≥T2b, biopsy Gleason score ≥7, and pre-treatment PSA >20 ng/mL). (14) Patients are classified into 1 of 3 high-risk groups, defined by the presence of 1, 2, or all 3 features. Probability of death from prostate cancer was highest among men with 3 high-risk features.
High-risk patients with aggressive tumors (PSA >20 ng/mL and Gleason sum >7), advanced local lesions (T3-T4), or patients with symptoms suggestive for metastatic disease, should have imaging studies. (17)
While not uniformly accurate, there are some imaging studies that help us to identificate the high rish disease:

- DRE provides some evidence of the cancer's size and pathologic stage.
- Transrectal ultrasonography (TRUS) is extremely useful for guiding needle biopsies.
- Computed tomography (CT) scans poorly the prostate and lack of sensitivity and specificity for detecting extraprostatic extension.
- Magnetic Resonance Imaging (MRI) provides additional information about the local lession, it has largely replaced CT in the local staging of prostate cancer.
- MRI has been used primarily to determine local disease extent. Body MRI has a role in identifying seminal vesicle involvement, but not extra capsular extension.
- Bone Scan, which is highly sensitive but relatively nonspecific because areas of increased radiotracer uptake are not always secondary to osteoblastic activity from metastases. (17)

An alternative to patients risk-grouping with similar but not identical risk features is use of multivariable models such as nomograms. These models incorporate data from all risk factors relevant to the probability of treatment failure and proportionately weigh their relative contribution in order to calculate a risk score. (48)
Eastham et al. demonstrate that high-risk patients were more likely to exhibit adverse pathologic features and to have biochemical progression. Nevertheless, roughly one-third of high-risk patients (22% to 63%, depending on the definition) had organ-confined cancers and roughly half (41% to 74%) remained progression-free 10 years after surgery alone. These results confirm that current definitions of high risk disease are unreliable in identifying patients who cannot be cured by local therapy. (48)

3.3 Objectives of treatment in high risk prostate cancer

The actual objectives of the treatment of high prostate cancer are:

1. To offer a radical treatment
2. Trying to decrease prostate cancer progression
3. To increase metastatic disease free interval
4. To provide a proper quality of life.

Men with high-volume lesions or high-stage yet clinically localized disease must receive multimodal therapy. More advances will require concerted efforts through clinical trials. (45)
Neoadjuvant Androgen Deprivation Therapy may indeed provide no additional benefit over surgery alone for patients with clinically localized prostate cancer. Recent studies have demonstrated the feasibility of neoadjuvant chemotherapy prior to RP in patients with high-risk prostate cancer. (17). If such a strategy was shown to be effective, future clinical practice could be altered significantly. A randomized phase 3 clinical trial, CALGB 90203, is currently investigating whether neoadjuvant chemo-hormonal therapy followed by RP reduces the risk of biochemical recurrence when compared to RP alone.

3.4 Actual treatment in high risk prostate cancer

Actually, the optimal treatment are:

- radical prostatectomy (RP) + radiation therapy (RT)
- radical prostatectomy + hormonotherapy
- radiation therapy + hormone therapy

There is no consensus regarding the optimal treatment of men with high-risk PCa.
Surgery is showing good results, but decisions on whether to elect surgery as local therapy should be based on the best available clinical evidence. (49)
On the other hand, it has been recently assessed the effect of RP and RT on the rate of distant metastases in patients with clinically localized prostate cancer on the study from Memorial Sloan Kettering Cancer Center comparing patients whom underwent surgery versus radiotherapy (50). Patients with clinical stages T1c-T3b prostate cancer treated with intensity-modulated RT (81 Gy) from 1998 to 2002 were compared with similar cohort of men treated with RP.
This study, showed that patients with higher-risk disease, treated with RP had a lower risk of metastatic progression and prostate cancer-specific death, than men treated with RT. The metastatic progression is infrequent in men with low-risk prostate cancer, treated with either RP or RT.
These results, despite being from retrospective review of patients treated at a single institution, certainly suggest that RP should be considered as a treatment option in men with clinically localized, high-risk prostate cancer. (50)

As mentioned above, the multimodal treatment is achieving good results, and to corroborate this, several randomised studies of radiotherapy combined with androgen-deprivation therapy (ADT) versus radiotherapy alone have shown a clear advantage for combination treatment, but no trial has ever proven combined treatment to be superior to RP.

4. Radical prostatectomy in high risk CaP

4.1 Introduction

Actually radical prostatectomy is accepted as an election treatment in both low and high risk prostate cancer with different evidence level, and even for very high risk prostate cancer. (Table 3)

INDICATIONS	LE
In patients with low and intermediate risk localised PCa (cT1a-T2b and Gleason score 2-7 and PSA ≤ 20) and a life expectancy > 10 years	1b
Optional	
Patients with stage T1a disease and a life expectancy >15 yr or Gleason score 7	3
Selected patients with low-volume high-risk localised PCa (cT3a or Gleason score 8-10 or PSA > 20)	3
Highly selected patients with very high-risk localised PCa (cT3b-T4 N0 or any T N1) in the context of multimodality treatment	3
Optional for selected patients with T3a, PSA < 20 ng/mL, biopsy Gleason score ≤ 8 and a life expectancy > 10 years.	3

Table 3.

The goals of RP are to remove the cancer completely with negative surgical margins, minimal blood loss, no serious perioperative complications, and complete recovery of potency and urinary continence. From an oncologic standpoint, obtaining negative surgical margins is paramount. A positive surgical margin has been associated with as much as 4-fold higher risk of biochemical recurrence, even after adjusting for other prognostic factors such as Gleason grade, extracapsular extension, seminal vesicle invasion, and lymph node metastasis. (48)
On the same way, there are good results in terms of morbidity and survival when radical prostatectomy is offered as a radical treatment.

4.2 Evidence of RP in HR.PC

RP in locally advanced PCa: cT3a

Is defined, as cancer that has perforated the prostate capsule. Surgical treatment has traditionally been discouraged, mainly because patients have an increased risk of positive surgical margins and lymph node metastases and/or distant relapse
In recent years, there has been renewed interest in surgery for locally advanced PCa, and several retrospective case-series have been published. In general, 33.5-66% of patients will have positive section margins, and 7.9-49% will have positive lymph nodes.
On the other hand, excellent 5-, 10- and 15-year overall survival (OS) and cancer-specific survival (CSS) rates have been published.
Therefore, it is increasingly evident that surgery has a place in treating locally advanced disease (45)

The problem remains on patient selection before surgery: Nomograms, nodal imaging with CT and seminal vesicle imaging with magnetic resonance or directed specific puncture biopsies of the nodes or seminal vesicles can help to identify those patients unlikely to benefit from a surgical approach. (17)

In addition, it is extremely important that radical prostatectomy for clinical T3 cancer requires sufficient surgical expertise to keep an acceptable morbidity level.

RP in High-grade PCa: Gleason score 8-10

In this group of patients, the incidence of organ-confined disease is around 26% to 31%. The PSA value and percentage of positive prostate biopsies may help to select men with high-grade PCa most likely to benefit from RP.

Rioja Zuazu J. et al. (38) analyzed the characteristics of the clinical Gleason 8-10 group of patients within their series of patients diagnosed with prostate cancer and treated by means of radical prostatectomy, and tried to ascertain which were the influence factors within this group, upon progression and progression free survival. They conclude, that Clinical Gleason Score 8-10 is a negative independent prognostic factor on the progression free survival, but its prognosis is better if they present a PSA prior surgery lower than 11 ng/ml and the pathological stage is a pT2. So, these kind of patients could be beneficed of RP.

RP in PCa with PSA > 20

Yossepowitch et al. (19) and D'Amico et al. (15) have investigated the results of RP in these patients. In all cases, very good results were seen, with a cancer- specific survival of up to 91% in 10 years in patients treated with RP.

More recently, Inman and co-workers (43) described the long-term outcomes of RP with multimodal adjuvant therapy in men with PSA > 50. Systemic progression-free survival rates at 10 years were 83% and 74% for PSA 50-99 and > 100, respectively, while CSS was 87% for the whole group. These results argue for aggressive management with RP as the initial step.

RP in cT3b-T4 N0

Provided that the tumour is not fixed to the pelvic wall, or that there is no invasion of the urethral sphincter, RP is a reasonable first step in selected patients with a low tumour volume.

In 2005, The Mayo Clinic reported a series of patients with seminal invasion, treated with RP + HT adjuvant. They had a progression free survival at 5, 10 and 15 years, of 85%, 73% and 67% respectively, and a cancer specific survival of 95%, 90% and 79%.

Despite this, management decisions should be made after all treatments, and should be discussed by a multidisciplinary team, and after balancing benefits and side-effects of each therapy modality by the patient, with regard to his own individual circumstances, decision has to be taken.

4.3 Optimal surgical technique for high risk cancer

Surgeons must understand the important anatomical and surgical principles that will allow them to improve their own technique, particularly when operating in the high-risk setting. Certain principles are important, and apply equally to open, laparoscopic and robotic surgical techniques.

Even in a patient with a high risk of extra prostatic disease, a portion of the neurovascular bundle can often be preserved. (17)

This approach has been facilitated by recent anatomical descriptions of the periprostatic anatomy. (51)

Dissection of the neurovascular bundles can be done in an intrafascial plane (directly adjacent to the prostatic capsule; complete nerve sparing), an interfascial plane (within the lateral prostatic fascia; partial nerve sparing) and extrafascial plane (outside the lateral prostatic fascia; nerve resection)

Deep dissection beneath Denonvilliers' fascia posteriorly should be performed routinely, as few nerves are present in this area and deep dissection will reduce the incidence of posterolateral margins.

Large, high-grade cancers, near the base of the prostate, or in the anterior transition zone often invade the bladder neck. For anterior cancers, begin division of the bladder neck a centimeter or more from its junction with the prostate. For large posterior tumors or those with seminal vesicle invasion, include the posterior bladder distal to the interureteral ridge in the specimen. (48)

5. Pelvic lymph node dissection

For patients with low risk disease, PLND is not necessary and is not recommended, because the chance of metastasis is low.

For patients with high and intermediate risk disease, extended PLND at least for external iliac, obturator and hypogastric lymph nodes should be performed during radical prostatectomy. Removing at least 10 lymph nodes is recommended to detect LNI. (52)

Prostate cancer lymphatic spread ascends from the pelvis up to the retroperitoneum invariably through common iliac lymph nodes. PC lymphatic spread can be divided in two main levels: pelvic and common iliac plus retroperitoneal lymph nodes. (53)

So the technique try to remove all lymphatic tissue between the external iliac vein and hypogastric vein above and below the obturator nerve, including the hypogastric and obturator lymph nodes.

Therefore may assert that an eLND should be performed in all high-risk cases, as the estimated risk for positive lymph nodes will be in the range 15-40%. (10)

However, despite the above, some authors like Bubley are not so categorical in affirming this.

Although it is generally accepted that eLND provides important information for prognosis (number of nodes involved, tumour volume within the lymph node, capsular perforation of the node) that cannot be matched by any other current procedure, consensus has not been reached as to when eLND is indicated and to what extent it should be performed. When making such decisions, many physicians rely on nomograms based on pre-operative biochemical markers and biopsies. (54)

5.1 Role of RT in high risk prostate cancer

Indications for RT after RP

As stated earlier, currently, a multimodal treatment is chosen to increase survival and reduce biochemical progression. In this sense the RT play an important role.

There are two important studies about this:

The EORTC Trial 22911 included 1,005 patients with positive surgical margins or pT3 disease (extracapsular extension and seminal vesicle involvement) and randomized them to adjuvant EBRT (50 Gy to the prostatic fossa and periprostatic tissue plus a 10–14 Gy boost to the prostatic fossa only) versus no immediate treatment. (55) The cumulative rate of loco regional failure was significantly lower in the irradiated group (P <0.0001). However, other clinically important endpoints were not improved. In particular, 5-year metastasis-free survival, cause-specific survival, and overall survival were not affected by adjuvant RT.

The Southwest Oncology Group (SWOG) trial 8794 included 425 patients with high-risk localized disease, who were randomized to receive either 60–64 Gy to the prostatic fossa or observation only. (56) Biochemical control, disease-free survival, cancer-specific mortality, and overall survival were significantly increased in the adjuvant irradiation arm at a median follow-up of 10.6 years.

Both the EORTC and SWOG randomized trials, provide evidence that adjuvant post-prostatectomy irradiation reduces the risk of biochemical recurrence and local clinical failure. It remains uncertain, whether administration of radiation immediately after PSA is detected, could provide equally effective long-term outcomes to patients receiving adjuvant therapy, while sparing such patients from unnecessary irradiation. (17) (48)

Salvage radiotherapy

The efficacy of radiotherapy in the setting of a rising PSA after RP is unproven, and its use is highly controversial. Stephenson et al. reported on a large retrospective analysis of salvage irradiation of 501 patients from 5 institutions. (57)

Positive surgical margins, Gleason scores <8, or PSADT >10 months. In such patients, PSA relapse-free survival outcomes were in the range of 70% to 80% at 3 years.

6. Survival

Regarding cancer-specific survival rate, and the overall survival rate, there are many studies, with different results (table 4).

First, in terms of morbidity, Berglund and colleagues (58) showed, that recovery from surgery, duration of catheterization, and the overall return of continence were essentially similar to those observed in the low-risk population.

Another important factor to consider when analyzing survival, is the overstaging sometimes happens in the T3. Therefore, Ward et al report a long-term experience with radical surgery in patients presenting with locally advanced (cT3) prostate cancer, as the best management of such patients remains a problem. They found that, significantly many patients with cT3 prostate cancer were over-staged (pT2) in the PSA era, and RP as part of a multimodal treatment strategy for patients with cT3 disease offers cancer control and survival rates approaching those achieved for cT2 disease. (31)

For short term survival, Loeb et al (35) reported a complication rate of 11% in 288 consecutive high-risk patients treated by RP, which was not different from the rate in a previous study from the same group that included 3,477 consecutive patients with prostate cancer (59) when analyzing intermediate-term cancer control, and quality-of-life outcomes after radical retropubic prostatectomy (RRP), and concluded that RRP offers excellent intermediate-term cancer control for selected men, of all ages, who present with high-risk or locally advanced disease. Both, continence and potency, were preserved in most patients, although the potency rates were significantly greater for the younger men. RRP with appropiate postoperative radiotherapy and/or hormonal therapy is a reasonable treatment option for selected men with high-risk or locally advanced disease. (35) (Table 4)

	↑Risk	N° Patients	% 5 years BR free survival	% 10 years cancer especif survival
Van de Ouden (29)	T3 clínic	136	39	72
Hsu (26)	T3 clínic	235	60	92
Ward (20)	T3 clínic	841	58	90; 15 y 79
Lau (23)	Gleason 8-10	407	49	85
Berglund (19)	PSA ≥15 or Gleason 8-10	281	65	NR
Loeb (21)	T2 and Gleason 8-10 or PSA ≥15 o T3	288	39-53	70-93
Van Poppel (27)	T3a y PSA ≤20 and Gleason ≤7	32	3mo:90	NR

BR: Bioquimical recurrence
NR: No results.

Table 4.

For long term survival, Van Poppel (60) showed in 2006, that in patients with locally advanced disease, the cancer-specific survival rate after RP at 5- and 10-years of follow-up, was 85-100% and 57-91.6%, respectively. The overall survival rate at 5 and 10 yr was, 75% and 60%, respectively. In patients with high-grade prostate cancer (Gleason score> or =8), the biochemical recurrence-free survival, after RP at 5 and 10 yr of follow-up was, 51% and 39%, respectively.

Van Der Ouden et al. determined the progression and survival rates, and investigate subgroups of patients who may not benefit from this treatment. Defining that Radical prostatectomy as monotherapy, in patients with locally advanced non-metastatic prostate cancer (T3) produces acceptable results, in those with well or moderately differentiated tumors. The results of progression and survival, are not significantly different from those patients with organ confined prostate cancer. (29)

Yossepowitch describe the results of RP in their patient's serie, classify patients in risk groups: (61) he studied pathological and clinical outcomes among high-risk patients treated with RP. To identify high-risk subsets, eight definitions from the medical literature were applied. Depending on the criteria, high-risk patients comprised 3% to 38% of the entire study population, highlighting the immense variability among available high-risk definitions.

High-risk patients were more likely to exhibit adverse pathological features (35%–71% with extra capsular extension, 10%–33% with seminal vesicle invasion, and 7%–23% with lymph node involvement), but roughly one third (22%–63%) had organ-confined cancers and nearly half (41%–74%) remained progression-free 10 years after surgery alone. (Table 5)

More recently the group from the Mayo Clinic, has reported their long-term result after radical prostatectomy versus external bean radiotherapy for patients with high-risk prostate cancer. (62) The 10-year cancer specific survival rate was 92%, 92% and 88% after RRP, EBRT plus ADT and EBRT alone. After adjusting for case mix, no significant differences in the risks of systemic progression or prostate cancer death were observed between patients who received EBRT plus ADT and patients who underwent RRP. However, the risk of all causes of mortality was greater, and statistically significant, after EBRT plus ADT than after RRP.

Criterion ↑R	N° patients	% confined organ	% free survival in 5 years	% cancer specific survival in 10 years
Gleason 8-10	274	35	53	88
PSA > 20	275	33	56	91
T3c(*year 1992)	144	22	49	89
Nomogram PFP 5 years ≤50%	391	28	53	92
PSA velocity >2 ng/mL/year	952	63	80	97
PSA≥ 20 o ≥T2c o Gleason 8-10	957	43	68	93
PSA≥15 o T2Bc o Gleason 8-10	1752	51	73	95

Table 5.

7. Local control

Local control, main objective with both techniques, is better achieved with surgery. Local relapse rates between 3-30%(63-65) Depends on clinical stage (pT2: 2-7%; negative margins 7%; pT3-4: 40%; positive margin 27%) While with Radiotherapy, local recurrence rate is for T1: 17-22% (Standford); 4.6% (Schelhamer); T2: 19%-35%.

The rate of positive biopsies is between 20-70%, although is difficult to classify its meaning, they highlight disease and progression. It depend on clinical stage (B=17%, C=59%) and Gleason score. A valuable biopsy is at 18 months after finishing treatment.

Frequency of positive prostate biopsies on patients whom underwent radiotherapy, is around 38% on average.

In the study (66) with 100 patients, with biopsy every 6 months showed following results T-1b: 21%; en T-2a: 24%; en T-2b-c: 28%.

There is no doubt regarding its prognostic value. Although the pioneers showing these results were Rhamy (1972) and Sewel (1975) Scardino has been reporting, and highlighting its value (67). At Baylor-Collegue (Houston) 147 patients treated with Au 198 and external bean radiotherapy, clinical stage A2, B, C with pelvic lymphadenectomy. They had a positive biopsy rate of 42%, 36%, 28% at 6, 12 and 18 months. The chance of local recurrence at 5 years for positive and negative biopsies is around 52% and 12%, and at 10 years of 72% and 30%.

8. Conclusions

Many cancers, categorized clinically as high risk, are actually pathologically confined to the prostate, and most men with such cancers who undergo RP, are free of additional therapy long after surgery.

For men with high-risk, clinically localized prostate cancer, decisions on whether to elect surgery as local definitive therapy should be based on the best available clinical evidence rather than on an individual practitioner's experiences and biases.

Patients classified with high-risk prostate cancer, by commonly used definitions, are at increased risk of PSA failure, need for secondary therapy, metastatic progression, and death from systemic disease. Nevertheless, such high risk patients do not have a uniformly poor prognosis after RP.

- If the prostate cancer risk has a high probability of progression to metastasis or death, we must offer aggressive treatment, which achieves high cure rate, and eliminate the illness onset.
- Radical prostatectomy is proving a very valid option with high success rate, for which we must select patients appropriately
- The success of RP in high-risk patients, with stage T3 resection depends entirely local tissue containing the tumor and include the resection of seminal vesicles and extended lymphadenectomy.

9. References

Reiter R.E., de Kernion J.K Epidemiology, etiologyand prostate cancer prevention. In Campbell-Walsh Urology, 8th ed. Volume 4, Section XI, Chapter. Pagina 328-85, Ed: Wein A.W., Kavoussi L., Novick A.C., Partin M.D. and Peters C.A. Saunders.

NCCN prostate Guidelines 2011

Andriole GL, Crawford ED, Grubb RL 3rd, et al; PLCO Project Team. Mortality results from a randomized prostate-cancer screening trial. N Engl J Med 2009 Mar 26;360(13):1310-9.

Schröder FH, Hugosson J, Roobol MJ, et al; ERSPC Investigators. Screening and prostate-cancer mortality in a randomized European study. N Engl J Med 2009 Mar 26;360(13):1320-8.

Börgermann C, Loertzer H, Hammerer P, et al. [Problems, objective, and substance of early detection of prostate cancer]. Urologe A 2010 Feb;49(2):181-9

Roobol MJ, Roobol DW, Schröder FH. Is additional testing necessary in men with prostate-specific antigen levels of 1.0 ng/mL or less in a population-based screening setting? (ERSPC, section Rotterdam). Urology 2005 Feb;65(2):343-6.

Carter HB, Kettermann AE, Ferrucci L, et al. Prostate specific antigen testing among the elderly; when to stop? J Urol 2008 Apr:174.

Makarov DV, Trock BJ, Humphreys EB, et al. Updated nomogram to predict pathologic stage of prostate cancer given prostate-specific antigen level, clinical stage, and biopsy Gleason score (Partin tables) based on cases from 2000 to 2005. Urology 2007 Jun;69(6):1095-101.

Shao YH, Demissie K, Shih W, et al. Contemporary risk profile of prostate cancer in the United States. JNatl Cancer Inst 2009 Sep 16;101(18):1280-3.

Yossepowitch O, Eggener SE, Bianco FJ Jr, et al. Radical prostatectomy for clinically localized, high risk prostate cancer: critical analysis of risk assessment methods. J Urol 2007 Aug;178(2):493-9 discussion 499.

D'Amico AV, Whittington R, Malkowicz SB, et al. Biochemical outcome after radical prostatectomy, external beam radiation therapy, or interstitial radiation therapy for clinically localized prostate cancer. Jama 1998;280:969-974

Gerber GS, Thisted RA, Chodak GW, et al. Results of radical prostatectomy in men with locally advanced prostate cancer: multi-institutional pooled analysis. Eur Urol 1997;32:385-390

Donohue JF, Bianco FJ, Jr., Kuroiwa K, et al. Poorly differentiated prostate cancer treated with radical prostatectomy: long-term outcome and incidence of pathological downgrading. J Urol 2006;176:991-995

Tsai HK, Chen MH, McLeod DG, et al. Cancer-specific mortality after radiation therapy with short-course hormonal therapy or radical prostatectomy in men with localized, intermediate-risk to high-risk prostate cancer. Cancer 2006;107:2597-2603

D'Amico AV, Chen MH, Roehl KA, Catalona WJ. Preoperative PSA velocity and the risk of death from prostate cancer after radical prostatectomy. N Engl J Med 2004;351:125-135

Bianco FJ, Jr., Kattan MW, Scardino PT. PSA velocity and prostate cancer. N Engl J Med 2004;351:1800-1802; author reply 1800-1802

Scardino P., Vicent P. Laudone. The Role of Radical Prostatectomy and pelvic lymph node dissection in an integrated program of treatment of high risk prostate cancer. Educational Course handout book. AUA, May 2011

Borque A., Sanz G. Current validity of nomograms for staging of prostate cancer. Arch Esp Urol, 59, 10(989-1000), 2006.

Ross, P.L; Scardino, P.T.; Kattan, M.W.: "A catalog of prostate cancer nomograms". J. Urol., 165: 1562, 2001.

Remzi, M., Fong, Y.K., Dobrovits, M. y cols.: "The Vienna nomogram: validation of a novel biopsy strategy defining the optimal number of cores based on patient age and total prostate volume". J. Urol., 174: 1256, 2005.

Partin, A.W.; Kattan, M.W.; Subong, E.N.P. y cols.: "Combination of prostate-specific antigen, clinical stage, and Gleason score to predict pathological stage of localized prostate cancer". JAMA, 277: 1445, 1997.

Borque A., Sanz G., Allepuz C., Plaza L., Rioja LA. The use of neural networks and logistic regression analysis for predicting pathological stage in men undergoing radical prostatectomy: a population based study. J Urol 2001; 166: 1672-8

Kattan, M.W.; Eastham, J.A.; Stapleton, A.M. y cols.: "A preoperative nomogram for disease recurrence following radical prostatectomy for prostate cancer". J. Natl. Cancer Inst., 90: 766,1 998.

Hodgson D, Warde P, Gospodarowicz M. The management of locally advanced prostate cancer. Urol Oncol 1998;4:3-12.

Fallon B, Williams RD. Current options in the management of clinical stage C prostatic carcinoma. Urol Clin North Am 1990 Nov;17(4):853-66.

Boccon-Gibod L, Bertaccini A, Bono AV, et al. Management of locally advanced prostate cancer: a European Consensus. Int J Clin Pract 2003 Apr;57(3):187-94.

Yamada AH, Lieskovsky G, Petrovich Z, et al. Results of radical prostatectomy and adjuvant therapy in the management of locally advanced, clinical stage TC, prostate cancer. Am J Clin Oncol 1994 Aug;17(4):277-85.

Gerber GS, Thisted RA, Chodak GW, et al. Results of radical prostatectomy in men with locally advanced prostate cancer: multi-institutional pooled analysis. Eur Urol 1997;32(4):385-90.

van den Ouden D, Hop WC, Schroder FH. Progression in and survival of patients with locally advanced prostate cancer (T3) treated with radical prostatectomy as monotherapy. J Urol 1998 Oct;160(4):1392-7.

Isorna Martinez de la Riva S, Belón López-Tomasety J, Marrero Dominguez R, et al. Radical prostatectomy as monotherapy for locally advanced prostate cancer (T3a): 12 years follow-up. Arch Esp Urol 2004 Sep;57(7):679-92.

Ward JF, Slezak JM, Blute ML, et al. Radical prostatectomy for clinically advanced (cT3) prostate cancer since the advent of prostate-specific antigen testing: 15-year outcome. BJU Int 2005 Apr;95(6):751-6.

Hsu CY, Joniau S, Oyen R, et al. Outcome of surgery for clinical unilateral T3a prostate cancer: a single-institution experience. Eur Urol 2007 Jan;51(1):121-8

Allepuz Losa C., Sanz Velez JI., Gil Sanz MJ., Mas LP., Rioja Sanz LA. J Urol 1995;154:1407-11

Van Poppel H, Ameye F, Oyen R, et al. Accuracy of combined computerized tomography and fine needle aspiration cytology in lymph node staging of localized prostatic carcinoma. J Urol 1994 May;151(5):1310-14.

Loeb S, Smith ND, Roehl KA, et al. Intermediate-term potency, continence, and survival outcomes of radical prostatectomy for clinically high-risk or locally advanced prostate cancer. Urology 2007 Jun;69(6):1170-5.

Heidenreich A., Bellmunt J., Bolla M., et al. European Guidelines on prostate cancer. Part 1: Screeing, diagnosis, and treatment of clinically localised disease. Euro Urol 2011; 59: 61-71

Grossfeld GD, Latini DM, Lubeck DP, Broering JM, Li YP, Mehta SS, et al. Predicting disease recurrence in intermediate and high-risk patients undergoing radical prostatectomy using percent positive biopsies: results from CaPSURE. Urology. 2002;59(4):560-565

Rioja Zuazu, J. Gleason Score 8-10 prostatic adenocarcinoma: prognostic influence in the biochemical progression free survival. Actas Urol Esp. 2008;32(8):792-798

Mian BM, Troncoso P, Okihara K, Bhadkamkar V, Johnston D, Reyes AO. Outcome of patients with Gleason score 8 or higher prostate cancer following radical prostatectomy alone. J Urol. 2002;167(4):1675-1680.

Lau WK, Bergstralh EJ, Blute ML, Slezak JM, Zincke H. Radical prostatectomy for pathological Gleason 8 or greater prostate cancer: influence of concomitant pathological variables. J Urol. 2002;167(1): 117-122

Manoharan M, Bird VG, Kim SS, Civantos F, Soloway MS. Outcome after radical prostatectomy with a pretreatment prostate biopsy Gleason score of ≥8. BJU Int. 2003;92(6):539-544.

D'Amico AV, Whittington R, Malkowicz SB, et al. Pretreatment nomogram for prostate-specific antigen recurrence after radical prostatectomy or external-beam radiation therapy for clinically localized prostate cancer. J Clin Oncol 1999 Jan;17(1):168-72

Inman BA, Davies JD, Rangel LJ, et al. Long-term outcomes of radical prostatectomy with multimodal adjuvant therapy in men with a preoperative serum prostate- specific antigen level >or = 50 ng/mL. Cancer 2008 Oct;113(7):1544-51

Hegarty J, Beirne PV, Walsh E, Comber H, Fitzgerald T, Wallace Kazer M. Radical prostatectomy versus watchful waiting for prostate cancer. Cochrane Database Syst Rev. 2010 Nov 10;(11):CD006590.

Thompson IM, Klotz L.Active Surveillance for prostate cancer. JAMA. 2010 Dec 1;304(21):2411-2.

Klotz L, Zhang L, Lam A, Nam R,Mamedov A, Loblaw AClinical results of long-term follow-up of a large, active surveillance cohort with localized prostate cancer. J Clin Oncol. 2010;28(1):126–131.

J.A. Eastham et al. / Urologic Oncology: Seminars and Original Investigations 28 (2010) 557–567).

Eastham JA, Evans CP, Zietman A. What is the optimal management of high risk, clinically localized prostate cancer. Urol Oncol. 2010 Sep-Oct;28(5):557-67.

Thompson I, Thrasher JB, Aus G, et al. Guideline for the management of clinically localized prostate cancer: 2007 update. J Urol 2007;177:2106-2131

Zelefsky MJ, Eastham JA, Cronin AM, et al. Metastasis after radical prostatectomy or external beam radiotherapy for patients with clinically localized prostate cancer: A comparison of clinical cohorts adjusted for case mix. J Clin Oncol 2009.

Walz J, Graefen M, Huland H. Basic principles of anatomy for optimal surgical treatment of prostate cancer. World J Urol 2007;25:31-38.

Kazzazi A, Djavan B. Current status of pelvic lymph node dissection in prostate cancer: the New York PLND nomogram. Can J Urol. 2011 Apr;18(2):5585-91.

Briganti A. et al. Prostate. 2011 May 2. doi: 10.1002/pros.21420.

Bubley GJ, Carducci M, Dahut W, et al. Eligibility and response guidelines for phase II clinical trials in androgen-independent prostate cancer: recommendations from the Prostate-Specific Antigen Working Group. J Clin Oncol 1999 Nov;17(11):3461-7.

Bolla M, van Poppel H, Collette L, et al. Postoperative radiotherapy after radical prostatectomy: a randomised controlled trial (EORTC trial 22911). Lancet 2005;366:572-578.

Thompson IM, Jr., Tangen CM, Paradelo J, et al. Adjuvant radiotherapy for pathologically advanced prostate cancer: a randomized clinical trial. JAMA 2006;296:2329-2335

Stephenson AJ, Scardino PT, Kattan MW, et al. Predicting the outcome of salvage radiation therapy for recurrent prostate cancer after radical prostatectomy. J Clin Oncol 2007;25:2035-2041

Berglund RK, Jones JS, Ulchaker JC, et al. Radical prostatectomy as primary treatment modality for locally advanced prostate cancer: A prospective analysis. Urology 2006;67:1253–6.

Kundu SD, Roehl KA, Eggener SE, et al. Potency, continence and complications in 3,477 consecutive radical retropubic prostatectomies.J Urol 2004;172:2227–31.

Van Poppel H, Vekemans K, Da Pozzo L, et al.: Radical prostatectomy for locally advanced prostate cancer: results of a feasibility study (EORTC 30001). Eur J Cancer 2006, 42:1062–1067.

Yossepowitch O, Eggener SE, Serio AM, et al. Secondary therapy, metastatic progression, and cancerspecific mortality in men with clinically high-risk prostate cancer treated with radical prostatectomy. Eur Urol 2008;53:950-959.

Boorjian S.A. Karnes R.J., Viterbo R., et al. Long-term survival after radical prostatectomy versus external bean radiotherapy for patients with high-risk prostate cancer. Cancer 2011; 117:2883-91

Pound CR, Christens-Barry OW, Gurganus RT, Partin AW, Walsh PC. Digital rectal examination and imaging studies are unnecessary in men with undetectable prostate specific antigen following radical prostatectomy. J Urol. 1999 Oct;162(4):1337-40

Petrovich Z, Lieskovsky G, Langholz B, Bochner B, Formenti S, Streeter O, Skinner DG. Comparison of outcomes of radical prostatectomy with and without adjuvant

pelvic irradiation in patients with pathologic stage C (T3N0) adenocarcinoma of the prostate. Am J Clin Oncol. 1999 Aug;22(4):323-31.
Obek C, Sadek S, Lai S, Civantos F, Rubinowicz D, Soloway MS. Positive surgical margins with radical retropubic prostatectomy: anatomic site-specific pathologic analysis and impact on prognosis. Urology. 1999 Oct;54(4):682-8.
Crook J, Robertson S, Collin G, Zaleski V, Esche B. Clinical relevance of trans-rectal ultrasound, biopsy, and serum prostate-specific antigen following external beam radiotherapy for carcinoma of the prostate. Int J Radiat Oncol Biol Phys. 1993 Sep 1;27(1):31-7.
Goad JR, Chang SJ, Ohori M, Scardino PT. PSA after definitive radiotherapy for clinically localized prostate cancer. Urol Clin North Am. 1993 Nov;20(4):727-36.

6

Radiotherapy in Prostate Cancer

Tatjana Arsenijević, Kata Dabić Stanković,
Miodrag Aćimović and Ljiljana Radošević Jelić
Institute for Oncology and Radiology of Serbia, Institute for Urology,
Serbia

1. Introduction

Therapeutic management of prostate cancer has become complex, multidisciplinary and stage-specific. (Heidenereich et al., 2011) Based on PSA level, histopathological grading and clinical staging, prostate cancer is classified as low-, intermediate- and high risk for disease recurrence. The risk status often plays a major role in deciding further therapy. (Kirby & Madhavan, 2010) It is usually impossible to state that one therapy is superior to another because of the lack of randomized controlled trials. However some recommendations can be made. (Heidenereich et al., 2011, Aus et al. 2001) Based on European Association of Urology recommendations in 2010, patients with low-risk (PSA ≤10 ng/ml, Gleason score <6 and cT1c-cT2a) or intermediate risk prostate cancer (PSA 10.1-20 ng/ml, Gleason score 7 or cT2b-c) are to be treated interdisciplinary with an urologist and a radiation oncologist. Treatment options for these patients vary from watchful waiting and active surveillance to radical prostatectomy or definitive radiotherapy. Multidisciplinary tumor board is needed when discussing neoadjuvant and adjuvant treatment options in high-risk prostate cancer patients (PSA>20ng/ml, Gleason score 8-10 or ≥cT3a) (Heidenereich et al., 2011, Choe & Liauw, 2010).
Radiotherapy is widely used as curative treatment modality for prostate cancer. There is a diverse array of radiotherapeutic strategies that can be effectively used to treat both organ-confined and locally advanced disease, alone or in combination with androgen-deprivation therapy. Furthermore, it has also a significant role in post-prostatectomy setting, as adjuvant or salvage radiotherapy.
In recent decades, radiotherapy in prostate cancer has undergone significant clinical and technological advances that aim to optimize cancer control outcomes while minimizing treatment morbidity. (Choe & Liauw, 2010, Hayden et al., 2010)

2. External-beam radiotherapy in prostate cancer

External-beam radiotherapy has a very long history in the curative treatment of prostate cancer. It is proven and most extensively used radiation modality. As a flexible, noninvasive, outpatient therapy, external-beam radiotherapy can be used in all stages of prostate cancer. (Hayden et al., 2010) It is based on daily delivery of radiation to a target volume using high-energy radiation beams from linear accelerators (or cobalt machines) over a course of 7 to 9 weeks.

In the last 30 years it has undergone a long, improving path from conventional, two-dimensional radiotherapy to intensity-modulated and image-guided radiotherapy and onwards. In low-risk prostate cancer its efficacy appears to be comparable to that of radical prostatectomy but with different toxicities (Choe & Liauw, 2010). For patients not suitable for surgery, external-beam radiotherapy will be the treatment of choice in most cases, alone or combined with androgen-deprivation therapy.

2.1 Conventional radiotherapy

Introducing high-energy radiotherapy machines it become possible to deliver tumoricidal doses to target volume while minimizing damage to the skin and adjacent organs. Historically, various techniques have been used, ranging from parallel anteroposterior-/posteroanterior (AP/PA) portals to lateral portals (box technique) or rotational fields to irradiate or supplement the dose to the prostate. (Chao et al, 2002) Due to the difficulty of localizing the prostate gland, a large volume was treated to ensure proper coverage. More of the surrounding tissues were included in the treated volume so the safely applicable dose was limited to 60-65Gy. (Choe & Liauw, 2010)

The treatment fields for prostate cancer were simulated and designed on plane films and using bony markers with the patient in the supine position. Rectum and bladder were marked by intraluminal injection of iodinated contrast. Small intestine was marked with barium contrast ingested per os one hour prior to simulation.

If the external-beam radiotherapy was applied to the prostate only (local technique), the field size was approximately 8x10 cm for T1 and T2 tumors, 10x12 cm or 12x14 cm for T3 and T4 prostate cancer. Patients younger than 71 years of age with clinical T1c, T2a, and Gleason score more than 7 and PSA 20ng/ml or more, as well as patients with T2b, c T3 and T4 were treated to the whole pelvis with the field size of 15x15 cm, or 15x18 cm to cover the common iliac nodes. The inferior margin of the field usually was 1.5 cm distal to the junction of the prostatic and membranous urethra that is at or caudal to the bottom of the ischial tuberosities. The lateral margins were approximately 1 to 2 cm from the lateral bony pelvis.

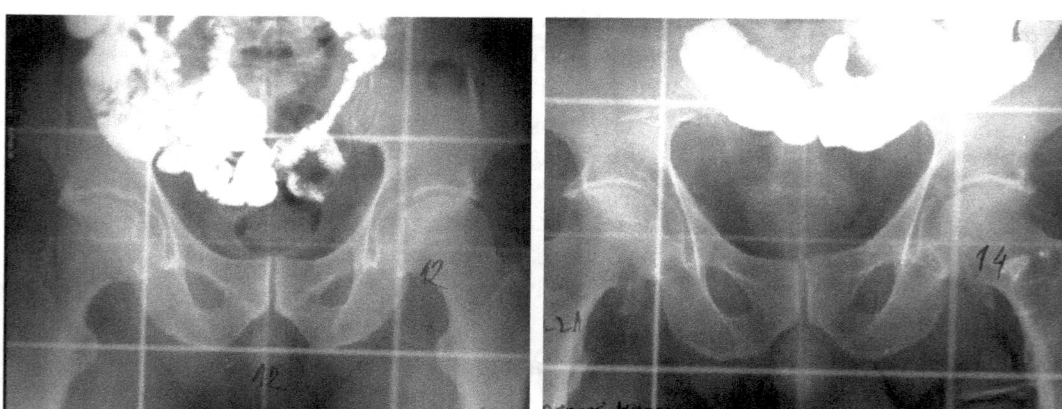

(a) (b)

Fig. 1. Simulation AP radiograph for field verification (a) size 12x12 cm and (b) 14x14 cm Low field border is on the lower border of ishiadic bone and the field centre on the symphisis. Barium contrast in bowels (With thanks to the Institute for oncology and radiology of Serbia, Belgrade)

The initial lateral fields included a volume similar to that treated with AP/PA portals. The anterior margin was 1.5 cm posterior to the projection of the anterior cortex of the pubic symphisis. Posteriorly, the fields included the pelvic and presacral lymph nodes above the S3 segment, which allowed some sparing of posterior rectal wall distal to this level.

Large treated volume was obtained since the average variation of prostate position relative to bony markers was approximately 8 mm in the superior and posterior positions, 7 mm in the inferior, 5 mm in the lateral and 4 mm in anterior position. The seminal vesicles are located high in the pelvis, and posterior to the bladder, which was very critical when reducing treated volume in T3 patients.

When indicated, the periaortic lymph nodes could be treated through extended AP/PA portals or separate periaortic fields placed above the pelvic fields. The superior margin of the periaortic field was at the Th12-L1 vertebral interspace with the width usually above 10 cm (determined by lymphangiogram or CT scan). (Chao et al., 2002, Dobbs et al., 1999)

Conventional external-beam radiotherapy required daily radiation delivery to target volume using high-energy beams (more than 10MV). In most institutions a standard fractionation was used with 1.8 to 2Gy per day. In radical approach, initially a dose of 45-50Gy was applied to the whole pelvis or to the prostate through two parallel opposed fields (AP/PA). Than addition of a boost dose was delivered, up to a total dose of 65-66Gy through lateral opposed fields, two anterior or two posterior oblique fields. (Chao et al., 2002, Dobbs et al., 1999)

2.2 Two-dimensional radiotherapy (2D-RT)

Once a decision is being made to treat prostate cancer with external-beam radiotherapy, the radiotherapy plan is defined either to limit treatment to the gland or to extend treatment field to include the periprostatic tissues, seminal vesicles and pelvic lymph nodes. (Hayden et al. 2010) CT or MRI of the abdomen and pelvis is used to assess the involvement of surrounding structures. MRI is particularly useful for distinguishing capsular invasion, seminal vesicle involvement and periapical extension. CT scanning for treatment planning is performed to every patient, which means that two-dimensional (2D) radiotherapy is a step forward comparing to conventional radiotherapy.

The patient is immobilized in supine position with skin tattoos over the pubic symphisis and laterally over the iliac crests to prevent lateral rotation. CT scans of pelvis are obtained with slice thickness of 4-5 mm. No oral, rectal or intravenous contrast is used. The CT section at the centre of the volume is used as the main planning slice to outline patient contour, target volume, rectum, and bladder. The margins of the target volume are determined by the tumor extent. The gross tumor volume contains entire prostate gland, but if there is a risk of seminal vesicles involvement, they must be included in target volume too. The gross tumor volume is outlined on the central slice only. To allow position variation, an additional margin is added to gross tumor volume (1-1.5 cm in all directions) defining planning target volume (PTV). For two-dimensional planning, PTV is outlined on multiple sections to ensure that the entire tumor is encompassed. The rectal outline must be transposed on to the central section so that the dose can be adequately calculated. Shaping the target volume by shielding blocks or multileaf collimators reduces the dose to normal tissues.

Treatment technique depends on the target volume size and shape. Three-field technique using an anterior and two posterior oblique or opposed lateral fields give a high dose to the prostate but spare the posterior rectal wall. Four-field (box) technique may result in better dose distribution when seminal vesicles are included in target volume, but increases the dose posteriorly.

The patient is than treated daily, 1.8 to 2Gy per fraction, on linear accelerator. The correct position is assured with skin tattoos. The field centre is marked with a tattoo also. All fields are treated isocentrically with shielding as instructed. The recommended dose is 64Gy in 32 fractions given in 6.5 to 7 weeks. (Dobbs et al., 1999)

2.3 Three-dimensional conformal radiotherapy (3D-CRT)

Introducing CT-based radiotherapy simulations by the mid 1980s and multileaf collimator in new aged linear accelerators, it became possible to arrange treatment fields to individually match prostate target volume minimizing high dose exposure to adjacent normal tissues. This led to dose escalation without inducing more toxicity and implementing three-dimensional conformal radiotherapy in clinical practice as a gold standard in prostate cancer radiotherapy treatment. Practically, the aim is to minimize treatment toxicity for patients with more favorable disease, and to maximize locoregional tumor control for those with less favorable disease. (Hayden et al., 2010, Dearnaley, 2001, Gazdda et al., 1996/97)

For 3D-CRT treatment planning a multi-slice CT scan and 3D planning system is used. In order to minimize random and systemic setup error, prior to CT scan, patient should be positioned and immobilized in a fashion that position obtained can be maintained and reproduced. This is secured by the use of alpha cradles, shells or by positioning the patient in supine position with leg restraints. In all this cases a midline and lateral laser lights are used for set up. These markers are tattooed on the skin over the pubic symphisis and laterally over the iliac crests. This is very important for daily positioning of the patient and prevention of lateral rotation. The position is later verified by portal image. (Dobbs et al., 1999, Hayden et al., 2010, Malone et al., 2000)

CT scan of pelvis is performed in a treatment position. Patient should empty the rectum and the bladder should be comfortably full both on the simulation and on the radiation. This standard should be followed because the variation in bladder and rectum distension results in significant prostate displacement. A great controversy still remains regarding prostate apex. MRI of pelvis and CT/MRI fusion is recommended to reduce inter-observer variability in contouring, improving target delineation accuracy, particularly the prostate apex. This fusion is also recommended were significant CT artifact is present i.e. from hip prosthesis.

Once the CT and/or MRI scans are obtained on each slice a target volume and organs at risk are delineated. Organs at risk are adjacent structures endangered by high radiation dose delivered to treated volume. These organs include bladder, rectum, femoral heads and small bowel when it is in the treatment field. (Fiorino et al., 2009)

In 3D-CRT of prostate cancer target volume consists of clinical target volume (CTV) and planning target volume (PTV). CTV includes prostate only, or prostate with seminal vesicles and lymph nodes depending on risk category of the disease. In low-risk prostate cancer, the risk of seminal vesicles involvement is less than 5%, so the CTV should be restricted to prostate only. But, for intermediate risk patients the risk of seminal vesicle involvement is higher (over 15%) hence the proximal third of the seminal vesicles (1 cm) should be included in CTV. For high-risk patients proximal 2 cm of seminal vesicles should be in encompassed with CTV. In cases were seminal vesicle involvement is proven, whole of them should be included in CTV. Any extracapsular extension is also delineated under the CTV, and even a margin of 2-5 mm (excluding rectum) should be considered in high-risk and T3 disease. (Hayden et al., 2010, Koh et al., 2003, Boehmer et al., 2006) According to RTOG guidelines in 2009, pelvic lymph node irradiation may be considered in high-risk patients judged by the treating clinician. The risk of lymph node involvement approaches the risk of distant metastases so the benefit of lymph node irradiation remains controversial. (Lawton et al., 2009)

PTV is a margin added to CTV to reduce the impact of set-up error and organ motion on CTV displacement. PTV also covers inter-observer variability in both delineating of mentioned structures and verification process. According to RTOG recommendation, a PTV is determined by institutional set-up and verification protocol, and measurement of institutional random and systemic errors of prostate position. (Lawton et al., 2009) In many institutions the acceptable CTV-PTV margin ranges from 5 do 10 mm. (Hayden et al., 2010) (Figure 2.)

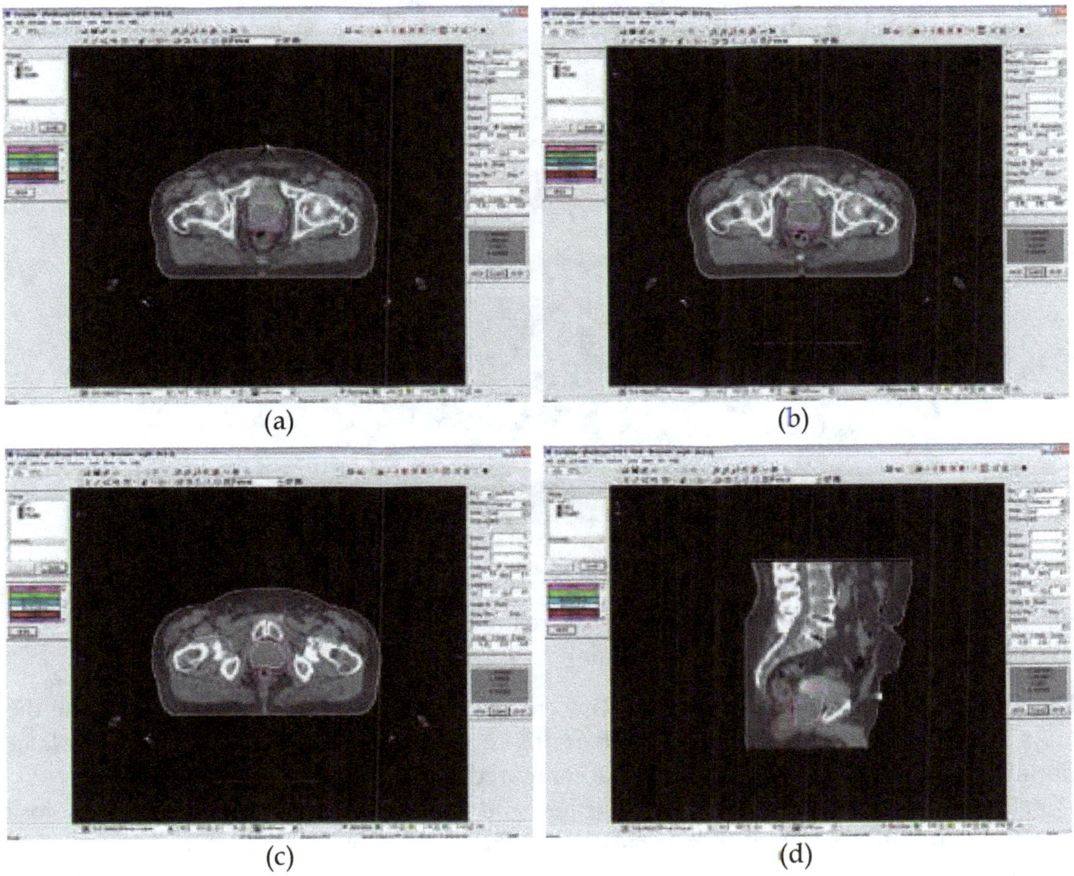

Fig. 2. Delineation of target volume (prostate-pink and seminal vesicles-purple) and organs at risk (bladder-green, rectum-red and femoral heads-light green and dark green) delineation. PTV margin-magenta (a, b, c). Sagital reconstruction (d). (With thanks to the Institute for oncology and radiology of Serbia, Belgrade)

When the delineation process is completed, the medical physicists arrange beam angles and adjust them to maximize target coverage and minimize high-dose exposure to normal organs. (Choe & Liauw, 2010) (Figure 3.)

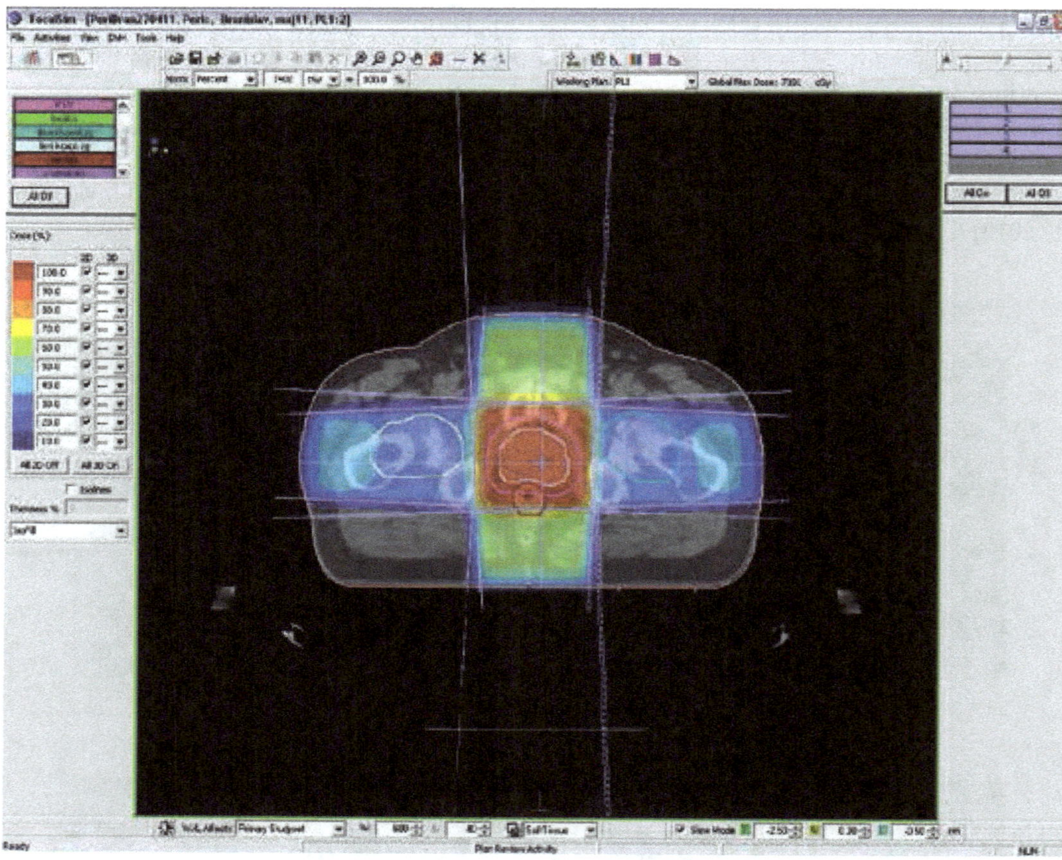

Fig. 3. Field arrangement for four-field (box) treatment (With thanks to the Institute for oncology and radiology of Serbia, Belgrade)

Digitally reconstructed radiograph (DRR) is created by computer program transforming the CT slices into a radiograph image. DRR represents the referent image to which the later portal films of treatment field position are compared. (Figure 4.)

Dose-volume-histogram (DVH) is also created and it shows the percent of prescribed dose to every delineated structure. For organs at risk the ALARA principle (as low as reasonably achievable) is recommended following the tolerant dose of each organ. But, although DVH gives valuable information on the dose to each structure, it is calculated on a single pretreatment pelvic organs position, and they are mobile. That is the reliability on a single pretreatment DVH is limited, and does not have to correlate with late toxicity (Fiorino et al., 2009) (Figure 5.)

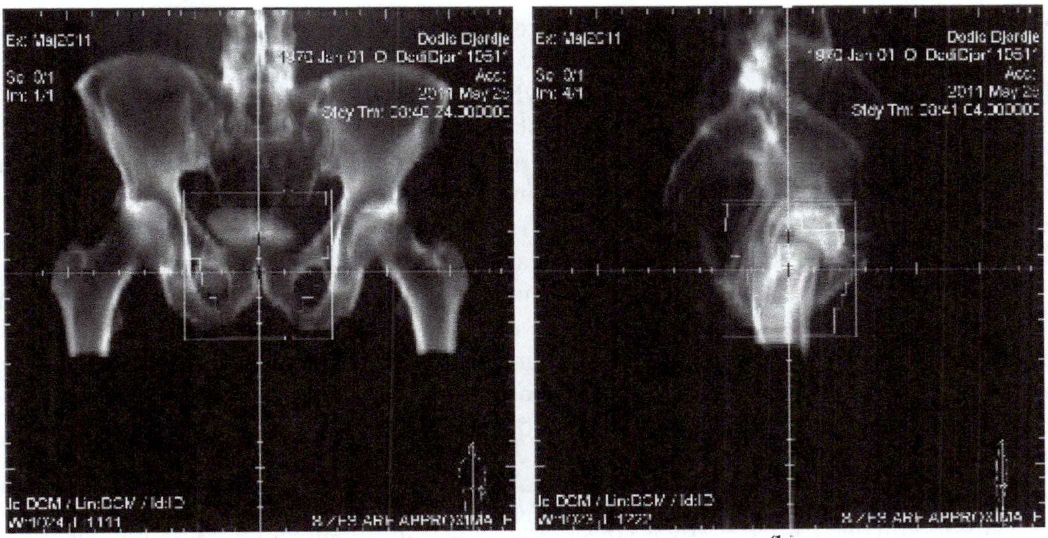

(a) (b)

Fig. 4. Digitaly reconstructed radiographs (DRR) for AP (a) and right lateral (b) field (With thanks to the Institute for oncology and radiology of Serbia, Belgrade)

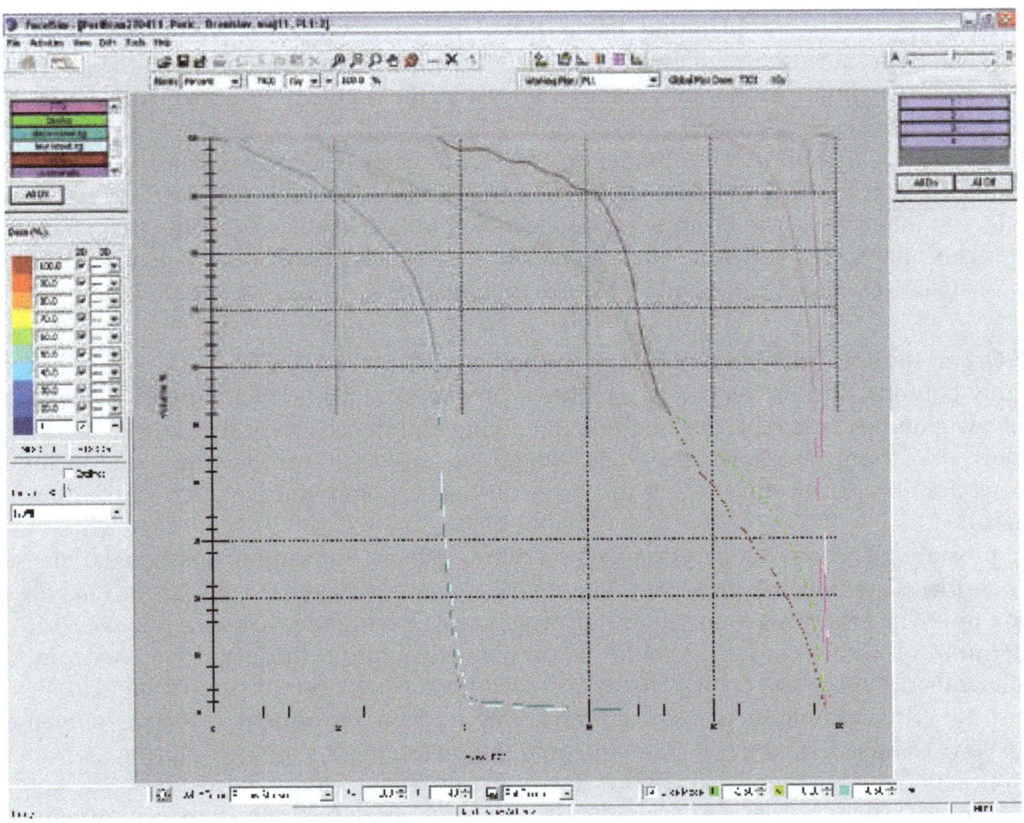

Fig. 5. Dose-volume-histogram (DVH) showing the doses delivered to each delineated structure (With thanks to the Institute for oncology and radiology of Serbia, Belgrade)

According to EAU guidelines in prostate cancer in 2010, for external radiotherapy, a dose of at least 74Gy to PTV is recommended for low-risk prostate cancer because the biochemical disease-free survival is significantly higher when compared to a dose of under 72Gy (69% vs. 63%; P=0.046). For intermediate-risk prostate cancer the dose is ranging from 76Gy to 81Gy, and for high-risk prostate cancer a combination with androgen deprivation is recommended regardless dose escalation since the risk of systemic relapse has to be covered. (Heidenereich et al., 2011)

The patient is treated daily, 1.8 to 2Gy per fraction, on linear accelerator in a position that matches the position taken during CT simulation. The correct position is obtained by immobilizing devices and by setting up the skin tattoo markers to treatment room wall lasers. Once the radiotherapy has started, portal films of arranged fields are taken on the accelerator, in treatment position and compared with digitally reconstructed radiograph (DRR) for set-up or other errors several times during radiotherapy course.

2.4 Intensity-modulated radiotherapy (IMRT)

Intensity-modulated radiotherapy is considered a grate improvement in radiation oncology. It is a form of 3D-CRT in which the optimization of the dose prescribed to the target volume is achieved by x-ray beam intensity changes. By using computer algorithms the intensity of the beam is changed in order to increase the dose difference between the target volume and organs at risk.

Radiotherapy treatment planning using IMRT is based on a CT slices on which the physician delineates target volumes as for the 3D-CRT, as well as organs at risk. For each delineated structure the tolerant dose in imputed in the mathematical algorithms and than the beam intensity is calculated as a function of beam angle. The beam angle is individually adjusted by inclination of the radiotherapy bed, collimator or gentry. (Valicenti et al., 2000)

Unlike 3D-CRT, in IMRT the dose from each beam is not delivered all at once. At each beam angle, the intensity of the beam is modulated by multiple smaller subfields that change in time. This allows a high degree of dose conformity around complex and irregularly shaped tumors (Choe & Liauw, 2010) and dose escalation up to 86Gy. (Zelefsky et al., 2002)

2.5 Organ motion tracking and image-guided radiotherapy (IGRT)

Highly conformal radiation therapy requires precise localization of the prostate. Since the prostate gland is a movable organ due to breathing and distention of rectum and bladder, a variety of strategies have been developed to account prostate motion including transabdominal ultrasound-based imaging, on-line CT and implantation of radiopaque markers.

The prostate gland can not be visualized on portal images, but radiopaque fiducial markers can be placed within the prostate. These markers can be visualized on portal imaging so prior to every treatment a correction of targeting can be made. (Choe & Liauw, 2010) A minimum of three markers should be implanted under ultrasound guidance in the ipsilateral apex, base and contra-lateral mid-gland one week prior to simulation. (Hayden et al., 2010) This technique is used to track interfraction movement (prostate movement between treatments), but it cannot account prostate movement during treatment (intrafractional movement). Nowadays there is a growing interest in real-time tracking of the prostate. There is a special system that uses a real-time tracking of the radiofrequency transponders implanted into the prostate and if they present outside of the predetermined margins the radiation stops.

These new technologies are still under investigation, but first results are optimistic. (Choe & Liauw, 2010) When IGRT is used prostate displacement caused by rectal distension is largely corrected. (Hayden et al., 2010)

2.6 Acute and late toxicity of external-beam radiotherapy in prostate cancer

Radiation-induced complications can be acute and late. Acute adverse events occur during treatment and late may develop months to years after treatment. When we irradiate the prostate, acute and late toxicity are a consequence of high dose given to the surrounding organs i.e. bladder, rectum and skin. The severance of these side-effects largely depends on the tissue volume irradiated and relates to the treatment technique.

During conventional radiotherapy of the prostate acute toxicity include acute proctitis followed by rectal discomfort, tenesmus and diarrhea, and rarely rectal bleeding. It is mostly mild and resolves after symptomatic therapy with hydration and antidiarrheal and anti-inflammatory medication. Skin reactions include erythema, dry and humid desquamation. According to RTOG scale (RTOG, 1999) acute toxicity has four grades of severity stated in table 1.

Grade	0	1	2	3	4
Dermatitis	No complications	Mild erythema or dry desquamation	Moderate erytherma or incipient moist desquamation, mild skid edema	Confluent moist desquamation more than 1.5 cm of the skin, moderate edema	Ulcerations or skin necrosis
Colitis	No complications	Asymptomatic	Abdominal pain, mucus and/or blood in stool	Abdominal pain, fever, peritoneal signs or ileus	Perforation
Diarrhea	No complications	Up to 4 stools per day	4-6 stools per day, night stools	More than 7 stools per day and/or incontinency or parenthеral substitution due to dehydrations	Hemodynamic collapse
Cystitis, dysuria	No complications	Mild dysuria	Moderate dysuria that need symptomatic therapy	Symptoms not relieved on symptomatic therapy	

Table 1. Acute toxicity in radical radiotherapy of prostate cancer-RTOG scale

The most frequent adverse event on the urinary tract is radiation cystitis producing dysuria, nocturia, frequency and urgency. It is low graded in most cases (7.7%) while severe urinary complications are seen in less than 0.5% of patients. According to RTOG study on over 1000 prostate cancer patients treated with external-beam radiotherapy, acute toxicity occurs in 70-90% of the patients with mild symptoms. Moderate symptoms are developed in 20-45% of the patients while 1-4% has severe or prolonged reactions. (Dearnaley, 2001)

Although acute toxicity is very unpleasant for the patient it usually resolves after the treatment. Late toxicity is of much more concern since it is unpredictable and very often irreversible. According to RTOG, late toxicity also has four grades of severity (table 2).

Mostly it is mild and does not influence quality of life, but sever late toxicity is reported in 4-8% of patients. Most common genitourinary side effects are chronic cystitis (5%), incontinency, urethral stricture (5%, mostly patients with previous transurethral resection of the prostate), bladder ulceration and impotency (30-40%). Late toxicity on rectum affects 3% of the patients and includes tenesmus, sphincter dysfunction, occasional bleeding, strictures or ulcerations. (Dearnaley, 2001)

Grade	0	1	2	3	4
Bladder	No complications	Mild epithelia atrophy, discreet teleangiectasia	Diffuse teleangiectasia, macroscopic hemathuria	Frequent urinating, dysuria and hemathuria, bladder capacity less than 150 ml	Bladder necrosis, capacity less than 100 ml, hemorrhagic cystitis
Skin	No complications	Mild skin atrophy, hyperpigment ation, hair loss	Moderate skin atrophy, teleangiectasis, total hair loss	Severe skin atrophy, severe teleangiectasia	Ulceration
Bowels	No complications	Mild diarrhea or increased bowel motion, or mild rectal bleeding	Moderate diarrhea, abdominal pain, rectal mucus or harder bleeding	Ileus or bleeding that requires surgical treatment	Necrosis, perforation, fistula

Table 2. Late toxicity in radical radiotherapy of prostate cancer-RTOG scale

Introducing 3D-CRT and IMRT the volume of bladder and rectum irradiated is limited, but the dose escalation can still induce significant toxicity. In trials of dose escalation, reported rates of acute toxicity are very similar to those of conventional radiotherapy. Late toxicity however is still considered high. MD Anderson trial has shown a significant gastrointestinal toxicity (grade 2 or more) in 25% of patients with escalated dose comparing to 13% in low dose group (78Gy vs. 70Gy). (Kuban et al., 2008) The Dutch trial reported 26% of late rectal toxicity grade 2, and Medical research council 33% in dose escalated group. (Al-Mamgani et al., 2008, Dearnaley et al., 2007) These results compare with reports of IMRT treatment with 81Gy (3% of patients experienced late rectal toxicity at grade 2 or grater) and treatment with IGRT with 79.8Gy (12% of patients with grade 2 rectal toxicity). (Hayden et al. 2010) For urinary toxicity none of these trials found significant correlation between late adverse events and radiation dose. Although improved radiotherapy techniques appear to enable dose escalation with less toxicity, the optimal dose that can eradicate the disease without the risk of toxicity is jet to be defined. (Choe & Liauw, 2010)

2.7 Results of external-beam radiotherapy of prostate cancer

Following external-beam radiotherapy, long-term clinically assessed local tumor control is good for patients with stage T1 cancers (83% at 15 years), but it is falling to 65-68% for T2 and 44-75% for T3 cancers. Reported incidence of positive biopsy after external-beam radiotherapy vary from 18 to 45% and increases with disease bulk from 15% for T1 disease, to 68-79% for men with T2 and T3 cancers. Regarding biochemical control, Hanks et al. reported a long-term biochemical control in 72% of T1 cancers, falling to 22% and 28% for bulky T2 and T3 cancers in a mean follow-up of 12.6 years.

PSA level and Gleason score are powerful predictors of outcome. In patients with low Gleason score the rate of biochemical control ranges about 75%, compared to only 18% for Gleason score 7 and 0% for Gleason score 8 or 9. In patients with pretreatment PSA more than 20 ng/ml only 28% remained biochemically free of progression at 4 years in the results of Hanks et al (Dearnaley, 2001)

Several randomized controlled trials and one meta-analysis shown that improved biochemical outcomes (biochemical failure free survival) are associated with dose escalation. (Kuban et al., 2008, Al-Mmgani et al., 2008, Dearnaley et al., 2007, Zietman et al., 2010, Viani et al., 2009). Radiation Therapy Oncology Group trials have even shown that higher radiation dose improves disease-specific and overall survival in high-grade prostate cancer. (Valicenti et al., 2000) Despite promising results of dose escalation there are still uncertainties regarding routine application of dose escalation especially. The subgroup of patients that will benefit the most from dose escalation is not clearly defined. These trials enrolled men in all risk groups of localized prostate. Only U.K. Medical Research Council trial divided patients in risk groups showing the benefit of dose escalation in all groups. But statistically significance was reached only in high-risk group. In the Dutch trial the benefit from dose escalation from 68 to 78Gy was also registered in intermediate and high-risk patients. These results led to a question whether a higher dose is required for low-risk prostate cancer. Although MD Anderson trial shown the benefit form dose escalation in high-risk group of patients, it also reported longer follow-up of 8.7 years that can indirectly demonstrate a benefit of dose escalation even in the low-risk group. While the improved biochemical outcomes are practically proven with dose escalation, there is still no sufficient evidence of improvement in cancer-specific survival and overall survival. (Choe & Liauw, 2010)

Regarding overall survival, radiotherapy is efficient method for many cases of localized prostate cancer. Five-year overall survival for T1 and T2 stage ranges about 70-80%, and 90% of local tumor control. Locally advanced stages have poorer prognosis with 5-year overall survival of 40-50%. High Gleason score is the most significant negative prognostic marker since it is associated with higher malignant potential. Cancer related death for high Gleason score tumors (8-10) is about 60-80% in 15 years. (Hadzi-Djokic, 2005)

3. Brachytherapy in prostate cancer

In the age of the developed imaging technology (CT, MRI, PET, US), and advanced biochemical markers (tumor-specific and nonspecific), a large number of tumors, including prostate cancer, are being diagnosed in the early stages. In early stages of prostate cancer (T1-T2 N0 M0, PSA <10ng/ml, Gleason Score <6, prostate volume <50ml, maximum urinary flow>15ml/s), in addition to the conventional, laser and robotic prostatectomy, hyperthermia, hormone therapy and brachytherapy is often applied.

In brachytherapy sealed sources of radiation are placed either in direct contact or in proximity of the tumor, so the interstitial brachytherapy for localized prostate cancer often represents the method of choice, and its efficiency is not far behind the effectiveness of surgery, with less morbidity. Brachytherapy allows local application of extremely high doses (up to 160Gy, even more). The effectiveness of prostate cancer brachytherapy is directly correlated with the total dose and precision of administration, which represents its advantage over transcutaneous radiotherapy.

Prostate cancer is usually multicentric, so the brachytherapy target is the entire prostate, and the total dose has to cover the area of about 2-5 mm beyond the prostate capsule. From the point of radiotherapy, particularly brachytherapy, the initial prostate cancer (prostate itself, with or without vesicles involved) represents the ideal target, with adequate spare of the urethra, rectum, bladder and perineal area. Moreover, brachytherapy can be applied within a combined radiotherapy (brachytherapy + transcutaneous radiotherapy) by the additional dose (*boost*), as well as in the case of local recurrence or rest after prostatectomy or transcutaneous radiotherapy.

Brachytherapy for prostate cancer is not a new therapy method, though in the history of medicine it experienced its ups and downs, mainly due to the previous imperfections of visualization techniques and applications, as well as, imperfection in radiation and dosimetric characteristics of the radiation sources, while today it is a routine method of treatment. With the introduction of transrectal ultrasound (TRUS), CT and development of new sources of radiation (^{103}Pd, and ^{192}Ir), techniques of radioisotope implantation (loading and afterloading) and computer systems for brachytherapy planning in routine clinical practice, interstitial brachytherapy for prostate cancer began to experience another upswing, but with markedly better results and lower morbidity.

Today, two modalities for interstitial brachytherapy are applied:

1. **low dose rate (LDR),** about 2Gy/day, with low activity ^{125}I sources (from 0.03 to 1.5GBq per seed, max. photon energy of 35.5 keV, the half-life about 60 days in the form of cylinders /height 4.5 mm, 0.8 mm diameter, encapsuled in titanium sleeve/) or ^{103}Pd (Blasko et al., 2000) (dose rate to about 5Gy/day; activity around 0.07GBq per source, the maximum photon energy of 21 keV, the half-life 17 days in the form of cylinder/ height 4.5 mm, 0.8 mm diameter /or spheres/ diameter of about 1 mm /) - a permanent implant;
2. **(high) dose rate (HDR)** about 0.2 to 3Gy / min with radioactive ^{192}Ir source in the form of cylinder /dimensions around 0.6 x3,5 mm / (initial activity of about 370GBq; time

half-life of 74.2 days, mean photon energy of about 380keV,) - a temporary implantation.

3.1 Low dose rate brachytherapy

Strictly speaking, from the point of view of radiobiology, the only differences (not great) in the indications for applying permanent (LDR) or temporary implantation (HDR) are mostly related to tumor grade. For example, with low-grade and low-risk tumors (eg Stage<T2a, PSA<10, Gleason Score 2-4) and slow-growing tumors, we expect greater efficiency in the application of permanent implants, while with tumors of high grade and higher risk, higher efficiency is expected from temporary implantation. Although there are relative differences in the indications for application of LDR or HDR brachytherapy, it seems that the predominant technique is the one with permanent implants (LDR). Selection of isotopes (^{125}I or ^{103}Pd) is in the favor of the cheaper iodine, so if otherwise not indicated it's considered that radioisotope ^{125}I is being used in LDR brachytherapy for treating prostate cancer. Permanent implants are rarely used in cases of rest or local recurrence after prostatectomy or transcutaneous radiotherapy. In this case a HDR brachytherapy with ^{192}Ir of initial activity over 370 GBq, by using afterloading device, is applied.

Prostate brachytherapy requires a multidisciplinary approach, which assumes collaboration between urologists, radiation oncologists (brachytherapists), anesthesiologists and brachytherapy physicists. Regardless of which brachytherapy modality is implemented in prostate brachytherapy, and with the aim to providing a top quality treatment, all steps are strictly determined:

1. Assessing the stage and spread of the disease (laboratory-biochemical, prostate morphology / palpatory findings, prostate size - US and TRUS /, histopathological verification and determination of Gleason Score, a CT/MRI, scintigraphy, determination of TNM disease stage)
2. Assessing the possibility of applications (talk with the patient, the patient's state, maximum urinary flow rate, the presence of residual urine, previous TUR, assessment of cardiovascular conditions, the possibility of implanting, anatomy of the pelvis, prostate size, type of implant LDR vs. HDR)
3. Preparing the patient prior to implantation - 24 hours in advance (admission of the patient, medical therapy, anti-coagulant and antibiotic, preparation of the patient, rectum cleaning)
4. Preparation of instrumentarium (selection and sterilization of instruments, calibration of stepper, network and TRUS) (Figure 6.)
5. Patient's positioning and anesthesia (in lithotomic position on the movable therapy table; spinal or general anesthesia)
6. Placing markers of critical radiosensitive structures (Folly catheter for marking the bladder and urethra)
7. Setting TRUS probes, template and steper, and prostate visualisation, and visualisation of urethra and rectum (in steps of max. 5 mm from base to apex (Grey et al., 2000), (Figure 7. a, c)
8. Pre-planning (determinatuion of the number and location of radiation sources and methods of implantation)
9. The application (placing the radiation source guides/needles; in the LDR technique inserting a radiation source - seeds) - TRUS-guided (Figure 8. b)

10. Verification and correction (cistoscopic, fluoroscopic, x-ray (Figure 7. c) - optional CT and/or MRI; in case of LDR brachytherapy adding of seeds, if necessary)
11. Computer reconstruction (seeds / LDR / - needles / HDR /, prostate capsule, the position of the urethra and rectum), optimization, plan analysis (the determination of DVH - Dose Volume Histogram, ie. minimum volume of prostate receiving 90%, 100%, 150% and 200% of the total dose, and the dose and volumes that receive critical radiosensitive structures), (Figure 7. d, e);
12. Irradiation; for HDR brachytherapy: deapplication of needles or observation of the patient (LDR)
13. Transport of patient to the patient room
14. Patient care (analgesic and antibiotics therapy, toilet)
15. Check-up (of dysuric problems and estimate the degree of proctitis) and discussion with the patient, the patient's discharge
16. Regular checks (during treatment /HDR/ and in 2, 3, 6, 12 and 18 months, then annually - the level of PSA, rectal examination, assessing the level of dysuric problems and evaluation of potency)

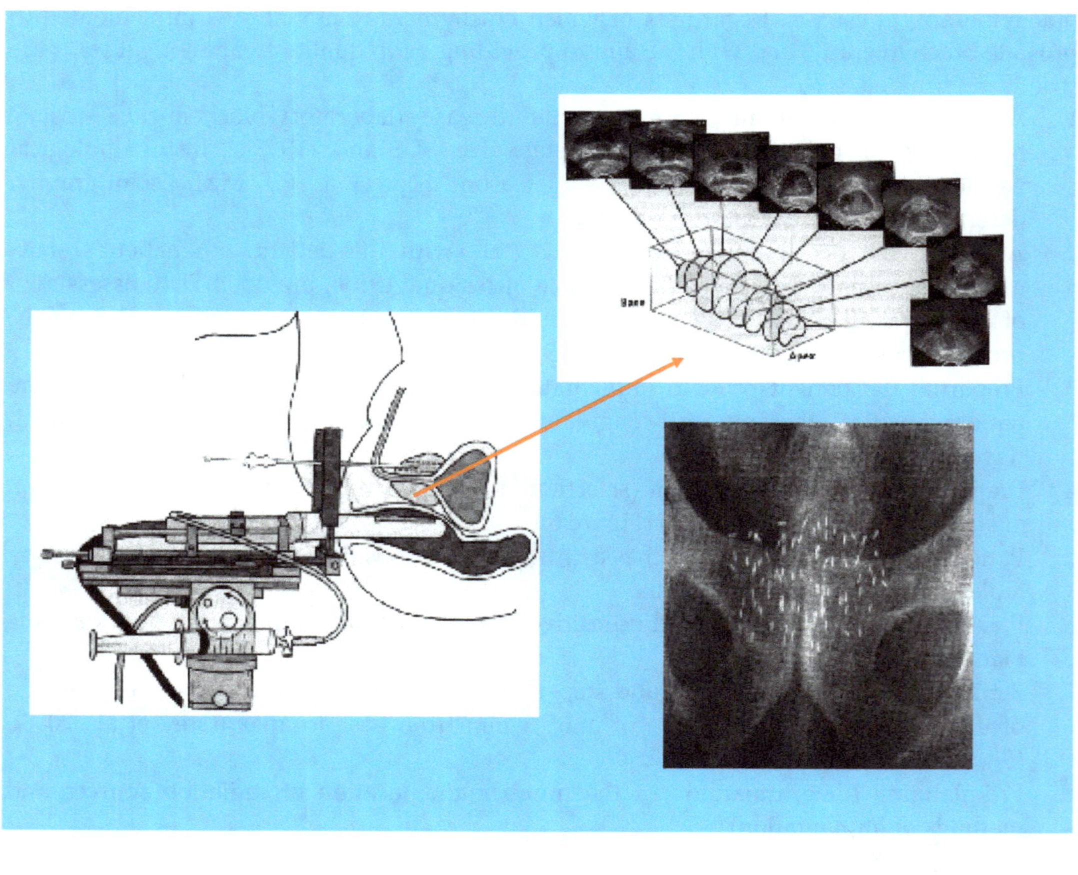

Fig. 6. Schematic representation of TRUS-guided brachytherapy with radioactive seeds.

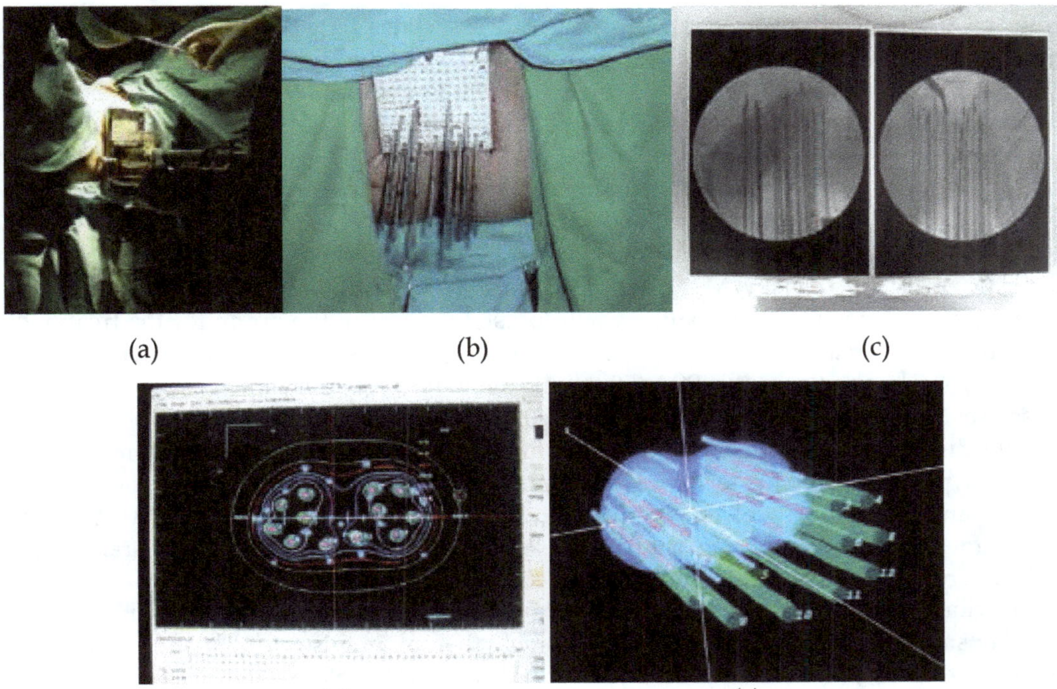

(a) (b) (c)

(d) (e)

(a) TRUS guided needles application
(b) Administrated needles / guides of ^{192}Ir source
(c) Radiographic verification of the needles' positions
(d) Isodose transversal view
(e) 3D treatment volume
(With the thanks of the General Hospital Medical System, Belgrade)

Fig. 7. Steps in HDR prostate cancer brachytherapy - real patient

When using permanent implantation (monotherapy) radiation sources (seeds) remain in the prostate of the patient. It is therefore recommended to the patient a minimal two-week sexual abstinence and avoidance of contact with pregnant women and small children for a minimum of 2 months. A typical therapeutic dose of radiation, when ^{125}I is implanted, is in the range 140-160Gy, and when ^{103}Pd is implanted to about 125Gy. In a case of a "boost" dose, for ^{125}I a somewhat lower dose of 80-120 is applied or to about 90-100Gy for ^{103}Pd. (Blasko et al., 2000, Beyer, 2001)

3.1.1 Results of low dose rate brachytherapy

Prostate cancer with its characteristics and different biological behavior represents a problem in the analysis of brachytherapy final outcomes in terms of overall survival or local control. We are aware that many patients with untreated prostate cancer can survive tens of years, ie. do not die from prostate cancer. Therefore to evaluate the effectiveness of treatment of patients with prostate cancer, as for overall survival and local control, the PSA level was adopted.

Greem and associates (Greem et al., 1997)provide representation of the results of treatment of patients with permanent implants (monotherapy), showing a five-year survival of NED (no evidence of disease) of 94%, 84% and 54% for low risk, medium risk and higher risk group of 403 patients, respectively . Blasko and associates (Blasko et al, 2000) show the results of a five-year biochemical PSA control: 94%, 82% and 65% for low risk, medium risk and higher risk respectively. Slightly worse, but comparable results are displayed by other authors: 85-94%, 33-82% and 5-65% for low risk, medium risk and high-risk group, respectively (Beyer, 2001). Based on these results, most urologists and brachytherapists exclude a group of patients at high risk from the LDR brachytherapy and consider them patients with advanced disease in which the tumor penetrated the prostate capsule. Association of American Brachytherapy Society has established a Low Dose-Rate Task Group (Merrick, G., Zelefsky, M., Sylvester, E., Nag, S., Bice, W) with the task of defining the general criteria for inclusion of patients with prostate cancer in the group for the treatment by permanent implants (LDR): expected survival > 5 years, clinical stage T1b-T2c and selected T3, Gleason Score<10, PSA<50ng/ml, without involved lymph nodes, no distant metastases, Karnofsky performance status> 70%. Criteria for exclusion are: inflammatory prostate disease, severe urinary obstruction, the middle lobe hyperplasia, extensive TUR defects, a prostate size greater than 60x50 mm, the extension of disease to the seminal vesicles and bladder, involved lymph nodes, previously conducted EBRT. Absolute contraindications are distant metastatic disease, the inability of anesthesia (general, spinal, epidural), no possibility of peaceful lying, expected survival <5 years.

It is obvious that the consistent application of these criteria for inclusion and exclusion would ensure consistent application of LDR brachytherapy in this roup of patients, with the results of treatment (five-and even ten-year PSA control NED> 85%).

3.1.2 Toxicity of low dose rate brachtherapy

Mild and transient acute urinary symptoms (LENT SOMA, 1995) (hematuria and dysuria grade G1-G2) often accompany LDR brachytherapy, while the acute symptoms on the rectum (proctitis, tenesms and bleeding) are rare and mainly a result of edema and hematoma. All of the symptoms can be associated to radiation or trauma during the application procedure.

As late symptoms of bladder neck irradiation, chronic irritative urinary symptoms may occur and in a small number of cases due to urethral scarring, obstruction or incontinence may occur. Late effects on the rectum are mild, and manifested by periodic bleeding and proctitis. Erectile function was preserved for over 70% of treated patients whose erectile function was satisfactory before the implementation of brachytherapy. In order to preserve erectile function, it is important to avoid positioning of seeds in the perineal area, outside the prostate apex, which prevents the occurrence of fibrosis and consequent devascuralisation of this region. Most patients (over 2/3) treated with permanent implants, estimate their quality of life as good, which is just as important as biochemical and clinical course of disease.

However, due to the relatively limited fixation of radioactive seeds (which are smooth on the surface) there is a possibility of their inter-prostate migration and the creation of "hot" and "cold" zones, as well as, their migration to other organs (rectum, bladder and pelvic veins and even lungs), which sometimes requires serious surgical treatment and drastically reduces the quality of patient's life.

3.2 High dose rate brachytherapy

HDR temporary prostate cancer brachytherapy with ^{192}Ir entered into clinical practice mainly in combination with transcutaneous radiotherapy about 20 years ago. Obviously, it was necessary to acquire certain technical and technological advances for its application

Soon, the advantages of HDR regime compared to LDR brachytherapy of prostate cancer were noticed, which are reflected in: the high precision of application, the possibility of subsequent dose optimization, more accurate dose planning and application, sparing the surrounding tissues and organs, more favorable radiobiological effect, the fact that after treatment there are no sources of radiation in the patient and therefore no possibility of source "seeds" migration into the bladder, rectum or surrounding larger blood vessels, there is no irradiation of staff, there is the possibility of extending indicational scope of application and easier possibility of combination with transcutaneous radiotherapy. However, when it comes to temporary HDR brachytherapy of prostate cancer as monotherapy, less obvious results and experiences are presented in the literature, so one can get the wrong impression that this modality of brachytherapy is either less efficient or at very least, least mystified. To clarify this problem to an extent, if not totally resolve, the association of American Brachytherapy Society has formed a High-Dose Rate Task Group (Hsu, C., Yamada, Y., Vigneaut, E., Pouliout, J.) with the aim to define general criteria for inclusion of patients with prostate cancer in the treatment group Temporary implants (HDR), which was formed following the general criteria for inclusion: clinical stageT1-T3 and selected T4, Gleason Score any, PSA no upper limit, no distant metastases (T1-3N0M0). Criteria for relative exclusion are: severe urinary obstruction, extensive TUR defects, the TUR within 6 months, vascular disease. Absolute contraindications are impossibility to anesthesia and no possibility of peaceful lying

Given all the above-mentioned recommendations, for inclusion and exclusion, and in particular those given by the American Brachytherapy Society, extended operational criteria and opinions can be formed related to the application of HDR brachytherapy in different patient groups, including recommendations on the total dose and method of its fractions, and as:

- monotherapy - with tumor stage T1-T2 N0 M0, Gleason Score <7 and prostate volume to 70 cc and T3 confined to the prostate (TD - 31.5 Gy/3 fr. To TD45/6 hypofractioned (Duchesne & Peters, 1999) or hyperfractioned / pause between the fraction of at least 6 hours or even up to 54Gy/9 fr./5 days (Yoshioka et al., 2006) (where the stage T3 N0 M0 may include seminal vessicles);
- boost in the combined radiotherapy approach (TD - 12 (Mate et al., 1998) -24 (Demanes et al., 2009) Gy/1-4 fr. EBRT ± 36-50Gy or 9-15Gy/1-2 fr. EBRT ± 65Gy);
- for recurrent disease confined to the prostate (depending on the previousl therapy TD> Gy/1-2 7-14 fr. to 8Gy/4 fr.)
- further: to have no contraindications (no indication for exclusion).

3.2.1 Results of high dose rate brachytherapy

Yoshioka et al (Yoshioka et al., 2006) presented the results of 111 patients (15 low, 28 medium and 68 high risk, according to the ASTRO criteria (ASTRO, 1997) treated with HDR temporary implantation (monotherapy), showing a three-year and five-year survival without signs of biochemical disease of 83% and 70%, and overall survival of 100% and 97%, respectively. For the 17 patients from high risk groups, in which biochemical relapse was observed, in 9 patients the presence of distant metastases were confirmed, of which 4 patients died. Given that this group of patients is not stratified based on risk, it is clear that the shown results after the HDR brachytherapy are comparable or even better than in patients treated with permanent implants (monotherapy) (Blaskc et al., 2000, Beyer, 2001, Greem et al., 1997).

3.2.2 Toxicity of high dose rate brachytherapy

Mild and transient acute urinary symptoms (dysuria and hematuria of grade G1) followed HDR brachytherapy in about 50% of patients in the first week or two, and persist for up to 6 months in less than 35% of treated patients, while grade G2 symptoms occurred in about 11 % of patients in the first weeks after treatment and after 6 months they completely disappeared. Pronounced symptoms of grade G3 (urethral stricture at the level of bladder base) are very rare (less than 2%), and they require a retention of urinary catheter, and usually occur immediately after irradiation, and disappear within ten days. Acute symptoms of grade G1 rectum (proctitis, tenesma and bleeding) are rare and mainly are result of edema and hematoma, and occur in less than 25% of patients in the first weeks and decrease to about 8% in the 6-month after conducted therapy. Acute complications of grade G3 were not observed.

All listed acute symptoms may be connected to radiation and trauma during application procedure, although problems have not been noted during the application itself.

The frequency and severity of late complications after HDR brachytherapy is similar to the permanent implant brachytherapy (LDR), except that complications associated with the migration of radiation sources do not occur.

When HDR brachytherapy (22-24 Gy/5-6 fr.) is applied in combination with transcutaneous radiotherapy (EBRT to 40Gy), the results of treatment (five-year survival NED/biochemical/and overall survival) of 63% in patients with high risk are comparable and slightly better than with the application of brachytherapy (LDR and HDR) as a monotherapy. (Deamens et al., 2009) In the same paper, the authors conclude that no benefit was noted when applying deprivate androgen therapy in relation to combined radiotherapy.

Acute and late effects on the bladder and rectum are more pronounced in cases of combined radiotherapy, which can be expected.

4. Postoperative radiotherapy in prostate cancer

Radical prostatectomy is proven treatment modality for prostate cancer control for a long time. Some authors report 10-year cancer-specific survival of 85-90% in localized prostate cancer after radical prostatectomy, and 82% at 15 years. Survival is better if the tumor is low grade i.e. low Gleason score and low stage.

The risk of surgical margins positivity is of great concern after radical prostatectomy. Positive margins are noticed in 28% of patients with T1-T2 prostate cancer and prostate apex is the most common site. For T3 cancers this percent is even higher-up to 52%.

High tumor stage (T3a and T3b) and a positive surgical margin are strong predictors of local recurrence, biochemical and clinical failure. In general, it is considered that the percent of local recurrence after radical prostatectomy ranges about 15% for T2 prostate cancers, and 50-70% for T3 tumors.

In order to analyze the impact of predictive factors on development of local recurrence, univariate and multivariate analyzes were performed. In univariate analyzes strong predictors of local relapse are high-grade cancer, positive surgical margins and involvement of seminal vesicles. In multivariate analyzes these predictors are high-grade tumor, positive surgical margin and elevate prostatic phosphatase.

Identification of patients that are candidates for adjuvant therapies after radical prostatectomy is still a great issue. The adequate treatment modality for these patients is an open question too. There is no consensus yet.

After radical prostatectomy, the application of radiotherapy can lower the incidence of local relapses, but its effect on distant metastases appearance is not confirmed. Alternative regimen is the use of androgen-deprivation therapy alone or in combination with radiotherapy which can also improve local control and eradication of distant metastases. (Hadzi-Djokic, 2005)

Three randomized trials (Bolla, Wiegel & Thompson), have shown an advantage in biochemical relapse-free survival with postoperative radiotherapy for men with positive surgical margins or pT3 disease. These trials compared postoperative radiotherapy with 60-Gy to the prostatic fossa to radical prostatectomy alone in men with high-risk prostate cancer. With the use of postoperative irradiation the 5-year biochemical progression-free survival was significantly improved, as well as clinical progression-free survival. Thompson's trial has also show an advantage of overall survival (10.3 years for irradiated patients after prostatectomy to 3.1 year for prostatectomy only). Bolla failed to demonstrate this advantage. That means that not all men with adverse prognostic factors will relapse. Also, not all men treated with postoperative radiotherapy will be cured. Combined treatment is also associated with greater toxicity than radiotherapy or prostatectomy alone. So what will the optimal treatment be? (Hayden et al., 2010, Bolla et al., 2005, Wiegel et al., 2009, Thompson et al., 2009) Eastham et al. managed to give actually 4 possible scenarios for post-prostatectomy setting: (1) there is no residual disease and adjuvant radiation is not necessary; (2) persistent disease is present in the prostatic fossa only and adjuvant irradiation may provide long-term cure; (3) there is a residual local disease as well as microscopic disseminated disease and adjuvant irradiation may eradicate local disease but will have no impact on the systemic component; (4) disease is only systemic and adjuvant local irradiation is not necessary.

Salvage radiotherapy in the setting of a rising PSA after prostatectomy is unproven and still controversial. This is most likely the result of inadequately selected patients for post-prostatectomy irradiation. Many of them already have systemic recurrence so a detail diagnostic workout is necessary. (Eastham et al., 2010)

The special issue is the use of adjuvant hormone therapy. Some studies show that the application of adjuvant hormone therapy reduces the risk of positive surgical margins, improves local disease control, eradicates micro metastases and prolongs time to progression and overall survival. On the other hand, neoadjuvant hormone therapy, prior to surgery, in order to downstage the disease, has not been proven for successes neither in preventing biochemical or clinical relapse nor in improving survival so in most centres it is deserted. (Dearnaley, 2005)

5. Androgen-derprivation therapy combined with radiotherapy of the prostate cancer

Radiotherapy is traditionally the treatment of choice in locally advanced prostate cancer. Unfortunately the results of radical radiotherapy regarding 10-years and 15-years overall survivals are not satisfactory (Zlotecki, 2001) (Table 3.)

Androgen deprivation therapy is used routinely in combination with radiotherapy for locally advanced prostate cancer, but recent studies show that it improves treatment result is localized and intermediate-risk disease.(Milecki et al., 2010).

Hormone therapy, that is in fact androgen deprivation, can be realized in several ways: orchyectomy, blockade of the hypothalamus-hypophysis-gonade path (with gonadothropin realizing hormone agonist) or by direct blockade of androgen receptors with androgen antagonists. (Anderson, 2003) Although, it is generally thought that androgen deprivation combined with radiotherapy influence the results of treatment in local and systemic way, it is uncertain whether that action is the result of radiosensitizing, systemic micro metastases eradication or both. Androgen deprivation leads to the shrinkage of the entire prostate gland reducing the irradiated volume to which the higher dose can be applied. In several studies this prostate shrinkage is ranging form 30% to 40%. Some authors say that it improves radiotherapy effectiveness by oxygenation of hypoxic cancer cells and that it even induces apoptosis and tumoricidal immune system response.

Study/Institution	Clinical T stage	10 Year Survival (%)	15 Year Survival (%)
Pattern of Care	T3-T4	33	23
RTOG 75-06	T3-T4	38	No results
Mallinckrodt	T3	38	No results
Stanford	T3	35	18
Stanford	T4	15	15
M.D. Anderson	T3	45	31

Table 3. 10 and 15-year survival rate for patients with locally advanced prostate cancer treated with radical RT

The role of androgen deprivation therapy is unclear in men with low risk prostate cancer but some patients still received it as primary or neoadjuvant treatment. The Radiation Therapy Oncology Group (RTOG) 94-08 randomized trial included almost 2000 men with T1b-T2 prostate cancer and PSA less than 20ng/ml. Androgen deprivation therapy was administered 4 months prior or concomitantly with radiotherapy. Overall survival at 8 years was 76% vs. 73% for combined treatment and radiotherapy only, respectively. The disease-specific survival was 98% for hormone and irradiation vs. 99% for radiotherapy alone. This study did not bring solid results, as well as many others, because some patients were clinically in a higher risk stage than deemed low risk according to National Comprehensive Network classification. Retrospective studies of Bolla et al. and Cietzki at al. are among few that have shown the advantage of radiotherapy combine with androgen-deprivation in low risk prostate cancer (Milecki et al., 2010)

For intermediate and high-risk patients many randomized studies were performed such as RTOG 85-31 (977 patients T1-T2, T3, N+, adjuvant hormone therapy vs. radiotherapy alone), RTOG 86-10 (456 patients, T2-T4, neoadjuvant/concomitant hormone therapy for 4 months vs. radiotherapy alone), EORTC 22863 (415 patients, T1-T4 prostate cancer, concomitant/adjuvant hormone therapy for 36 months vs. radiotherapy alone). In 5-years follow-up all of them have shown a statistically significant difference in improved local disease control, reduction of distant metastases and longer progression free survival in hormone therapy-radiotherapy group. (Jelić et al., 2005) (Table 4.)

	N	Stage	Therapy	Therapy duration	Local control	PFS (%)	OS (%)	Follow-up
RTOG 85-31	977	T1-T2, N+,T3	Adj vs. only RT	>24m vs. 0	+	53 vs. 20 $p<0.0001$	Gs 8-10 66 vs. 55 $p=0.03$	5 years
RTOG 86-10	456	T2-T4	Neoadj/conc vs. only RT	4m vs. 0	+	33 vs. 21 $p=0.004$	Gs 2-6 70 vs. 52 $p=0.015$	5 years
EORTC 22863	415	T1-T4	conc/adj vs. only RT	36m vs. 0	+	85 vs. 48 $p<0.001$	79 vs. 62 $p=0.01$	5 years
RTOG 92-02	1554	T2c-T4	Neoadj/conc /adj vs. Neoadj/conc	28m vs. 0	+	46.4 vs. 28.1 $p<0.001$	Gs 8-10 81 vs. 70.7 $p=0.044$	5 years
RTOG 94-13	1323	T1c-T4	Neoadj vs. adj	4m vs. 4m	+	NA	NA	4 years

Table 4. Hormone therapy and RT. Randomized studies

Bolla M. recommends concomitant and adjuvant hormone therapy for three years in combination with radiotherapy for patients with locally advanced, intermediate or high-risk prostate cancer. (Bolla, 2003)

Although it is shown that androgen deprivation before, concomitantly and/or after radiotherapy significantly improves local disease control, minimizes progression and prolongs overall survival in locally advanced prostate cancer on intermediate and high-risk, there is not enough evidence for recommendation of optimal time to start hormone therapy, the type of hormones and the duration of the treatment which in clinical trials lasts from 3 months to 3 years. (ESMO, 2003)

6. Radiotherapy in metastatic prostate cancer

For patients in which prostate cancer develops quickly with bony and/or other metastases and elevation of PSA, androgen deprivation is considered a therapeutic method of choice. It includes orchyectomy or TAB. Radiotherapy is considered only as palliative for painful bony metastases or threatening pathological fracture.

Radiotherapy of bony metastases is mostly performed as local therapy to involved bones but sometimes it can be applied as half-body or total-body irradiation. For solitary or localized bony metastases radiotherapy is applied through simple fields (two opposed fields, single direct field etc). A higher daily dose of 2.5 Gy or 3 Gy is given. Single dose of 8 Gy (single shoot), 20 Gy in 5 fractions or 30Gy in 10 fractions are considered to have the same results regarding pain relief and survival.

Half-body irradiation is performed when there are many disseminated bony metastases and probably as many occult. The dose of 8 Gy is applied to lower half, and 6 Gy to upper half of the body. If we treat the whole body, the gap between irradiation of upper and lower half of the body is four weeks. (Samija et al., 1996)

On the other hand, for patients with extensive locoregional prostate cancer, radiotherapy can be applied to pelvis with a total dose of 50-60Gy in order to reduce pain, hemathuria, urethral obstruction or lymphedema (Jelić, 2005)

7. New radiation techniques

The biological effect of ionizing radiation to cancer cells and normal tissues it based on the fact that the cancer cells are more susceptible to radiation because the lack of normal repair mechanism. Hypofractionated radiotherapy can reduce the duration of treatment since larger dose is given per day and the cumulative dose is adjusted to a lower dose. The randomized trials that compared hypofractionation with conventional RT did not have long enough follow-up and used to low total dose for current standards. But the investigation is still on. The extreme form of hypofractionation is stereotactic body radiotherapy (radiosurgery). This method uses only few fractions but with very high doses applied to a target volume in a very precise fashion. Although these techniques are attractive for theoretical advantage in radiobiology, the risk of late toxicity is considerable.

Another possible radiotherapy approach to enhance radiotherapeutic ratio for prostate cancer is to utilize charged particles such as protons and carbon ions. The clinical benefit is still unclear but the optimism is based upon the fact that charged particles deposit most of their energy at a given depth followed by a dose fall-of with almost no dose deposition beyond the point of maximal dose called Bragg peak which can lead to increased normal tissue sparing. For proton therapy, a dosimetric analysis did not show a significant improvement in conformity to spare normal tissues over photon IMRT. Clinical outcome and toxicity is also similar. Carbon ion has the same dose distribution as proton beams with Bragg peak and following dose fall-of. But the relative biological effectiveness of carbon ion is four times higher than protons and photons that can lead to improved local tumor control without causing more toxicity. However these technologies are still developing and results are yet to be seen. (Choe & Liauw, 2010)

8. Conclusion

Radiotherapy is widely used as curative treatment modality for many cases of prostate cancer. There is a diverse array of radiotherapeutic strategies that can be effectively used to treat both organ-confined and locally advanced disease, alone or in combination with androgen-deprivation therapy. In recent decades it has undergone significant clinical and technological advances that aim to optimize cancer control outcomes while minimizing treatment morbidity.

9. References

Al-Mamgani, A., Van Putten, WL., Heemsbergen, WD. et al. (2008). Update of Dutch multicenter dose-escalation trial of radiotherapy for localized prostate cancer. *International Journal of Radiation Oncology Biology Physics*, vol 72, pp. (980-988)

American Society for Theapeutic Radiology and Oncology Consensus Panel, Consensus statement: Guidelines for PSA following radiation therapy. (1997). *International Journal of Radiation Oncology Biology Physics*, vol. 37, pp. (1035-1041)

Anderson, J. (2003). Treatment of Prostate Cancer. The Role of Primary Hormonal Therapy. *EAU Update Series*, vol. 1, pp. (32-39)

Aus, G., Abbou, C., Bolla, M. et al. (2001). Guidelines on prostate cancer. *European Urology*, vol. 40, no. 2, pp. (97-101)

Beyer, D. (2001). The evolving role of prostate brachytherapy. *Cancer Control*, vol. 8, pp. (163-170)

Blasko, J., Grimm, D., Sylvester, E. et al. (2000). Paladium 103 brachytherapy for prostate carcinoma. *International Journal of Radiation Oncology Biology Physics*, vol. 46, pp. (839-850)

Blasko, J., Grimm, D., Sylvester, E. et al. (2000). The role of external beam radiotherapy with I-125/Pd-103 brachytherapy for prostate carcinoma. *Radiotherapy and Oncology*, vol. 57, pp. (273-278)

Boehmer, D., Maingon, P., Poortman, P. et al. (2006). Guidelines for primary radiotherapy of patients with prostate cancer. *Radiotherapy and Oncology*, vol. 79, pp. (259-269)

Bolla, M. (2003). Treatment of Locally Advanced Prostate Cancer. The Clinical Use of Radiotherapy. *EAU Update Series*, vol. 1, pp. (23-31)

Bolla, M., van Poppel, H., Collette, L. et al. (2005). Postoperative radiotherapy after radical prostatectomy: a randomized controlled trial (EORTC trial 22911). *Lancet*, vol. 366, pp. (572-578)

Chao, KSC., Perez, C., & Brady, LW. (2002). Prostate, In: *Radiation oncology management decision*, pp. (447-467), Lippincot-Williams&Wilkins, ISBN 0-7817-3222-0, Philadelphia

Choe, KS., & Liauw, SL. (2010). Radiotherapeutic strategies in the management of low-risk prostate cancer. *The Scientific World JOURNAL: TSW* Urology, vol. 10, pp. (1854-1869)

Common Toxicity Criteria Version 2.0, DCTD, NCI, NIH, DHHS. (1999). Cancer Therapy Graduation Programme. RTOG: Late radiation morbidity scoring system.

Deamens, J., Brandt, D., Schour, L. et al. (2009). Excellent results from high dose rate brachytherapy and external beam for prostate cancer are not improved by androgen deprivation. *American Journal of Clinical Oncology*, vol. 32, pp. (342-347)

Dearnaley, DP., (2001). Radiotherapy and combined modality approaches in localized prostate cancer. *Prostate Cancer. Educational Book. ECCO 11*, pp. (137-140), Lisbon

Dearnaley, DP., (2005). Radiotherapy in locally advanced prostate cancer. *EJC Education Book. ECCO 13*, pp. (317-330), Paris

Dearnaley, DP., Sydes, MR., Graham, JD. et al. (2007). Escalated-dose versus standard-dose conformal radiotherapy in prostate cancer: first results from MRC RT01 randomized controlled trial. *Lancet Oncology*, vol. 8, pp. (475-487)

Dobbs, J., Barrett, A., & Ash, D., (1999). Prostate, In: *Practical radiotherapy planning*, pp. (271-280), Arnold, ISBN 0-340-70-631-7, Great Britain

Duchesne, G., & Peters, L. (1999). What is the alpha/beta ratio for prostate cancer? Rationale for hypofractionated high-dose-rate brachytherapy. *International Journal of Radiation Oncology Biology Physics*, vol. 44, pp. (747-748)

Eastham, JA., Chirstopher, PE., & Zietman, A. (2010). What is the optimal management of high risk, clinically localized prostate cancer? *Urologic Oncology*, vol. 28, pp. (557-567)

ESMO Minimum Clinical Recommendations for Diagnosis, Treatment and Follow up of Prostate Cancer. (2003). *Annals of Oncology*, vol. 14, pp. (1010-1011)

Fiorino, C., Valdagni, R., Rancati, T. et al. (2009). Dose-volume effects for normal tissues in external radiotherapy: pelvis. *Radiotherapy and Oncology*, vol. 93, pp. (153-167)

Gazdda, MJ., Lawrence, R., & Coia, MD. (1996/97). *Radiation treatment planning and techniques. Cancer Management: A Multidisciplinary Approach. Medical, Surgical & Radiation Oncology*, pp. (593-604), Huntington, New York

Greem, P., Blasko, J., Ragde, H. et al. (1997). Transperineal ultrosund guided 1251/103Pd brachytherapy for early stage prostate cancer: Update on clinical experience at seven years. *International Journal of Radiation Oncology Biology Physics*, vol. 39, pp. (219)

Grey, J., Merricks, S., Beyer, D. et al. (2000). Comparartive analysis of prostate brachytherapy pre-planing. *Radiotherapy and Oncology*, vol. 55, pp. (42-43)

Hadži-Đokić, J. (2005). *Lokalizovani karcinom prostate*, Elit. Medica, Beograd

Hayden, AJ., Catton, C., & Pickles, T. (2010). Radiotherapy in prostate cancer: a risk risk-adapted strategy. *Urologic Oncology*, vol. 17, no. 2, pp. (18-24)

Hayden, AJ., Martin, JM., Kneebone, AB. et al. (2010). Australian & New Zealand faculty of radiation oncology genito-urinary group; 2010 consensus guidelines for definitive external beam radiotherapy for prostate carcinoma. *Journal of Medical Imaging and Radiation Oncology*, vol. 54, pp. (513-525)

Heidenereich, A., Bellmunt, J., Bolla, M. et al. (2011). EAU guidelines on prostate cancer. Part 1: screening, diagnosis and treatment of clinically localized prostate cancer. *European Urology*, vol. 59, pp. (61-71)

Jelić, Lj., Stojanović, S., & Popov, I. (2005). Radiotherapy in prostate cancer treatment. *Acta Chirurgica Iugoslavica*, vol. 2, no. 4, pp. (93-102)

Jelić, Lj., & Stojanović, S. (2005). Radioterapija karcinoma prostate, In: *Lokalizovani karcinom prostate*, Hadži-Đokić J., pp. (109-118), Elit. Medica, Beograd

Kirby, R., & Madhavan, SG. (2010). Prostate cancer. Renal and urology II, In: *Surgery*, vol. 28, no. 12, pp. (594-598)

Koh, H., Kattan, MW., Scardino, PT. et al. (2003). A nomogram to predict seminal vesicles invasion by the extent and location of cancer in systemic biopsy results. *Journal of Urology*, vol. 170, pp. (1203-1208)

Kuban, DA., Tucker, SL., Dong, L. et al. (2008). Long-term results of the M. D. Anderson randomized dose escalation trial for prostate cancer. *International Journal of Radiation Oncology Biology Physics*, vol. 70, pp. (67-74)

Lawton, CA., Michalski, J., El-Naqa, I. et al. (2009). RTOG GU radiation oncology specialists reach consensus on pelvic lymph node volumes for high risk prostate cancer. *International Journal of Radiation Oncology Biology Physics*, vol. 74, pp. (383-387)

LENT SOMA scales for all anatomic sites. (1995). *International Journal of Radiation Oncology Biology Physics*, vol. 31, pp. (1049-1091)

Malone, S., Szanto, J., Perry, G. et al. (2000). A prospective comparison of three systems of patient immobilization for prostate radiotherapy. *International Journal of Radiation Oncology Biology Physics*, vol. 48, pp. (657-665)

Mate,T., Gottesman, J., Hatton, J. et al. (1998). High-dose-rate afterloading Ir-192 brachytherapy: Feasibility report. *International Journal of Radiation Oncology Biology Physics*, vol. 41, pp. (522-533)

Milecki, P., Martenka, P., Antczak, A. et al. (2010). Radiotherapy combined with hormonal therapy in prostate cancer: the state of art. *Cancer Management and Research*, vol. 2, pp. (243-253)

Thompson, IM., Tangen, CM., Paradelo, J. et al. (2009). Adjuvant radiotherapy for pathological T3N0M0 prostate cancer significantly reduces risk of metastases and improves survival: long term follow-up of a randomized clinical trial. *Journal of Urology*, vol. 181, pp. (956-962)

Valicenti, R., Lu, J., Pilepich, M. et al. (2000). Survival advantage from higher-dose radiation therapy for clinically localized prostate cancer treated on Radiation Oncology Group trials. *Journal of Clinical Oncology*, vol. 18, pp. (2740-2749)

Viani, GA., Stefano, EJ., & Alfonso, SL. (2009). Higher than conventional radiation doses in localized prostate cancer treatment: a meta-analysis of randomized controlled trials. *International Journal of Radiation Oncology Biology Physics*, vol. 74, pp. (1405-1418)

Wiegel, T., Bottke, D., Steiner, U. et al. (2009). Phase III postoperative adjuvant radiotherapy after radical prostatectomy compared with radical prostatectomy alone in T3 prostate cancer with postoperative undetectable prostate-specific antigen: ARO 96-02/AUO AP 09/95. *Journal of Clinical Oncology*, vol. 27, pp. (2924-2930)

Zelefsky, MJ., Fuks, Z., Hunt, M. et al. (2002). High-dose intensity modulated radiation therapy for prostate cancer: early toxicity and biochemical outcome in 772 patients. *International Journal of Radiation Oncology Biology Physics*, vol. 53, pp. (1111-1116)

Zietman, AL., Bac, K., Slater, JD. et al. (2010). Randomized trial comparing conventional-dose with high-dose conformal radiotherapy in early-stage adenocarcinoma of the prostate: long-term results from photon, radiation oncology group/American college of radiology. *Journal of Clinical Oncology*, vol. 28, pp. (1106-1111)

Zivkovic, M., & Deponte, V. (1996.) Palijativna radioterapija, In: *Radioterapija*, Samija, M., Krajina, Z., Purisic, A., pp. (363-378), Nakladni zavod Globus, Zagreb

Zlotecki, RA. (2001). External-Beam Radiation in the Management of Carcinoma of the Prostate. *Cancer Control*, vol. 8, pp. (503-510)

Yoshioka, Y., Konishi, K., Oh, R-J. et al. (2006). High-dose-rate brachytherapy without external beam irradiation for locally advanced prostate cancer. *Radiotherapy and Oncology*, vol. 80, pp. (62-68)

7

Renewing Perspectives on Men's Prostate Cancer Literacy and Engagement Along the Disease Continuum

Margareth Santos Zanchetta[1], Margot Kaszap[2], Marko Monteiro[3], Franklin Gorospe IV[4] and Roger Pilon[5]

[1]*Ryerson University, Faculty of Community Services*
Daphne Cockwell School of Nursing, Toronto, ON
[2]*University Laval, Faculty of Education, Quebec, QC*
[3]*State University of Campinas, Dept. of Science and Technology Policy, Campinas, SP*
[4]*Humber Institute of Technology and Advanced Learning, School of Health Sciences*
Nursing Program & University Health Network - Toronto General Hospital, Toronto, ON
[5]*Laurentian University, School of Nursing, Sudbury, ON*
[1,2,4,5]*Canada*
[3]*Brazil*

1. Introduction

In this chapter, we intend to familiarize readers with the complex scope of the experience of being a man with prostate cancer in current societies and dealing with scientific and popular health knowledge related to prostate cancer. We discuss issues of taking care of one's male body, being an older learner learning while facing a chronic degenerative disease, as well as the questions that social and health care professionals may encounter from men in providing meaningful health care. The provision of health care to men seems controversial, due to the lack of national policies on men's health in most countries as well as scarcity of men's health promotion programs in multicultural societies.

This chapter presents a brief overview of the state of knowledge about masculinities and gender, health literacy, and age - all major social determinants of health for men. The authors of each section present scientific knowledge produced in their qualitative research to contextualize other scholars' ideas and arguments. At the end of each section are clinical vignettes and reflection questions related to the contents of each section.

2. Men, masculinities, health and prostate cancer: Complex technology, body control, and decision making

In this section we address the issue of control that may coexist with other needs facing men, from prostate cancer detection through rehabilitation. Being in control relates to both the social enactments of masculinities and to how men understand current trends in health and technology. Control has been discussed as an important signifier of virility in different cultural contexts (Almeida, 1996; Bourdieu, 2001) and as a factor in men's perception of their bodies and assessment of the emotional and physiological care they receive. For men, losing control is seen as a negative experience, which may lead to negative experiences of preventative methods or care (Courtenay, 2000). Control is also a powerful metaphor for how current medicine, through increasingly technological interventions in the body, is being shaped by technoscience (Clarke et al., 2003; Steinberg, 1997). This "virile" [our emphasis] biomedical agenda should be tempered by attention to what some call "subjective variables," which we call "social or cultural factors". These factors include how men experience different types of masculinities and how these experiences and values inform men's attitudes toward health (Zanchetta et al., 2010). Social/cultural factors are relevant to every aspect of health and disease, and taking them into account will open professionals' perception to the complexity and richness of gender-related experiences of health practices.

2.1 Control in men's studies

The issue of control in the context of men's health is rooted in the upsurge of so-called men's studies in international academic literature, an upsurge that followed debates about gender in what is now known as the second wave of feminism (Butler, 1990; Scott, 1989). Men's studies tried to consider seriously the feminist claim that gender was not only about women, but should involve a close analysis of the relationships between genders. In addition, power relations emerged as a concomitant issue in debates about control. Such relations were not only analyzed in terms of how men relate to women, but also how men relate among themselves, and any claims that biology determined gender practices and power relations were to be vigorously denied. Gender was to be seen as socially constructed, not necessarily derivative of one's biological make-up. Men's studies scholars believed gender relationships are pervasive in our understanding of the world and that, therefore, our practices are deeply influenced by gendered understandings (Courtenay, 2000; Monteiro, 2000, 2001).

Studies of masculinities or men's studies became an important, separate subfield in the early 1980s and 1990s, especially in North America, Western Europe, and Australia (Carrigan et al., 1985; Cornwall & Lindisfarne, 1994; Gilmore, 1990; Kimmel, 1987). Masculinity was then increasingly incorporated into critical discourse on gender and power, instead of being an unquestioned universal category within discourse, culture, and politics (Monteiro, 2000). Authors began to discuss the unequal distribution of power between men and women, and among men themselves. The idea of hegemonic masculinities (Connell, 1995) became central to studies of masculinities, for example, because it enabled both deconstruction of masculinity as a uniform category that could be applied to all men and a discussion of power inequalities that affected men. Without construing men as merely victims of social expectations, these discussions opened up talk about plural masculinities in the study of men.

2.2 Masculinity, health, and prostate cancer

When discussing diversity among men, it then became important to address the challenges involved in becoming a man. Different masculinities are not purely biological or self-evident; they emerge in a process that is at the same time social, cultural, historical, etc. With the process of becoming a man seen as a process of men incorporating certain expectations, social roles, and practices (Bourdieu, 1997, 2001), masculinities can then be seen as also problematic, complex, and sometimes burdensome to men and their health. When men are viewed as a diverse group, with some men having better access to social prestige and power than other men and women, dynamics of gender and gender inequality become clearer and richer. Also, viewing men as diverse enables exploration of links between gender dynamics and health, a research agenda in progress.

Researchers pursuing this agenda has begun to explore the close relationships between masculinities and health (Courtenay, 2000), in the sense that gender perceptions and gender-related differences aid in explaining differences in health risks, and how health practices play a role in gender differences. Taking care of oneself, for example, might be considered effeminate in some contexts, leading to higher incidence of easily preventable diseases. When men embody masculinities that promote risky behavior as proof of virility, sexual conquests or failure to use condoms may put men (and their sexual partners) at higher risk for sexually transmitted diseases. In the case of prostate cancer, both the fear of bodily fragility (before and after treatment) and a masculinity that discourages care may be relevant to understanding how men experience their bodies and diseases (Mahalik et al., 2007).

Lohan (2007) suggests that, rather than focusing on men's studies and concepts such as hegemonic masculinities, researchers should embrace critical studies on men, a research area more attuned to feminist critiques of gender and power relations in society, in order to assess which factors explain how gender and health connect. Critical studies on men not only incorporate culture and behavior, but contextualize discussions of men's health in a wider explanatory framework including psychological, biological, and other factors. This context can be relevant to increasingly technological health interventions that regard differences (such as race and gender) in different terms than traditional health interventions. As biological difference becomes understood in genetic terms, for example, and as health research incorporates these advances in genetics, researchers of men's health will need to rethink how health, biology, and bodily differences are being lived in real life by men.

Men's experiences with health and prostate cancer should not be understood in a merely cultural register, however. Although cultural factors, such as the idea of "men don't cry" [our emphasis], are very important in understanding how men experience prostate cancer and care (Chapple & Ziebland, 2002), embodied factors, such as side effects of surgical and other interventions, reduce men's sense of their own virility (Chapple & Ziebland, 2002). Understanding embodied factors demands an understanding of masculinities that goes beyond social construction and embraces the complex interaction of many factors. Masculinities contradict each other, vary locally and nationally, and comprise complex hierarchies, for example (Connell & Messerschmidt, 2005; Wall & Kristjanson, 2005). They are also deeply infused with technology in varied contexts (Mellstrom, 2004).

2.3 Control in men's health-related experiences

Men's need and search for control, and attempts to be in control, suggest avenues to understanding the context for possible associations of cultural, embodied, and technological factors in men's experiences with prostate cancer. Such complex associations, because they help to constitute men's emotional and embodied experiences with disease and gender, may be crucial to understanding how men experience disease and recovery differently and thus how successful prevention and treatment can be. Control is multifaceted for men: Control over one's body and its diseases; control over other men, over women, over one's feelings, and over the public sphere, are some examples. As part of performing masculinities successfully, men generally avoid situations where they may lose control. Such situations may include preventive care and other actions that may improve health or prospects for survival (Kimmel, 1995; Lohan, 2007). Control is also at stake in current medical interventions, where advances in genetics, nanotechnology and other fields potentially enable control over every bodily process (Channel, 1991; Hogle, 2005). Proponents of this "virile" [our emphasis] approach to health and disease, we argue, need to pay attention to the complexity of men's lived experiences and gender differences in order to enhance the approach's effectiveness.

2.4 Control and the delivery of health care

Control is a general trend in how health and disease are being tackled by modern, techno-scientific medicine. The trend, called "bio-medicalization" (Clarke et al., 2003) describes how techno-science is becoming the dominant framework through which the concepts of health and the body are understood, as well as how health interventions are researched and used (Hogle, 2005; Lenoir, 2002a; Lenoir, 2002b). Bio-medicalization frames many health-related actions, from how we perceive the body visually, to the increasing use of technologies that make body interiors available for display and intervention (Taylor, 2005; Van Dijck, 2005), to ways of designing bodily interventions that are increasingly mediated by technology (Lenoir, 2004). This trend toward the incorporation of technology in health is increasingly evident as genetics becomes a dominant language to describe and understand diseases, including diabetes (Hedgecoe, 2002), cancer (Chung et al., 2002; Fujimura, 1996; Monteiro, 2009), and many others (Fullwiley, 2007). Not only has prostate cancer begun to be reinterpreted as a genetic disease, along with cancer in general, but the search is ongoing for genes to classify prostate cancer, diagnose it early, and refine surgical interventions (Shen & Abate-Shen, 2010). As prostate cancer becomes "molecularized" (Monteiro, 2009), its amenability to intervention is also transforming (Monteiro, 2011).

With a new, biomedical and techno-scientific approach to health and disease, control over bodily processes has been sought in ways unimaginable in the past. From increasingly precise interventions in the body, to the search for genes that would enable early diagnosis and even modeling of future behavior (Monteiro & Keating, 2009), control is at the center of how health is understood and practiced today. This effort to control bodily processes through increasingly sophisticated technology may, however, ignore the particularities of gender and masculinities, as discussed above. Nonetheless, an approach to prostate cancer that relies increasingly on techno-science to classify, diagnose, and surgically intervene can offer exciting new ways to approach the disease. Improving outcomes and enabling new methods for treatment and diagnosis will hopefully help circumvent some of the barriers towards self-care present in traditional masculinities, which usually see self-care as contrary to an ideal of the male body as impenetrable. New genetic tests could replace existing methods for examining the prostate, which many men find invasive. Establishing molecular bio-markers for prostate cancer that could reliably establish risk for the disease, for example, may enable early diagnosis, early treatment, and higher survival rates. Bio-markers would avoid, for example, uncomfortable examinations and unreliable prostate-specific-antigen (PSA) tests. However, an assumption of technological progress overlooks the many pitfalls such technology-based treatments could face. For instance, given discussion on the centrality of socio-cultural factors in explaining how men relate to their bodies and to health, it is not certain whether men will accept the idea of knowing in advance their risks for cancer. They may fear of loss of control over their health or fear becoming cancer "patients in waiting" at an early age before any cancer symptoms appear (Rajan, 2006). Mere knowledge that one carries genes that make one susceptible to cancer does not necessarily lead men to adopt preventive behavior. Indeed, it is clear that men avoid such behavior due to social expectations (Mahalik et al., 2007). Also, risks inherent in currently available prostate-cancer treatments are problematic for many men, in spite of any other considerations relating to their knowledge about preventing and monitoring cancer (Chapple & Ziebland, 2002).

When powerful trends to reinterpret health and disease in terms of new technologies (genetic or otherwise) dominate, researchers run the risk of ignoring the rich debate over socio-cultural factors that affect gender and health/disease. Although new technologies offer wonderful prospects for diagnosis and treatment, social factors such as gender, behavior, and culture should not be underestimated in terms of their contributions to understanding health and risk behaviors. Control, an attribute of hegemonic masculinity, is often associated with science and technology (two very male-dominated fields in some respects). This traditionally Western logic should be enriched with an understanding of how culture, society, and history explain health, disease, and treatment.

This debate about control, genetics, and technology is meaningful to social and health professionals who care for and advise men and their significant others throughout the prostate-cancer trajectory. Professionals should reflect on their beliefs about masculinity and prostate cancer, and their professional practice. Knowing that control is central to many men's experiences of masculinity, professionals should take a cautionary approach when presenting decision aids and discussing options about which they ask men to make immediate decisions. Caution is recommended mainly when men make decisions without professional guidance, because men may postpone reflection in favor of taking immediate action, thereby trying to demonstrate autonomy and willingness to decide. Men have been highly influenced by medicalization of erectile dysfunction in advertising for sexual-performance-enhancing drugs, advertising that focuses on the social importance of erections to virility. Therefore, professionals need to expand their understanding of the values and meaning that men attribute to diseases that threaten their sense of masculinity, and therefore their sexual and emotional health.

2.5 Informing professional practice

Knowledge of multiple aspects of culture, society, and history is important to help social and health professionals decode behavior expected of men as engaged partners in their own treatment and rehabilitation. Societies are becoming more and more multicultural, giving men opportunities to learn new meanings of being a man, and new attitudes to men's health, men's self-care, men's sexuality, and facts and myths related to prostate cancer (Zanchetta et al., 2010). For professionals, it is difficult to gather scientific evidence on men's behaviors, due to men's resistance to participating in clinical and behavioral studies (Deslauriers & Deslauriers, 2010). Again, gender-related discourse and perceived lack of control over data-collection encounters may affect men's participation in studies. To counteract resistance, researchers recommend allowing men to feel in control of their disclosure of personal information, such as feelings, fears, disagreeable symptoms, threatening thoughts, and awareness of uncertainties (Deslauriers & Deslauriers, 2010). Such research fieldwork strategies may also be helpful for assessment and follow-up interviews in clinical contexts, where professionals can use a conversational style with men, instead of a professional authoritative style of asking direct and probing questions. Despite a culturally and socially constructed trend of men being attracted to technology (Lerman et al., 2003;

Mellstrom, 2004) and technological advances in prostate-cancer-risk identification, early detection, treatment, and rehabilitation, men still perceive that technological interventions reduce their capacity to control the responses of their bodies and emotions to such interventions (Chapple & Ziebland, 2002).

Widespread public access to prostate cancer information in popular and scientific media has uncovered current discourse surrounding uncertainty about prostate cancer among researchers and health care professionals. Certainly, men are less likely to trust the health care system's assurance that current technologies are helpful and to rely on information from health care professionals in their decision making. Regardless of men's personal level of education and health literacy, they should be supported in enhancing their ability to perceive and differentiate levels of risk when making informed decisions about treatments. Gender-related experiences are, again, important to consider in the clinical context, because men's health experiences tend not to be solitary. Men's experiences are, instead, influenced by the roles of women (mothers, wives, partners, daughters, nieces, aunts, etc.) and other caring figures (fathers, same-sex partners, coaches, etc.) in their lives. Together, caring figures influence men's decisions to seek medical help, adhere to treatments, and most important, transcend the limitations and changes imposed by prostate cancer. Such a collective view of men's health experiences challenges current organizational policies requiring that personal information remain private and neglects the social and cultural fact that men are human beings, who (in less publicly demonstrative ways than women) are influenced by intimate others in seeking health and well being (Zanchetta et al., 2010).

2.6 Reflecting on control in men's experiences with prostate cancer screening

Below are some true stories with fictitious names as clinical vignettes and reflection questions to help readers identify control as a key concept in men's experience of prostate cancer and reflect on how control plays out in clinical practice. No answers are provided, because we want to stimulate readers' recall of their own experience so that they can construct appropriate answers to the reflection questions.

2.6.1 Clinical vignettes

- John, a 56-year-old accountant, was urged by his wife to get screened for prostate cancer. After months of postponing his decision, he agrees to make an appointment for an annual physical. During the history taking, he tells the doctor that he feels fine and does not understand why he should have a physical. John says, "If it isn't broken, why fix it?"
- Charles, a 50-year-old engineer, comes to the clinic for his annual physical and discusses prostate screening with his family doctor. They discuss the merits of DRE versus PSA testing. His doctor explains both screening tests. Charles is reluctant to have a DRE test, given the invasive nature of the procedure. In spite of the information his doctor provides about the limited sensitivity and specificity of the PSA test, Charles decided to have the PSA test done, because he believes that it will be less invasive than the DRE test.
- Silvio, a 50-year-old computer designer, is a newcomer to Canada who speaks and understands English at an intermediate level. After arriving, he looked for a family doctor to monitor a recurrent inflammation in his prostate as well as have his annual PSA test. Due to pain and urinary troubles, the doctor ordered an abdominal

ultrasound. Silvio remembers that he barely understood his doctor`s explanations about the ultrasound. He had it in a hospital without any problems but is worried about the presence of blood in his urine for the last 5 days, which he does not understand. He believes that the doctor "saw something" during the ultrasound. He feels lost, with no clues about his situation and really wants to do something about that. Unfortunately, he must wait three to four weeks for a follow-up medical consultation.

2.6.2 Questions

- Why is control important when it comes to men's health?
- What strategies could health care professionals consider that might promote men's empowerment as active participants in planning preventative health actions for prostate cancer and its treatment?
- What barriers might contribute to men feeling a loss of control over early detection of prostate cancer?

3. A contemporary view of educating elders for health: Insights for educational practice in clinical and community settings

This section focuses on the relationship between older people and health education, as it relates to men with prostate cancer. Men's knowledge and understanding of learning about health, both in a biomedical and socio-cultural sense, is essential during the prostate cancer trajectory. Davis et al. (2008) discuss the importance for health care professionals of recognizing factors that contribute to elder's low health literacy, which may be increasing. Health literacy is a central to successful communication between health care professionals and elderly patients. It is not only essential for elderly patients to be equipped with appropriate knowledge of the disease process so as to be actively involved in their care, but health education must support patients to become more autonomous. Education for empowerment, as pioneered by Paulo Freire, requires a health education process centered in dialog between educators and learners (Wallerstein & Bernstein, 1988). Educating today's older people about cancer requires new educational strategies, particularly new education technologies that simplify complex cancer information and facilitate learning. Older people are active users of computers and the internet; misconceptions to the contrary must not shape health care professionals' beliefs about older people's ability to learn about their health (Alpay et al., 2004).

3.1 Older patients' acquisition of formative learning

A discussion involving knowledge and learning implies talking about "alphabetization" and literacy, or even about various literacy levels and literacy backgrounds. Traditionally, literacy was defined in general terms but, currently, we tend to differentiate among a range of literacy concepts. The new term "alphabetization" belongs to the old literacy paradigm in which we assessed individuals in terms of their ability to read, write, and use numbers. The goal was to rank individuals according to their literacy level, what we now call the "degree of alphabetization." Today, some literacy researchers work within a new literacy paradigm: as a social practice reflecting the literacy background of the person (Barton et al., 1998, 2000). Kaszap and Clerc (2008) clarify both alphabetization and literacy concepts and suggest how to use them.

The degree of *health alphabetization* may indicate - at a specific time in one's life - competence in searching for, identifying, collecting, understanding, critiquing, and interpreting health information. This information is used to create and communicate messages about one's health status, to make choices in preventing disease, to recover or preserve health, to solve problems related to one's health using language (written, oral, visual, audible, tactile, etc.) in a variety of contexts in day-to-day life (at the world, community, school, and individual levels). Health alphabetization can frequently be measured by tests, and other reporting and self-appraisal methods. On the other hand, the concept of *health literacy* comprises several assets (translation of Kaszap & Clerc, 2008, as cited in Kaszap & Zanchetta, 2009). First, it sums all health information acquired from family, school, social, cultural, and professional sources (formal and informal) during a continuous, gradual learning process. Second, it sums all the values, beliefs, fears, habits, attitudes, and behaviors that each person holds in all the aspects of life related to health. Third, health literacy comprises one's specific background: (a) health culture and health knowledge, (b) the type of health education to which one was exposed, individual's attitudes, behaviours, and feelings, values and beliefs; (c) practices in searching for health information, reading and decoding it, and communicating it (in oral or written form), and (d) using numerical information and health information to solve health problems in everyday life.

Seen from the above-described point of view, measurement of health literacy is neither feasible nor possible. However, it is a state, or even a set of personal practices, that can be described more or less accurately. Seen this way, health literacy can be more or less broad, more or less adequate - or inadequate- for a situation or a context. Zanchetta (2002) describes the origin of men's prostate cancer literacy as follows:

All men reported that during childhood, school and family constituted the sources of available health information during the formation of their informational background on health matters. Health information in childhood was synonymous with consuming healthy food, having good hygiene, and receiving vaccinations at school. (p. 191)

Men's learning experiences with prostate cancer build on lifelong learning about health and its incorporation into daily life. Zanchetta (2002) proposes a definition of health literacy about prostate cancer based on survivors' experiences:

Older men live and deal with health information through the handling of the imprints of their beliefs, and representations, as well as life, learning, and illness experience. For this, a supportive environment is primordial to enable them to regain the sense of illness, the decision-making power upon one's body and destiny, as well as to redefine the social roles by reconstructing partnerships with the social and informational network. (p. 294)

The definition above shows that the construction of health literacy is multidimensional and involves social factors, such as life stories, cumulative experience, social learning, autonomy, and social interactions. Seminal studies have demonstrated a strong relationship between low literacy and poor health (Brown et al., 1993; Davis et al., 1991; Francis, 1991; Mayeaux et al., 1996; Weiss et al., 1992, 1994; Weiss & Coyne, 1997) and proposed health literacy as a new social determinant of health (Rootman et al., 2007; Zanchetta et al., 2011). Therefore, we suggest that inadequate health literacy may impede other social determinants of health, which in turn may worsen one's ability to use health information in making decisions.

Considering the above-mentioned factors, we propose a conceptual framework (Figure 1) that shows alphabetization as an integral part of health literacy, within the social determinants of health. Together with a supportive environment, health literacy may influence individuals' response to particular health situations and contexts as well as their awareness of existing resources and ways to accessing them. Perlow (2010) reports that low health literacy has major impacts on health disparities and adverse health outcomes throughout the lifespan, including hospitalization, chronic disease, and higher health care costs.

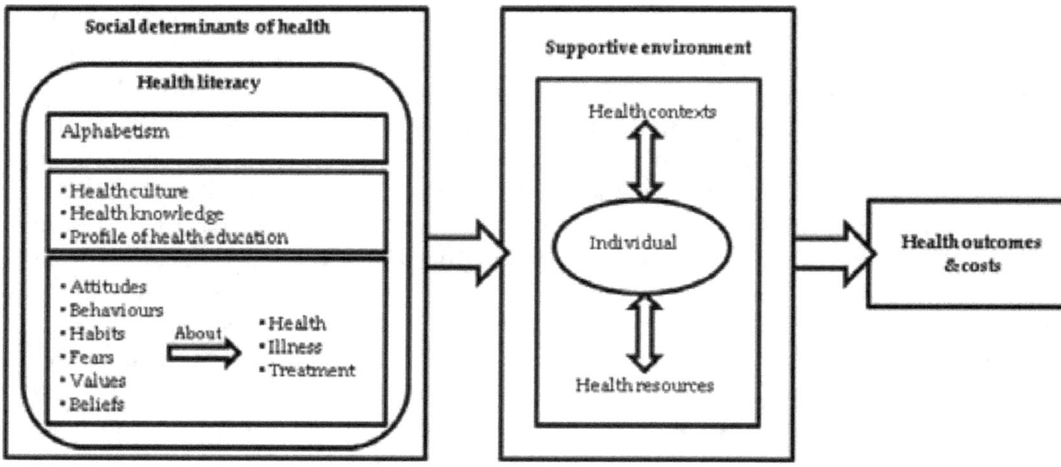

Fig. 1. The health literacy conceptual framework

With the growing elderly population in developed and developing countries, health costs (financial, human, material, physical, emotional, etc.) are anticipated to grow. The emerging worldwide movement of supporting patients to be autonomous, aware partners in health care is also leading education and health professionals to rethink the role of health educators. To promote health literacy, health educators are facing demands to renew and expand their toolboxes of educational aids and to adopt teaching innovations to sustain the mobilization of learning potential among older patients. The next section presents some considerations for health educators to think about.

3.2 Strategies in health education

Over time, health education has been done mostly in a traditional way by health professionals, according to health curricula. In this approach, information is given on disease, and treatments are explained in a "you have to" way. This approach is basically one-way knowledge transmission, from professionals to patients and not vice versa. Using this traditional approach, professionals scarcely have time to learn what health literacy patients already have. Patients do not have time to discuss their fears, values, and conceptions. The traditional approach to health education has brought with it serious problems. For example, recent research tells us that inadequate literacy often reveals misconceptions about different aspects of health, such as patient's erroneous understanding of how a body change in enduring diseases, long term effects of drugs or other treatments (Buston & Wood, 2000; Kaszap et al., 2000, 2006), and false beliefs about popular treatments (e.g., magical peas or liniments) with supposedly spectacular effects on blood pressure (Kaszap et al., 2000). With older men, health educators should take such health-related misconceptions and false beliefs into account and propose new strategies for health education.

Health education should not merely be transmission of information, because recipients of transmitted information may filter it through faulty premises; for example, misconceptions about bodies, health, and treatments and false beliefs about natural products that supposedly have miraculous effects on various diseases. Before delivering health information, health professionals should seek to understand the literacy backgrounds of older men: what they know, their beliefs, fears, habits, conceptions, and behaviors concerning their health, illness, medications, and treatments. Torres et al. (2008) reveal the importance of such exploration to understand and address the deeply rooted web of ideology, norms, and practices that influence health decision making and behavioral responses. Kruger et al. (2007) argue that professionals must ask elders questions about their functional and emotional health status. Health professionals should understand older men's "supportive environments" (Zanchetta, 2002, p. 294), comprising their families and their social and information networks. Without this baseline information about older men, health professionals will not be able to teach them appropriately, to enhance their understanding of diseases and treatment, to persuade them to follow medication and treatment regimes, or to prepare them to choose among treatment options (Kaszap & Drolet, 2009).

Transmitting information does not imply that its recipients agree with it and will immediately act upon it. New knowledge needs to be constructed. Knowledge construction means, therefore that, when new knowledge is offered, it needs to be discussed, even challenged, before it can be accepted and integrated in an individual's own existing knowledge system. Construction of health-related knowledge requires time, but taking this time will save time and money in the long run: time lost in repeated explanations, time and money lost in preventable hospitalization and preventable health deterioration. Moon (2011) explains that elder experience transformative learning with success but as a process which takes time and need support. Knowledge construction happens within relationships between older individuals and health professionals when professionals explore with elders their health backgrounds - their values, beliefs, fears, habits, attitudes, conceptions, and behaviors; and when professionals respect each patient's learning style: their individual ways of listening, asking questions and answering them. Knowledge construction also happens when explanations are meaningful (neither too technical nor childish) and use appropriate terminology, examples, or visual aids, such as photos and drawings. Concomitantly, lack of trust in relationships between health professionals and older individuals may jeopardize their engagement in teaching-learning initiatives, due their fear of disclosing personal information about their health problems (Kaszap & Drolet, 2009). Professionals need to find out about older men's misconceptions and false beliefs by asking questions about their health, illness, and treatment. By 'misconceptions', we mean erroneous explanations from erroneous understandings. By 'false beliefs', we mean beliefs based on superstitions and popular knowledge, not on scientific proof. All together, they are erroneous premises. These erroneous premises should be challenged and deconstructed prior to proposing new knowledge. Deconstructing knowledge means that professionals need to ask questions about an older man's conceptions or beliefs to be able to understand why the older man thinks the way he does. Where did he get that explanation? Then professionals need to start a dialog about both sides of the argument and give examples and explanations based on scientific knowledge. Professionals need to drive the discussion in a way that older men will adopt the scientific position because, when older people do not properly understand their disease and the needed treatments, when they are not adhering with their treatments or medication, they become severely ill and need to be hospitalized.

3.3 Evolution from existing to new educational technologies

Despite well documented challenges in educational initiatives with older learners, some researchers interested in promoting older learners' health literacy are incorporating new technological tools into health teaching to enhance learning. Most older individuals are willing to learn about new technology, even to use and master it, especially if they are under 80 years old and in good mental health (Kaszap et al., 2002; Gil-Gómez et al., 2011; Jensen et al., 2010; Mackert et al., 2009; Saposnik et al., 2010; Wallington, 2008). It seems to be just a matter of having help in learning how to use new technology and having enough time to understand and practice it. Kaszap et al. (2000), in a study exploring the experiences of rural and urban older individuals with various technologies, documented elders' preference for information-gathering contexts (see Figure 2). They preferred private contexts (such as a visit to a professional's office) for gathering information on personal matters and group

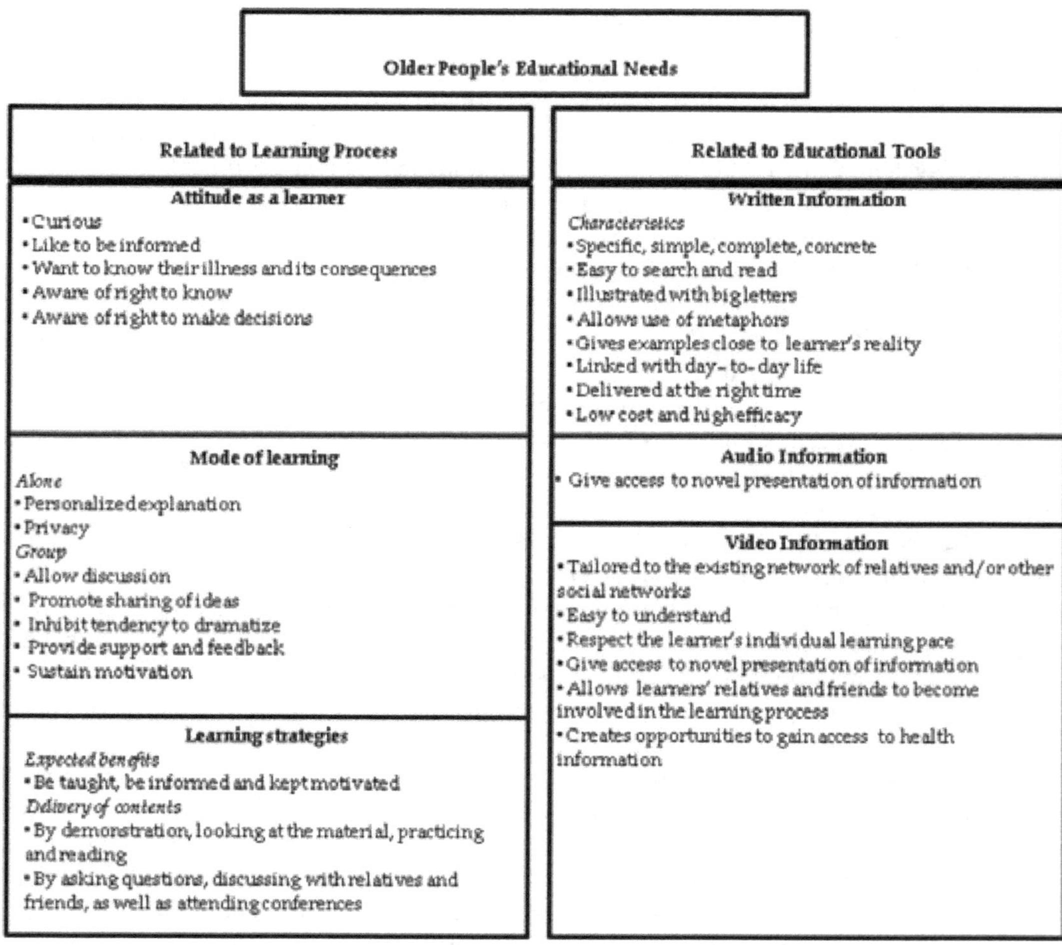

Fig. 2. Older individuals' views on different aspects of health learning

contexts (among relatives and friends, even strangers) for gathering general information about health, illness, and treatment, because belonging to a group allows discussion, idea sharing, support, and maintains motivation for continuous learning. Golding (2011) reports that older men in community settings learn when education is social, local, practical, situated, and in groups, particularly isolated men. Prins et al. (2009) argue that social interactions are needed to support elders, and Bergsma (2004) adds that personal and social change are possible through empowerment education.

In libraries nowadays, it is common to see elders looking for information on the Web, writing emails, or chatting on Skype. Community initiatives to develop computer literacy among older learners are undoubtedly opening new avenues for learning about health, for both already and newly computer-literate elders. Twenty-first century elders are becoming more familiar with technologies such as cell phones, videos, and computers. Even interactive video games (Nintendo Wii and Wii balance board) have been introduced to older patients for curative and rehabilitation purposes (Gil-Gómez et al., 2011; Saposnik et al., 2010). Elders are open to, and like, new experiences in the context of playing and exercising in rehabilitation and homecare settings. In the news, we see older people bowling via Wii to improve their balance after surgery and using Wii-based yoga and light exercise to regain vitality after hospitalization. Technological possibilities now exist that encourage elders to access information and take care of themselves in a variety of contexts. Health educators should support them through teaching older people to make use of these new opportunities for learning about health, illness, and treatments. Along with face-to-face discussion, virtual chatting can enhance older people's lives, despite any health conditions.

3.4 Rethinking prostate cancer and prostate health education

To prevent prostate cancer and deal with the disease throughout its trajectory, both prostate cancer information and prostate cancer literacy are important. The complexity of scientific knowledge make prostate cancer education with men of all ages and education levels a real challenge, in particular with older men having low degrees of alphabetization, whose social and information networks are crucial supports for decision making (Zanchetta, 2002). According to Kaszap and Drolet (2009), health literacy appraisal should explore a person's ability to acknowledge his/her own prior knowledge, current fears, beliefs, values, misconceptions, attitudes, habits, and behaviours - all of which build the foundation for constructing new knowledge. Innovations in clinical practice will certainly be needed to reveal the dynamic relationships between health knowledge, health literacy, the internet as a source of health information along with professional guidance (Jensen et al., 2010), especially for older people who are hard to reach (Macker et al., 2009), and the advantages of other technology used in rehabilitation and prostate cancer education. Levasseur and Carrier (2010) stress that rehabilitation and health literacy share goals: both see as important individuals' overall capacities for self-care, enhancing functioning, facilitating individuals' participation in their own health care, client-centered care, and equity in access to services, for example. Inspired by Zanchetta (2002) and knowledge construction theories (Jonnaert, 2009), education about prostate health can be expanded to include all men, regardless of their conceptual and experiential knowledge.

Older individuals may actively participate in transformative learning initiatives if time and supportive social interactions to foster learning are available to them (Moon, 2011; Prins et al., 2009). Support can include helping older individuals understand how to find information on the internet and how to mobilize a supportive network of groups or individuals in the community (Wallington, 2008). Health educators should use age-specific tools and elder-client-centered instructions to promote older people's health literacy (Morrow et al., 2007). Educational materials should be prepared for specific purposes and complex information delivered in forms other than writing (Roberts & Partridge, 2011), such as story telling (Wilkin & Ball-Rokeach, 2006). Discussions should using common terminology and repeat contents taught through learner-teach-back techniques. Professionals should apply medical information to topics familiar to elders (Prasauskas & Spoo, 2006), for which professionals need to understand older patients' literacy backgrounds. No more than four essential points should be provided at a time, with any written information reflecting learners' colloquial language, framed by learners' own health culture, and stating expected health behaviors (Prasauskas & Spoo, 2006).

It may take time for health professionals to learn about each elder's fears, beliefs, habits, behaviours, and conceptions of health before it is possible to discuss disease and their treatment (Orel et al., 2005). However, learning older men's communication styles and literacy backgrounds will help professionals to begin talking about prostate cancer treatment and to gain clients' trust, without inspiring too much fear. Health professionals should let older men absorb the fact that they have prostate cancer before discussing solutions - absorbing such information also takes time. The educational process should occur in several steps; otherwise it will be perceived as challenging older men's sense of masculinity. Such caution in communication is particularly relevant for physicians, who are advised to inquire, in all consultations, about older men's functional and emotional health status (Kruger et al., 2007). Finally, it is important that older men themselves examine their assumptions (about, for example, masculinity) before constructing new knowledge and accept the need to make changes in their lives; for example, they may need to change their food choices to supplement medical treatment of their prostate cancer (Mróz et al., 2011).

3.5 Reflecting on men's accounts of prostate cancer health education

In the clinical vignettes presented below we present the experiences of some older men in learning about prostate cancer, including why they sought information and how engagement in learning helped them move toward better prostate health.

3.5.1 Clinical vignettes

- Claudio, a 59-year-old flooring installer, receives a diagnosis of prostate cancer. He tells his urologist that he has no symptoms and feels just fine. Because he feels well, he is not concerned about the diagnosis and decides that he will not let this diagnosis affect him in any way. He is not interested in discussing treatment options and decides to leave the physician's office.
- When Constantin, a 67-year-old newspaper columnist, receives the diagnosis of prostate cancer, he tells his oncologist that his father had prostate cancer and experienced serious side effects from the treatment. Constantin does not want to go through what his father experienced and decides refuse any and all prostate cancer treatment offered to him. In fact, he is so concerned about possible side effects that he does not even want to discuss treatment options with the oncologist.
- When Bernardo, a 69-year-old retired parole officer, receives a diagnosis of prostate cancer, he is initially surprised. However, within a few days he tells his wife that he has gained the distinction of joining the brotherhood of prostate cancer. Bernardo is, has lived a full life and refuses to let the prostate cancer diagnosis define who he is. Bernardo has a great sense of humor and subscribes to the adage that laughter is the best medicine.

3.5.2 Questions

- What are some principles of adult learning that can guide health professionals in teaching older men about prostate cancer?
- Identify strategies that could foster learning among older men about their health and their bodies.
- What teaching strategies should health professionals consider when promoting literacy about health and prostate cancer among older men?

4. Information strategies and health behaviors related to levels of prostate-cancer literacy

In Section 3, we contextualized health literacy within the perspective of men's experiences with prostate cancer. In this section, we present the results of a qualitative study with 14 Francophone Canadian men. The study documented men's strategies for dealing with prostate cancer information and their self-rated levels of health literacy (Zanchetta, 2002). The study demonstrated that levels of health literacy were not influenced by older men's self-reported general literacy (Zanchetta et al., 2007) and that, despite differences in their levels of health literacy, older men reported similar strategies for dealing with prostate cancer information: comparison, deduction, and hypothesis formation (Zanchetta et al., 2007). These information strategies revealed the importance of communication through social, intimate, and interpersonal interactions in enhancing older men's health literacy.

4.1 Older men's construction of health literacy

Older men's health literacy is influenced by several factors, such as seeking health-related information to promote and maintain health, leading to personal empowerment (World Health Organization, 1998), reading and numeracy skills, comprehension, and decision making (Oldfield & Dreher, 2010); opportunities to obtain health-related information; concepts of masculinity (Peerson & Saunders, 2010; Zanchetta et al., 2010); and congruency between health-related information and personal views of masculinity (Zanchetta, 2002).

To guide decision making in collaboration with physicians, men with prostate cancer face great challenges in learning about and understanding their disease (Barry, 2010). Two of these uncertainties relate to prostate cancer's trajectory and the complex information patients receive about their prognosis and treatment options (Nanton et al., 2009). These uncertainties influence men's ability to participate in decision making about their care. In Zanchetta et al.'s (2007) study, men's various information strategies allowed them to participate in making decisions about their complex care. Low health literacy rates are another prominent challenge. Low health literacy rates limit men's understanding of prostate cancer information (Easton et al., 2010). Another challenge to the health literacy of men with prostate cancer is the lack of consensus among health care professionals about the most effective decision aids and the safest methods for screening and monitoring (Gwede & McDermott, 2006). Nor does consensus exist among health professionals on whether prostate cancer screening improves health outcomes (Krist et al., 2007) or what harmful consequences prostate cancer treatment has for men's physical and sexual functioning (Barry, 2010).

All of the above challenges, added to contradictions in information from health care professionals, contribute to men's confusion in trying to understand scientific discourse about prostate cancer and the impact of treatment on men's sexual function. Men's goal for learning about prostate cancer becomes clear: They seek information they can use to survive the disease, not scientific understanding of the disease process (Zanchetta et al., 2007). Erectile dysfunction, one potential consequence of prostate cancer treatment, represents failed masculinity (Knight & Latini, 2009) for men who adopt traditional masculinities. This representation undermines their motivation to learn about prostate cancer and its treatment.

4.2 A new understanding of older men's construction of prostate cancer literacy

Through a discourse analysis technique called "abduction in communication" (Boudon, 1998, 1999, 2000), reasons why men with disparate levels of education (from three years of home schooling to doctorate) used similar information strategies were identified. Three analytical assumptions guided the analysis that revealed the similarity of these cognitive processes: (a) men's attempts to connect general health information with prostate cancer information would disclose the *modus operandi* of becoming prostate cancer literate, (b) men's key motivations for learning would determine the strategies they used to construct information strategies, and (c) external factors initially considered negative, non-collaborative, and obstructive would motivate men to construct more information strategies. The results of the analysis are (presented in the rest of Section 4.2 and in Figure 3 to 6) portray how older men's use of prostate cancer information and their discourse about prostate cancer was framed by ideas of space, distance, and possibility. Men's use of information responded to their need to deal with notions of truth, lies, and the possibility of errors; plausible and non-plausible uses of information; possible and impossible decisions; fact and illusion, and so on. In addition, men dealt with how long they might live; whether they would remain in their own homes as they grew older or move to retirement homes or seniors' apartments; and where they might ultimately die.

4.2.1 Core information strategies men use to become prostate-cancer literate

Despite differences in men's self-reported levels of schooling and self-rated health literacy, with survival as an ultimate goal for learning, men looked for new informational support among peers, other individuals, relatives, media, and health professionals. Men mainly used hypothetical reasoning to decode the prostate cancer information they acquired from health professionals and informal sources (newspapers, television, internet, books, pamphlets, etc.). Men's struggles to become prostate cancer literate included reflecting on life and death as well as using the cognitive processes of hypothesizing, deducting, and comparing. To do that, they combined prostate cancer information they gathered from medical journals and their physicians with information from their own illness experiences. Figure 3 presents the general analytical categories and shows how the interpretative poles oscillate between the positive and negative impacts of decoded information related to the dimensions of health, diagnosis of prostate cancer and illness, men's socio-cultural identity, the external world, and the imprints of life and prostate cancer-related information. One of the key strategies men used to decode information was to compare information from different sources about the accuracy of medical prognoses, changes in lifestyle due to cancer, recovery expectations, and expected difficulties in end-of-life situations. As men felt more certain about the predictability of medical prognoses, some men's attitudes changed. Although some remained socially isolated, others enrolled in prostate cancer support groups, became more committed to their own health, or to men's collective health. Certainty also brought to older men a greater will to live and a peaceful acceptance of possible death from prostate cancer.

In the figures 3 to 6, the arrow going from bottom left to top right of each figure means the paradigm of understanding from a negative to a positive pole.

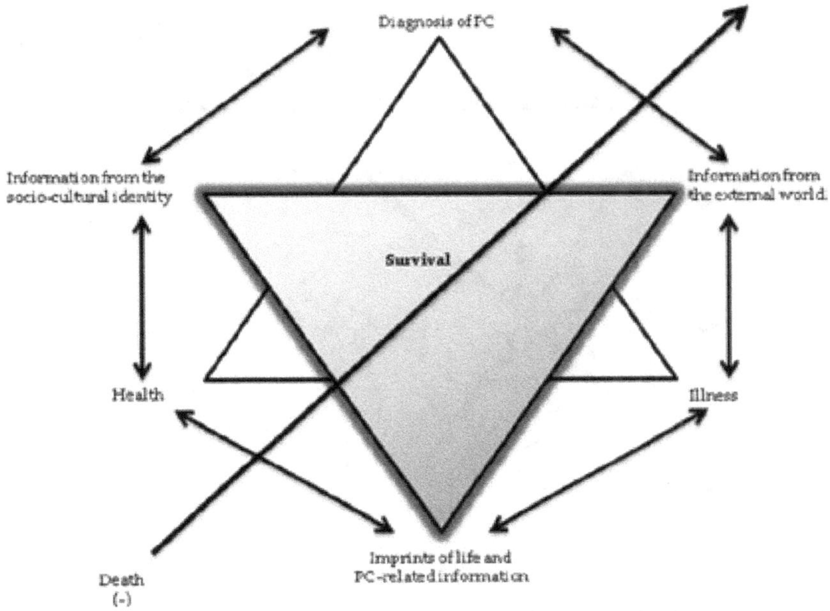

Fig. 3. General analytical categories related to core information strategies

4.2.2 Strategies for dealing with prostate cancer-related information within the paradigm of health literacy

Older men also used their new prostate-cancer health literacy to create multiple possibilities for living with prostate cancer. They used their accumulated knowledge to transform previous representations about life after prostate cancer and the disease itself. From their contacts with other individuals in their social networks, men learned how to survive better and longer with prostate cancer. Particularly relevant in this transformation were information exchanges with other prostate cancer survivors, sharing information with undiagnosed men, and new information provided by significant others.

Analysis of men's accounts of exchanges of information also revealed controversies about whether information gathered through the process mentioned above actually contributed to men's prostate cancer literacy. First, older men seemed to be more interested in communicating information and personal experiences with prostate cancer than in the process of learning itself. Second, partial, imprecise, or superficial information about prostate cancer could either stagnate or propel older men's learning about prostate cancer. Third, the hypotheses (deductive and inductive) those men generated after contact with prostate cancer information impelled them to either confirm or refute the hypotheses. In doing so, older men built the core of their interpretative logic and thereby created meaning out of their experiences with prostate cancer. The information strategies thus fueled men's determination to transform all future contact they had with prostate cancer information. Figure 4 presents how men compared their situations with those of other individuals living with cancer and, whether they had low or high levels of health literacy, formed hypotheses, made comparisons, and decisions.

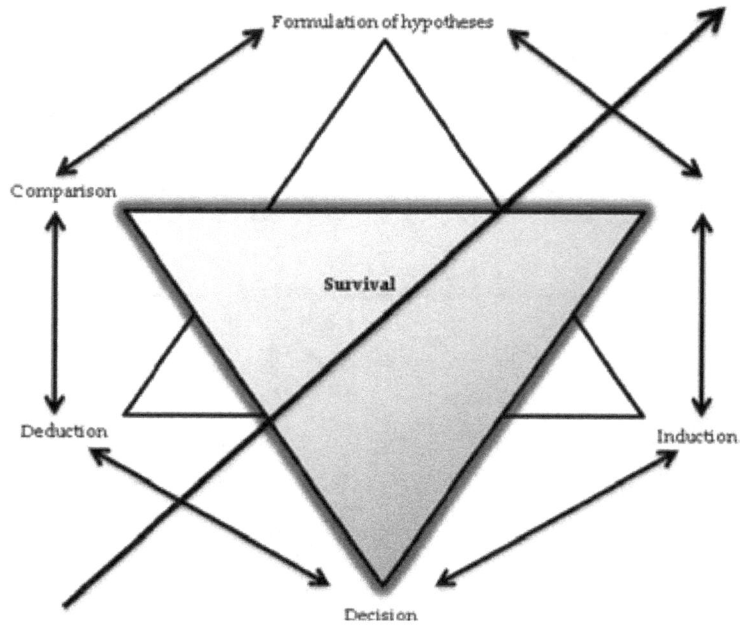

Fig. 4. Strategies for dealing with prostate cancer-related information

4.2.3 Strategies men use to make sense of prostate cancer information

Men's use of hypothesizing and of deductive and inductive reasoning varied in intensity and frequency, depending on older men's self-rated level of health literacy and the uncertainty they faced about their medical conditions. Men's use of these analytical techniques was congruent with their tendency to assess information logically by seeking to understand events and facts and by decoding large amounts of (sometimes contradictory) prostate cancer information. The intensity and frequency of men's hypothesizing, deduction, and induction seemed to be associated with the importance they attributed to the process of decision making, regardless of its domain. The cognitive processes of hypothesizing and deducting also influenced men's acceptance or refusal of prostate cancer information, because men selected information based on their values. Selecting, valuing, and incorporating prostate cancer information, and other information indirectly related to prostate cancer, can be explained by men's increasing interest in information seeking. Men's main focus was learning what to do to ensure their survival and how to do it. This focus led men to value what could help them understand clinical facts. Men sought to find, in each piece of prostate cancer information, anything that could contribute to a pragmatic plan for surviving cancer. Men valued information that was personally relevant to them and could contribute to decision-making. In this information-selection process, men's participation in information networks and the information support that they received from significant others were important.

Men's constant hypothesizing seemed to be an attempt to understand and compare information from multiple sources, information that created doubts in their minds. With these doubts, men constantly struggled to reduce abstraction and uncertainty in the information they gathered. The difficulty with abstraction related most often to descriptions of cellular processes and cell-level responses to treatment, as expressed by levels of PSA, prostate cancer recurrence, and metastasis. Without being able to understand this complex information, men could not evaluate its pertinence and quality.

Men needed to evaluate this information to construct meaning by comparing it to their own health experiences, as well as with health and prostate cancer information they had already gathered. Figure 5 displays the key factors that influenced the way older men lived with prostate cancer information.

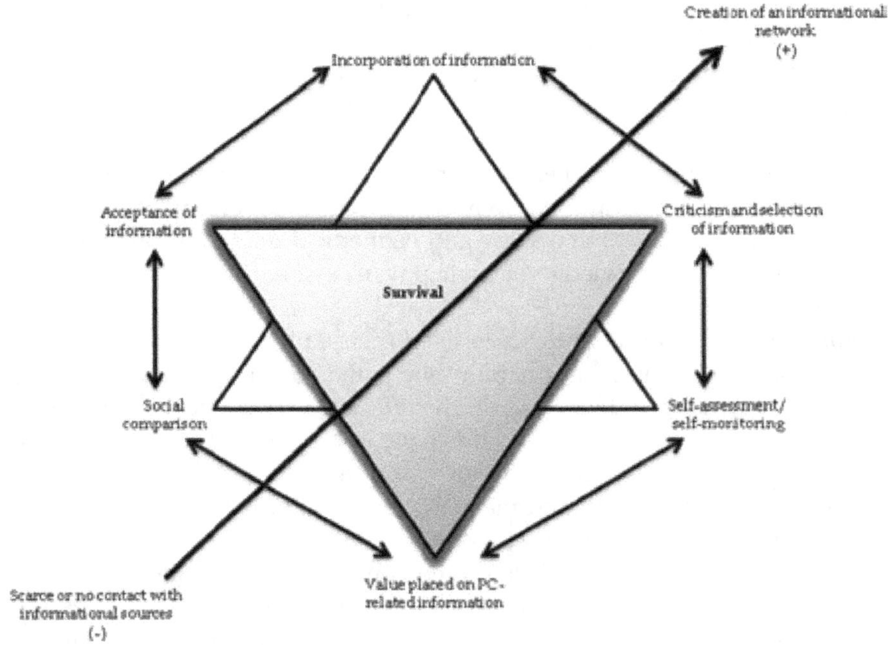

Fig. 5. Key factors influencing the way men live with prostate cancer-related information

4.2.4 Key factors underlying older men's information strategies

For older men, the utility of all information men found relevant was its contribution to solving problems, filling knowledge gaps, and helping men learn how to live with prostate cancer. The relevance individual men attributed to information revealed differences among older men in their critical attitudes to the information they gathered. Men either focused on analyzing the information's technical content or applied the information to political and collective aspects of men's experiences with prostate cancer.

These critical attitudes revealed how men came in contact with and joined information networks to explore their social environments. Men who had little or no contact with sources of health information other than their urologists lived in cognitive isolation. On the other hand, men who gradually constructed networks comprising health professionals (other than urologists) and lay people slowly incorporated new knowledge into their lives through collective learning and exchanging experiences, knowledge that supplemented and complemented information from their urologists.

Incorporation of information into men's lives was a goal shared by men with prostate cancer and other individuals who were directly or indirectly involved with their new lives after medical recovery. Before being able to decode prostate cancer information, some men confronted the reality that other men and women live with cancer that was more or less severe than theirs. This confrontation raised men's awareness of the potential impact of prostate cancer on their own lives. Comparing their lives to the lives of others allowed men to ascertain the relevance of prostate cancer information and incorporate it into their daily lives, specifically into self-assessment and self-monitoring. Men valued information that responded to their pragmatic needs, rather than theoretical information that was difficult to decode. Once they found enough information to answer their questions, men stopped searching.

The quality of prostate cancer information was another factor men used to evaluate the credibility of information sources and whether or not to accept information from them. When men perceived new information to be high quality, even if it contradicted information that they deemed valuable, they were open to comparing it to contradictory information. The issues of quality, criticism, and acceptance explained men's unwavering acceptance of medical diagnoses of prostate cancer, their strong tendency not to seek second medical opinions, and their unconditional acceptance of medical therapies recommended by their physicians. Moreover, other issues were at play in this process: men's lack of knowledge about the disease and its medical treatment, trust in the technical competence and scientific knowledge of their physicians, and what value men placed on prostate cancer information.

Figure 6 displays the dynamics of how men lived their daily lives (outside of hospitals and clinics) with the prostate cancer information they gathered through information networks. Men's prostate cancer literacy depended on the effects of experiences with prostate cancer within or outside such networks. Men would create and be part of information networks to build their individualized knowledge about prostate cancer. Being part of information networks helped them understand and make meaning out of their own illness experiences. Men's understanding of the disease was a shared construction of experiences of others in their immediate social environment. This shared construction filled men's knowledge gaps and resolved misunderstandings, allowing men to construct new social roles inspired by their awareness of the need to share knowledge and gain empirical skills to manage prostate cancer. Therefore, men tended to transmit information about the prevention and early detection of prostate cancer, as well as how men already touched by the disease had improved the quality of their lives.

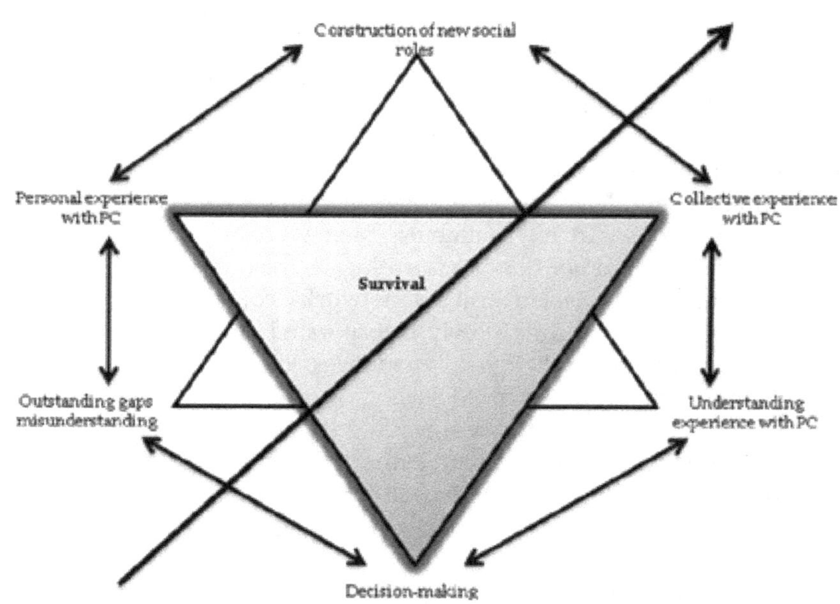

Fig. 6. Dynamics of living with prostate cancer-related information

4.3 Ultimate goals in constructing information strategies for becoming prostate-cancer literate

As described above, the process of becoming prostate-cancer literate unfolded along the life-death continuum; levels of health literacy (from low to high); levels of contact with information networks (from no contact to creation of one's own information network); and illness experiences within or outside information networks. Men's information strategies came out of the desire to preserve their moral integrity, self-image, and to maintain their social roles (as husbands, fathers, grandfathers, friends, and peer counsellors). Awareness of loss, regret, deception, and hope encouraged older men to remain in their social roles, while sharing their wisdom about how to live well[1] with prostate cancer (Zanchetta, 2004). Living well with prostate cancer included creating a new body free of embarrassing conditions (e.g., urinary incontinence), a new masculinity, and a new perception of control. Living well also included redefining one's sense of successful adaptation and, most important, adopting new familial and other social roles while being aware of one's own vulnerability (Kelly, 2009). Men's experience with uncertainty throughout their prostate cancer trajectory was affected by their knowledge about the disease, the disease's stage, and the availability of informal support networks (Nanton et al., 2009). These factors may, in turn, have affected men's desire to survive prostate cancer.

One of older men's primary goals was to understand their illness experiences, an understanding which would enable them to tackle their other primary goal: to regain decisional power over their own bodies and destiny. Guided by hope of surviving prostate cancer, older men decided either to make their journey solitary or collective - experiences shared with family, friends, peers, and strangers. It was between these two extremes of experience with prostate cancer that construction of new social roles, even new social identities, occurred. These new roles and identities preserved the integrity of men's masculine self-images, despite suffering related to loss of sexual functioning.

Men reborn out of collective prostate-cancer journeys distinguished between sharing their own experiences and transmitting information about prostate cancer. They also discerned with which strangers to talk about their experiences of prostate cancer and with which strangers to share its private issues. In contrast, men emerging out of solitary prostate-cancer journeys felt unprotected from the dehumanizing health care system and its professionals. They felt restrained in their freedom to share their cancer experiences with others and believed that silence among men about prostate cancer was natural. Despite these differences in men's preferences for living with prostate cancer, we can identify in the participants' accounts the same underlying rationale. Men's decisions about disclosing their experience with prostate cancer were explained by the intensity of their wishes, as fathers and husbands as well as friends, to protect their loved ones from worry.

4.4 Contributions of this research to the practice of social and health professionals

The research findings described in Section 4 may challenge clinicians' perception that academic education level is the only indicator of patients' ability to understand health information and that less educated patients will be unable to do so. For example,

---

[1] Because none of the research participants was free of prostate cancer, it is beyond the scope of this section to discuss men's perspectives on being free of the disease, feeling safe, or having the disease under control.

sometimes physicians' communication style (e.g., rapid transmission of brief information, underestimating men's capacity to capably make decisions) can push men to adopt a critical, reflective attitude toward the information physicians transmit. In the research described above, this paradox supported older men's determination to educate themselves about prostate cancer and general health. Therefore, social and health professionals should view men's process of becoming prostate cancer literate as a collective, affective, and social process involving other men, women, and other significant others. Medical information about treatment options and their impacts on sexual health is less important to men with prostate cancer than prostate cancer's impacts on men's social identity.

4.5 Reflecting on men's accounts of constructing prostate cancer literacy

In Section 4, we discussed how men construct their prostate cancer literacy throughout the disease process. Below are some accounts to guide readers' reflection about the multiple dimensions of literacy that underpin the process of becoming prostate cancer literate. There are no correct answers to the reflection questions. We hope that reflecting on your own experience as health care professionals will help you answer the questions.

4.5.1 Clinical vignettes

- Michael, a 56-year-old underground miner, was recently diagnosed with prostate cancer. He arrives at an appointment with his oncologist to discuss treatment options. Michael is presented with two options: hormone therapy and orchiectomy. The oncologist discusses the potential outcomes of each of these options. Michael is quite concerned about hormones' possible side effects, such as hot flashes, growth of the mammary glands, and reduction in sexual stamina. Neither option is particularly appealing to Michael. He decides that he needs time to consider the treatment options and discuss them with his wife of 30 years.
- Frank, a 67-year-old retired postal worker, shares with his doctor his experience of participating in a support group for men undergoing prostate cancer treatment. At first he thought this group might be a good source of support as he navigated the often complex world of prostate cancer treatment. After attending a few meetings, however, he discovered that all the men in the support group do is complain. He was also surprised that their complaints were not about discomfort or side effects that they had experienced as a result of their treatments but, instead, about their difficulties getting information and answers to their questions.
- Raymond, a 51-year-old registered nurse, was diagnosed with prostate cancer six months ago. He began hormone therapy two months ago. As a health care professional, his is well acquainted with medication side effects. During a routine follow-up visit with his urologist, Raymond reports that he has been experiencing numerous side effects which he believes are related to the hormone therapy. In addition, and perhaps more concerning, is the fact that his sex drive has severely diminished and he is now experiencing erectile dysfunction. His symptoms are so intense that he finds himself unable to work. He reports that he has been doing some reading on alternative and more natural methods of treatment and wants to discuss discontinuing his hormone therapy. He tells the urologist that his quality of life is so affected by the hormone therapy that he is not willing to continue living like this.

Questions

- What new facilitators for learning can professionals give men, to help them decode prostate cancer information?
- How should professionals incorporate discussion about issues of masculinity when teaching men about modalities of screening, monitoring, treatment, and rehabilitation?
- What are the advantages, for professionals, of learning about how men construct personally relevant meaning from prostate cancer information?
- What innovations should be introduced into prostate-cancer-teaching practices to move from a treatment-focused teaching toward a gender- focused approach?
- Which simple strategies could you create to assess the health literacy of men with prostate cancer in your clinical practice?

5. Health literacy: Impact on survival of the prostate cancer patient, significant others, and clinicians

Health professionals demonstrate growing interest in the functional aspect of health literacy (Oldfield, & Dreher, 2010), despite their concomitant concern about how to assess and deal with it in daily professional practice. According to Peerson and Saunders (2009), "Because health literacy involves knowledge, motivation and activation, it is a complex thing to measure and to influence" (p. 285). Professionals' interest in health literacy focuses on individuals' understanding of health messages, which can enable them to participate more actively in their treatment and be successful in self-management of their illnesses. For years, research on the multiple factors related to health literacy has been guided by several conceptual and theoretical models: information seeking (Bagley-Burnett, 1992; Lenz, 1984), information needs (Derdiarian, 1987), uncertainty in illness (Mishel, 1990), and unaided decisions in health care (Pierce, 1996). Relevant psychological features of information-seeking behavior were explored in some seminal studies. These features are anxiety, resulting in the tendency to attribute responsibility for decision making to others; avoidance or receptivity to learning about one's disease; motivation to seek disease-specific information; and attributing the cause of cancer to fate or personal fault (Lavery & Clarke, 1999; Siegel & Raveis, 1997; Walker et al., 1996). Furthermore, studies have shown that representations of a disease tend to shape individuals' preferences for the type, amount, nature, and use of health information (Fieler et al., 1996; Gollop, 1997a, 1997b; Griffiths & Leek, 1995; Ko et al., 1997; Meischke & Johnson, 1995). Other studies opened new avenues for understanding individuals' preferences for the content of health information: the *how, when, why, who,* and *where* of prognosis, treatments, management, and control of illness (Chalmers et al., 1996; Davison & Degner, 1997; Fieler et al., 1996; Hack et al., 1994; Shaw et al., 1994).

5.1 Health literacy as a survival tool for the patient

If patients' ultimate goal in obtaining health information is to survive, health literacy plays a key role in individuals' sense of self-determination (Zanchetta, & Moura, 2006) and in their ability to deal with illness uncertainty (Zanchetta, 2005). Despite the impressive number of studies related to learning about health issues, few researchers have explored the influences of health learning on individuals' illness experiences within the context of their community life. This learning experience, framed by community features, seems to be particularly critical to older individuals living with cancer, because they report decreased social and community involvement as well as shrinking social networks (Houldin & Wasserbauer, 1996). Cutilli and Bennett (2009) demonstrated that men perform worse than women on health-literacy-assessment tests, due to factors such as education, language, income, information-seeking behavior, and type of health insurance. For older men, such predictors of low performance on health literacy assessments are particularly relevant, because marital status, education, and perceived health status predict health-information seeking (Elder et al., 2010). Low literate individuals tend to have difficulty understanding health information and using the health care system. The reasons for this difficulty include (a) limited comprehension of written and verbal health information, (b) not trusting written health information and preferring to gather health information through personal communication, (c) inability to understand health terms and concepts, (d) insufficient information about the health system, and (e) feelings of shame and embarrassment in revealing their limitations (Health Canada, 1999). The paramount issue, low health literacy, seems to be related to cultural, cognitive, and social aspects of having access to, understanding, and using health information (Oldfield & Dreher, 2010). In particular, low literate individuals who have low levels of numeracy and general knowledge may have difficulty dealing with treatment-related information containing ratios, probabilities, or percentages. Such information, about cures, treatment complications, and/or side effects, is usually given to patients in the contexts of decision making or informed consent. Certainly, one's ability to understand complex health information can either undermine or enhance one's interest in gathering health information.

Studies have also demonstrated that older men consider information on self-management of their diseases too superficial (Walker et al., 1998), especially because of aging-related problems such as cognitive impairment and decrease in vitality. The search for, processing of, incorporation of, and meaning attached to health information seems to be directly affected by older men's level of disease awareness (Morasso et al., 1997), which may decline with cognitive impairment. The nature of prostate cancer treatment demands that health professionals provide clinical education that responds to older men's knowledge deficits and addresses the physical and psychological problems men experience after treatment (Miaskowski, 1999). For example, men who undergo cryosurgical ablation of the prostate may face complications, such as urethrorectal fistulae, bladder-outlet-obstruction incontinence, impotence, and urinary tract infections. Radical prostatectomy may lead to anxiety, bladder spasms, pain, high risk of hemorrhage, and pulmonary embolisms. The complications surrounding external beam radiation include fatigue, diarrhea, and cystitis. Finally, hormone therapy leads to impotence, hot flashes, gynecomastia, and high risk of pathologic fractures (Giddens, 2004). The impact of such complications can affect men's self-image, and dealing with complex medical information can become challenging for older men. To become health literate, they must make sense of health information, find congruency between their past and new knowledge (Craig, 1987), and incorporate health information into their daily lives in a meaningful way.

Interestingly, incorporation of new knowledge about prostate cancer and other medical issues differs according to men's self-reported level of health literacy and unfolds within the multiple, interconnected dimensions of their lives. Zanchetta (2002) showed that health information is incorporated into daily life only if it is congruent with the following factors: men's individual identities; their social trajectories within a specific masculine identity, health-education experience, and life stories; representations of aging, body, cancer/prostate cancer, and health/illness. Table 1 summarizes key definitions of health literacy applicable to learning about prostate cancer in a clinical context.

As consumers of prostate cancer information, men with prostate cancer reveal common strategies for using information (Zanchetta, 2004). Older men tend to perceive prostate cancer as an innocuous disease and react nonchalantly to prostate cancer diagnosis. They usually receive partial information and lack comprehension of clinical conditions and/or the evolutionary stages of prostate cancer. Nonetheless, they enjoy reading, which leads to an interest in reading books about other men's experiences with prostate cancer, the prostate gland, prostate-cancer survival, prognosis, and treatments. They also enjoy learning about principles of chemotherapy, preparation for undergoing chemotherapy and its effects, and modes of adaptation to prostate cancer. They do not believe information displayed in medical pamphlets, due their lack of identification of the pamphlet's authors. Frequently, older men assess their own clinical conditions and the effectiveness of their treatments by tracking changes in their PSA test results. They tend not to seek second opinions from urologists other than their own to either confirm the need for therapy or the quality of scientific evidence in health information. However, men correlate the health information they have with new information they find. Finally, because older men value their physicians' professional competence and trust them, men do not gather health information from other (formal or informal) sources (Zanchetta, 2002).

Conceptual definitions of health literacy – ability to:
Access, read, or listen to; process; and appraise textual, graphic, and numeric health information.
Build new meanings from health information.
Understand health messages and communicate them in users' social environments.
Navigate the health care system.
Use textual, numeric, and graphic health information to inform decision making, reduce health risks, and enhance quality of life.
Use health information to access health care in a medical culture that requires self-defense and health vigilance.
Evaluate and communicate health information to improve one's own and one's family's life.
Solve health problems by using multiple forms of language (written, oral, visual, tactile, etc.), at multiple levels (individual, family, community, world) and in multiple contexts (home, work, school).
Use all family, school, social, cultural, and professional assets gathered through continual learning (formal or informal), through regular contact with information, knowledge, attitudes, and health behaviors in all aspects of life.

Source: Kaszap & Zanchetta (2009)

Table 1. Conceptual definitions of health literacy

Zanchetta (2002) observed, during a community information session with a total of 50 participants (women, and men with and without prostate cancer) about the epidemiological, treatment, and rehabilitation aspects of prostate cancer, that most men's questions were about technical procedures. These questions indicated lack of comprehension, difficulty with basic interpretation of the medical content of health information, and knowledge gaps, and thereby revealed the participants' world of living with prostate cancer. Table 2 gives the questions men asked, in their original form and grouped into themes. In the same study, men's learning needs were raised by two chairmen of a prostate cancer support group, who had compiled the accounts of several other men. The chairmen said that becoming literate about prostate cancer is not a linear, one-dimensional process. According to them, men become aware of their lack of knowledge about prostate cancer and motivated to seek information about it for the following reasons: (a) acknowledgment that, for men, ageing is usually accompanied by prostate problems, (b) symptoms of excessive prostate enlargement launch information seeking about early signs/symptoms of prostate cancer, (c) men's new awareness of their vulnerability to disease after receiving a prostate cancer diagnosis, (d) receiving information about treatment side effects and their impacts on men's lives, (e) men's perception and experience of treatment and its side-effects, (f) recurrence of prostate problems after treatment, and (g) psychological and social impacts of treatment of prostate cancer.

Theme	Questions
Epidemiology	Why do the rates of prostate cancer increase? What are the environmental risk factors? Are the risk factors presented in the slides in conformity with their degree of importance? Is there something that one can do about the family risks factors? What is the most dangerous type of cancer? Rectal, bladder, or prostate?
Screening procedures	When must one begin PSA testing? What do you recommend as preventive action? After what age must one have an examination? After the age of 50, what is the suggested interval between examinations?
Causes	Is there any link with stress? Does drinking alcoholic beverage cause prostate cancer? Does bleeding during the biopsy transmit cancer? Is it true that sitting for long periods may cause prostate cancer? Could a vasectomy cause prostate cancer? Could hormone therapy cause prostate cancer?
Knowledge issues	What is serum testosterone? Is there another type of testosterone? What is its source of production? What does a gland full of granulomatosis mean? What are the meanings of the letters and degrees used to classify cancer?

Theme	Questions
Diagnostic procedures	Can a prostate cancer diagnosis be made using a blood test? If the cancer is in its beginning stage, can a biopsy indicate its presence?
Self-assessment	Does prostate irritation mean prostate cancer? Does the presence of blood in the sperm indicate prostate cancer?
Technical procedures	What does a rectal examination indicate? What justifies the removal of the testes? Does an examination exist that allows us to see the whole prostate? During a rectal examination, does the physician feel just a part of the prostate? Can a physician identify prostate cancer simply by looking at the prostate? How can one see the prostate with an echography? How is the result of an echography analyzed with the PSA? What can one do after having lymph nodes removed? Is radiation therapy applied through the rectum? Is chemotherapy as efficient as surgery? What is the likelihood of bleeding after radiation therapy?
Interpretation of PSA titration levels	What are the normal limits of the PSA test? Does the PSA have another type of utility? Could it indicate another type of disease?

Table 2. Scope of men's questions about prostate cancer

Men may also learn about prostate cancer through the collective experience offered in prostate cancer support groups. In these support groups, men learn from each other as well as from invited speakers; exchange information and experience; offer and obtain mutual help, advice, and support; and advocate for their rights as health consumers and citizens. Despite these multiple opportunities, some men still believe that other men come together in prostate cancer support groups to complain and cry "like a woman" (F. S. and W. K., personal communication, Kingston, Canada, March 2004). Such a misconception may explain why men from ethnic minorities tend not to enrol in prostate cancer support groups and why some men only attend them after treatment, despite their physicians' recommendations or referrals. In other cases, doctors referred men to prostate cancer support groups after treatment, which may imply that these men decided on treatments with only partial knowledge of their consequences and later regretted their decisions (D. G., personal communication, Montreal, Canada, June 2001).

Other ethno-cultural influences also influenced study participants' behavior related to prostate cancer. First, most of the Caucasian men (who self-identified as being of European descent) were socially expected to keep silent about disease and any suffering. Second, their mothers taught them to promote their own health and take preventive action against diseases, mainly through nutrition (Zanchetta et al., 2004). Given such expectations of stoic silence, men need professional mentoring and assistance to acknowledge that time is required to deal effectively with the diagnosis of prostate cancer, adequately comprehend medical information, consider available alternatives, and reflect on the potential outcomes of their decisions. Such an investment of time will ultimately generate a greater sense of control over men's life choices and a greater degree of normalcy in their lives.

5.2 Impact of men's prostate cancer literacy on their significant others

The impact of a prostate cancer diagnosis on couple and family dynamics is frequently reported in the scientific literature. However, other than shared stress, other experiences of men's significant others with prostate cancer information remain poorly explored. Men themselves report feeling embarrassed in revealing to their wives that prostate-biopsy results confirm their urologists' suspicion of prostate cancer (Zanchetta, 2004). Another gap in the literature concerns partners' unidentified or unmet information needs (Sinfield et al., 2008). For partners, becoming prostate-cancer literate would facilitate their participation in decision making as well as collaboration in all stages of treatment - as information gatherers, care providers, promoters of adherence with treatments, and even advocates for health and social services. As most of partners of men with prostate cancer are women, likely also elderly and living with their own diseases, we can expect that men's partners are knowledgeable consumers of health services who are able to sustain their partners' struggles to learn about prostate cancer. Because close interpersonal relationships influence illness experiences and transform the solitary cancer journey into a joint experience (Illingworth et al., 2010), partners can discover, learn about, and transcend limitations to redefining the meaning of prostate cancer.

Another impact of prostate cancer literacy is men's decision to share their illness experiences with their sons. This decision relates to genetic predisposition to cancer, early detection, and screening procedures (Zanchetta, 2002, 2004). However, a "code of silence between men" can prevent disclosure of diagnosis. In Zanchetta's (2002) study, decision to inform sons and sons was explained from two opposite perspectives. Fathers who shared their illness experiences with their sons did so because of feelings of fatherhood and its perceived inherent responsibilities, and a concomitant desire to protect their sons. These fathers were concerned about the possibility of another case of prostate cancer in the family, felt confident in talking about prostate cancer, valued talking about illness experience to improve their own well-being, and perceived themselves as being open minded. Fathers who did not share their illness experiences with their sons felt unable to discuss parental subjects with their children, did not want to upset their sons with the daily problems caused by prostate cancer, felt that their sons were not concerned about prostate cancer, and had difficulty revealing personal experiences that provoked feelings of frustration and regret.

5.3 Surviving multiple professional challenges to sustain men's prostate cancer literacy

Health professionals utilize evidence-based practice to bridge the theory–practice gap and to guide patient care with the best available evidence (Paley et al., 2007). The goal of health and social professionals in the prostate cancer care continuum (screening, detection/diagnosis, treatment, rehabilitation) is to provide instrumental care and information that combines effective medical and social science with optimal technology, allied to a humanistic approach. However, to provide services that respond to the specific needs of men, according to the World Health Organization (2002), professionals need to acknowledge gender-specific roles and biological distinctions as well as differences among men in needs, power, access to resources, obstacles, and opportunities. Gender equity is needed in the delivery of health services to overcome the structural oppression that grants women access to a humanist approach in health care relationships, but denies men access to the same humanist approach. Zanchetta et al. (2010), in discussing the role of health and social professionals in supporting men's preventative prostate health behaviors, warn that "men today also define their relationships according to trustworthiness. For this reason, professionals should learn how to build trusting relationships with men, to facilitate a new men's culture of seeking preventive care for diseases that threaten men's self-identity" (p. 266). Although Kelly (2009) found that health professionals acknowledge the need to establish trusting relationships with men and aim to overcome communication barriers with them, men in the same study reported that not being taught to deal with physical changes after undergoing prostate cancer treatment led them to feel betrayed by the health care system.

Prostate cancer can significantly impact every aspect of a man's life. Jonsson et al. (2009) conclude that men with prostate cancer "are placed in a new life situation, against their will" (p. 273). These patients move through their illness experience with feelings of fear and uncertainty. Although scientific advances continue to enhance preventative, screening, diagnosis and treatment options, patients continue to experience the prostate cancer journey as separate silos of care. Patient-centered care is one approach that could reconnect these silos into a care continuum. Patient-centered care, which has gained momentum in the last two decades, is an approach to providing health care in which the patient is the focal point. According to the Picker Institute (2011), the eight guiding principles of professional practice in organizations committed to patient-centered care are (a) respect for patients' values, preferences, and expressed needs, (b) coordination and integration of care, (c) information, communication, and education, (d) physical comfort, (e) emotional support and alleviation of fear and anxiety, (f) involvement of family and friends, (g) continuity and transition, and (h) access to care.

The application of these principles coexists with challenges that professionals may face to satisfactorily implementing patient-centered care to ultimately sustain men's prostate cancer literacy. The first challenge is the unresponsiveness of professional practice to the needs of male patients. Despite the patient centered-care movement, patients are continually *cared for* not *cared with;* for instance, professionals present patients with complex treatment options, seeking yes or no decisions about life-changing, high-risk treatments but allowing little time for men to reflect, learn about, and discuss options. Professionals who provide direct care, such as nurses, are faced with the difficult choice of dividing their time among a complex array of institutional demands. These other priorities ultimately result in less time for teaching their patients about health. Professionals are driven by their technical expertise, leading to the transfer of knowledge from 'expert health care professional' to 'patient'. Is this prevalent practice effective? Does men's motivation to seek care rest on the attainment of 'patient knowledge'? Or does their need to survive underpin all the other tasks that men living with prostate cancer must undergo? Ethnic-minority men are less likely than Caucasians to share health information with care providers that they obtained elsewhere. Those whose first languages are not

English tend to complain about disrespect and racial discrimination and are thus less likely than Caucasians to advocate for tests and treatments (Elder et al., 2010). Older men with co-morbidities do not extensively seek information on prostate cancer and its treatment, relying more on the technical expertise of health professionals (Nanton et al., 2009). How do health professionals deal with all these simultaneous and synergistic factors?

The second challenge is twofold: first, it concerns the complexity of the health teaching needed for men to become partners in their care; second, it concerns the similarly complex health teaching needed for men to become decision-making partners. A prostate cancer diagnosis may give a man the opportunity to revisit his life priorities and to learn more about health and how to face health threats (Mishel et al., 2002). For this reason, promotion of health literacy goes beyond simple provision of information; instead, men's lived experience must be taken into account to facilitate their discovery of health information within their unique masculine contexts of living, learning, and applying knowledge. Throughout the prostate cancer trajectory, health education will offer men reassurance, knowledge, and understanding about how to balance the changes they are expected to face.

For prostate cancer screening, Gaster et al. (2010) suggest an "Ask-Tell-Ask" approach that fosters open, interactive dialog between health professionals and men. *Ask* initiates discussion that enables the health professional to explore a man's need for information; *Tell* provides a patient-focused response by the health professional, tailoring information to the patient's needs; and *Ask* allows for reflection and summation of the dialog. This approach facilitates therapeutic interaction between health professional and patient, actively focusing on the patient's own perspective and situation. It enables the patient to move beyond receiving the information toward understanding, internalizing, reflecting, and ultimately, discovering prostate-cancer-care information as it intertwines with sense of himself as a person. No matter what the presentation tool (simple paper or Web-based decision-making aid), the Ask-Tell-Ask approach engages men in learning about prostate cancer screening and making decisions about it (Krist et al., 2007).

Application of patient-centered care to prostate cancer promotes reciprocation and interactivity, allowing patients to be active partners with health professionals in the delivery of care. The one-way, linear communication in traditional prostate cancer care is less effective in engaging men with their own care (Gaster et al., 2010). Individualized teaching may better satisfy men's knowledge needs. Feldman-Stewart et al. (2009) found that men most often asked questions about treatment: first, because of their need to understand and, second, because of their desire to make decisions and plan. Even if men living with prostate cancer did want a lot of information, the amount of and details of information they asked for varied enormously, due to personal reasons. For example, with recent technological advances in the treatment of prostate cancer, men have the opportunity to consider various treatment options. Open prostatectomy procedures can now be performed by surgeons with success rates similar to those with laparascopic or robot-assisted prostatectomy (Lallas & Trabulsi, 2010). Despite these options, patients' feelings of vulnerability when facing complex information about treatment options can be overpowering. Health professionals ask men with prostate cancer to make life-altering decisions about complex, high-risk treatments they know little about. Men are expected to reduce their experience of prostate cancer to a simple *yes* or *no* consent to treatments. When health professionals focus only on outcomes of the procedures, they leave behind the process by which the outcomes are achieved. In contrast, men not only focus on the outcomes of care, but more important to them, the process of care (Jayadevappa et al., 2010). The way that health professionals deliver prostate cancer care can significantly influence men's active engagement in their care (Martinez et al., 2009). Knowledge of disease progression and response to treatments is key for men living with advanced or recurrent prostate cancer, because they need instrumental knowledge to deal with uncertainty about how long their bodies will be able to respond to therapies (Nanton et al., 2009).

Being a partner in care means being a decision maker. Stacey et al. (2010) report that men want more opportunity to decide than they are allowed. Their vehemence remains unchanged if they are not offered decision aids or the opportunity to discuss the details of treatment with health professionals. This vehemence applies equally to the informed consent process, which usually requires more in-depth information and clearer explanations to support men's understanding. Moreover, men want more information on potential harms of therapies, since health professionals tend to present more often the benefits. As discussed in Section 5.2, men's partners should be considered in the process of decision-making. To include men's partners, Illingworth et al. (2010) propose that health professionals talk to men about their significant others and all spheres of their lives. These authors emphasize the central role of men's interpersonal relationships in their experiences with prostate cancer.

Finally, the last challenge for professionals relates to collaboration within their own professions and with other health and social professions. It is known that limited professional links between family physicians and urologists erect structural barriers for health care delivery to older men (Greene & Adelman, 2003). It is beyond the scope of this section to suggest that other members of multidisciplinary cancer-care teams change their practice, due to ethical principles. However, we would like to highlight that Zanchetta (2004), at the time an oncology nurse interested in health literacy, made some recommendations to nurses to counteract misconceptions about older men's health literacy. These recommendations may inspire other professionals. Aiming to awake and enhance nurses' awareness of their opportunity, and responsibility, to expand professional knowledge about men's health literacy, Zanchetta (2004) recommended that nurses (a) be aware that functional health literacy is a result of a broad, socially constructed process, rather than a set of abilities comprising reading, counting, and recognition of words, (b) be particularly attentive to the nature and extension of individual men's social networks, (c) encourage men to collaborate with nurses in creating educational materials, (d) invite physicians to co-create educational materials that respond to knowledge gaps and misunderstandings about prostate cancer, (e) redesign, with men, innovative strategies to communicate others' experiences with cancer, and (f) record their clinical observations of the differences among men's information behaviors.

Enhancing the quality of prostate cancer care involves more than advances in science and technology. It requires engaging patients in treatment-related decisions and fostering a health care environment that facilitates health literacy among patients. The patient-centered care approach enables health care professionals to focus on patients as well as their significant others, as they journey through the prostate cancer trajectory. Engaging patients through patient-centered care allows their collaboration with health care professionals to fulfil the goal of *caring with the patient*.

5.4 Reflecting on the complexity of patient-centred care and survival in prostate cancer

Our aim in the following exercise is to present some insights into the complexity of patient centred care and men's experience of prostate cancer literacy as a survival tool. While reading each clinical vignette, we suggest that readers consider how difficult it is for men to decode medical information in order to make decisions, as well as how challenging it is for professionals to promote men's health and prostate-cancer literacy.

5.4.1 Clinical vignettes

- Juan, a 49-year-old elementary school teacher, comes into the clinic for a follow-up appointment with his urologist/oncologist after undergoing a prostatectomy and radiation therapy. He has been having his PSA level monitored regularly since he was diagnosed and underwent surgery and treatment. Juan's doctor tells him that his PSA level remains unchanged following radiation therapy and that they will continue to monitor it over time. Juan is not satisfied with this report and wants the doctor to tell him conclusively whether his cancer is cured. The doctor responds that time will tell.
- Hassan, a 55-year-old car salesman, is diagnosed with prostate cancer. His urologist discusses possible treatment options, including surgery and radiation. Hassan was recently remarried, to a much younger woman, and explains that their sex life is quite active. They have been discussing the possibility of having a baby. Hassan is concerned that prostate-cancer treatment could lead to erectile dysfunction, which could end his happy, active sex life. He is unwilling to take a chance that his sex life will be affected and that he could jeopardize his chance of having a baby with his new wife.
- Roberto, a 45 year-old Crown attorney, receives a diagnosis of prostate cancer. He is devastated. His father died of advanced prostate cancer at the age of 55. Roberto reports that he has a strong faith in God and that he plans on praying for a miracle. He refuses any and all treatment that is offered to him, because he believes that, through prayer, he will be healed. Roberto's physician attempts to convince him that, if he refuses treatment, he risks the same outcome as his father. The physician tells Roberto that, because he is a young man and the cancer was detected early, the outcome could be favorable if he considers treatment.

5.4.2 Reflection questions

- What factors contribute to men's difficulty in understanding prostate cancer information and utilizing the health care system?
- What impact can men's experience of prostate cancer have on significant others, and how can that impact be attenuated by new professional attitudes and practices?
- What changes in professional practice relating to prostate cancer literary will acknowledge the importance of different perceptions of masculinity?
- How could education, social, and health professionals collaborate to develop age- and gender-appropriate, sensitive educational tools?
- How do you foresee education about prostate cancer focusing on aspects of men's lives other than sexuality?

6. Conclusion

In this chapter, we presented a multidisciplinary view of men's health literacy in prostate cancer, drawing from the disciplines of medical anthropology, education, and nursing. We intended to expand readers' vision of health literacy beyond measurable personal skills toward a view of health literacy as a personal asset that individuals build throughout social interactions within the multiples spheres of their lives. We also intended to portray men's experience of prostate cancer as an experience that goes beyond failures and improvement in sexual performance to a much broader and more significant masculine experience. Health literacy for older men with prostate cancer can preserve their moral integrity, social identity, and self-perception of masculinity. Health education for men with prostate cancer should expand their awareness of health challenges, guide them in correctly interpreting prostate cancer information, and create new ways of enjoying life after prostate cancer. Uncertainties, challenges, and doubts are shared with significant others, who may also have difficulty talking openly about the impacts of prostate cancer, present and future, on the men they love and care for. For this reason, significant others should also be educated about prostate cancer. To create collaboration among men, health educators, social and health professionals, and significant others to improve men's prostate cancer literacy, it will be necessary to redesign current communication approaches. Communication needs to be innovative, creative, and sensitive to men's social networks, age, cultures, general literacy, and, of course, gender. Men differ in the way they understand and live their own masculinity. Not all men are equally health literate; health literacy depends on the collective project of health education. The kind of prostate cancer literacy that we envision is one that will liberate men from any sense of powerlessness and hopelessness, enabling men to transcend any limitations imposed by prostate cancer.

7. Acknowledgements

We acknowledge Yasmin Taher and Mohamed Mohamed for their support as research assistants and Ms Margaret Oldfield for editing the manuscript's text.
Funding: Faculty of Community Services Publications Grant, Ryerson University and Faculté des sciences d'éducation, Université Laval.

8. References

Alpay, L. L.; Toussaint, P. J.; Ezendam, N. P. M.; Rovekamp, T. J. M.; Graafmans, W. C. & Westendorp, R. G. J. (2004). Easing Internet Access of Health Information for Elderly Users. *Health Informatics Journal.* Vol.10, No.3, (September), pp. 185-194, ISSN 1741-2811

Almeida, M. V. de (1996). *The Hegemonic Male: Masculinity in a Portuguese Town,* Berghahn Books, ISBN 157181891X, London, United Kingdom

Bagley-Burnett, C. (1992). Measuring Information-seeking Behaviors. In: *Instrumental for Clinical Nursing Research,* M. Frank-Stromborg (Ed.), 151-169, Jones & Bartlett, ISBN 0867203404, Norwalk, Connecticut. United States

Barry, M. J. (2010). Shared Decision Making Supported by Patient Decision Aids for Prostate Cancer Screening and Treatment. *Psicooncología,* vol.7, No 2-3, pp. 257-267, ISSN 16967240

Barton, D.; Hamilton, M. & Ivanic, R. (2000). *Situated Literacies: Reading and Writing in Context*, Routledge, ISBN 0-415-20670-7, London, United Kingdom

Barton, D. & Hamilton, M. (1998). *Local Literacies: Reading and Writing in One Community*. Routledge, ISBN 0-415-17150-4, London, United Kingdom

Bergsma, L. J. (2004). Empowerment education: The Link Between Media Literacy and Health Promotion. *American Behavioral Scientist*, Vol.48, No.2, (October), pp. 152-164, ISSN 1552-3381

Boudon, P. (2000). Entre Rhétorique et Dialectique: La Constitution des Figures d'argumentation [Between Rhetoric and Dialetic: The Constitution of the Figures of Argumentation]. *Langages*, Vol. 34, No.137, pp. 63-86, ISSN 0458-726X

Boudon, P. (1999). *Le Réseau du Sens: Une Approche Monadologique pour la Compréhension du Discours* [The Network of Meaning: An Approach to Understanding the Monadological Discourse] Allemagne: Éditions scientifiques européennes, Peter Lang, ISBN 3906761959, Bern, Switzerland

Boudon, P. (1998). L'abduction et le Champ Sémiotique. Le Tiers Communicationnel, 255-284, Harmattan, Montréal, Canada

Bourdieu, P. (1977). *Outline of a Theory of Practice*, Cambridge University Press, ISBN 0 521 29164, Cambridge, United Kingdom

Bourdieu, P. (2001). *Masculine Domination*, Stanford University Press, ISBN 0-8047-3818-1, Stanford, United States

Brown, P.; Ames, N.; Mettger, W.; Smith, T. J.; Gramarossa, G. L.; Friedell, G. H.; & McDonald, S. S. (1993). Closing the Comprehension Gap: Low Literacy and the Cancer Information Service. *Journal of the National Cancer Institute*. Monographs. Vol. 14, (November), pp. 157-163, ISSN 1052-6773

Buston, K. M. & Wood, S. F. (2000). Non-Compliance amongst Adolescents with Asthma: Listening to What They Tell Us about Self-Management, *Family Practice*, Vol.17, No.2, (April), pp. 134-138, ISSN 0263-2136

Butler, J. (1990) *Gender Trouble: Feminism and the Subversion of Identity*, Routledge, ISBN 0415900425, New York, United States

Barry, M. J. (2010). Shared Decision Making Supported by Patient Decision Aids for Prostate Cancer Screening and Treatment. *Psicooncología*, vol.7, No 2-3, pp. 257-267, ISSN 16967240

Barton, D.; Hamilton, M. & Ivanic, R. (2000). *Situated Literacies: Reading and Writing in Context*, Routledge, ISBN 0-415-20670-7, London, United Kingdom

Barton, D. & Hamilton, M. (1998). *Local Literacies: Reading and Writing in One Community*. Routledge, ISBN 0-415-17150-4, London, United Kingdom

Bergsma, L. J. (2004). Empowerment education: The Link Between Media Literacy and Health Promotion. *American Behavioral Scientist*, Vol.48, No.2, (October), pp. 152-164, ISSN 1552-3381

Boudon, P. (2000). Entre Rhétorique et Dialectique: La Constitution des Figures d'argumentation [Between Rhetoric and Dialetic: The Constitution of the Figures of Argumentation]. *Langages*, Vol. 34, No.137, pp. 63-86, ISSN 0458-726X

Boudon, P. (1999). *Le Réseau du Sens: Une Approche Monadologique pour la Compréhension du Discours* [The Network of Meaning: An Approach to Understanding the

Monadological Discourse] Allemagne: Éditions scientifiques européennes, Peter Lang, ISBN 3906761959, Bern, Switzerland

Boudon, P. (1998). L'abduction et le Champ Sémiotique. Le Tiers Communicationnel, 255-284, Harmattan, Montréal, Canada

Bourdieu, P. (1977). *Outline of a Theory of Practice*, Cambridge University Press, ISBN 0 521 29164, Cambridge, United Kingdom

Bourdieu, P. (2001). *Masculine Domination*, Stanford University Press, ISBN 0-8047-3818-1, Stanford, United States

Brown, P.; Ames, N.; Mettger, W.; Smith, T. J.; Gramarossa, G. L.; Friedell, G. H.; & McDonald, S. S. (1993). Closing the Comprehension Gap: Low Literacy and the Cancer Information Service. *Journal of the National Cancer Institute*. Monographs. Vol. 14, (November), pp. 157-163, ISSN 1052-6773

Buston, K. M. & Wood, S. F. (2000). Non-Compliance amongst Adolescents with Asthma: Listening to What They Tell Us about Self-Management, *Family Practice*, Vol.17, No.2, (April), pp. 134-138, ISSN 0263-2136

Butler, J. (1990) *Gender Trouble: Feminism and the Subversion of Identity*, Routledge, ISBN 0415900425, New York, United States

Carrigan, T.; Connel, R. & Lee, J. (1985). Towards a New Sociology of Masculinity. *Theory and Society*,Vol.14, No.5, (November), pp. 551-604, ISSN 0304-2421

Chalmers, K.; Thomson, K. & Degner, L. F. (1996). Information, Support, and Communication Needs of Women with a Family History of Cancer. *Cancer Nursing*, Vol.19, No.3, (June), pp. 204-213, ISSN 0162-220X

Channel, D. F. (1991) *The Vital Machine: A Study of Technology and Organic Life*, Oxford University Press, ISBN 0195060407, New York, United States

Chapple, A. & Ziebland, S. (2002). Prostate Cancer: Embodied Experience and Perceptions of Masculinity. *Sociology of Health and Illness*, Vol.24, No.6, (October), pp. 820-841, ISSN 0141-9889

Chung, C. H.; Bernard, P. S. & Perou, C.M. (2002). Molecular Portraits and the Family Tree of Cancer. *Nature Genetics*, Vol.32, (December), Supp:533-540, ISSN 1061-4036

Clarke, A. E.; Shim, J. K.; Mamo, L.; Forsket, J. R. & Fishman, J. R. (2003). Biomedicalization: Technoscientific Transformations of Health, Illness and U.S. Biomedicine. *American Sociological Review*, Vol.68, No.2, (April), pp. 161-194, ISSN 0003-1224

Cutilli, C. C. & Bennett, I. M. (2009). Understanding the Health Literacy of America: Results of the National Assessment of Adult Literacy. *Orthopaedic Nursing*, Vol.28, No.1, (January-February), pp. 27-32, ISSN 0744-6020

Connell, R. (1995). *Masculinities*, University of California Press, ISBN 0520089995, Berkeley, United States

Connel, R. W. & Messerschmidt, J. W. (2005) Hegemonic Masculinity: Rethinking the Concept. *Gender and Society*, Vol.19, No.6, (December), pp. 829-859, ISSN 1552-3977

Connor, A.; Layne, L. & Thomisee, K. (2010). Providing Care for Migrant Farm Worker Families in Their Unique Sociocultural Context and Environment. *Journal of Transcultural Nursing*, Vol.21, No.2, (April), pp. 159-166, ISSN 1552-7832

Cornwall, A. & Lindisfarne, N. (1994) (Eds.). *Dislocating Masculinity: Gender, Power and Anthropology*, Routledge, ISBN 0-203-39343-0, London, United Kingdom

Courtenay, W. (2000). Constructions of Masculinity and Their Infuence on Men's Well-Being: A Theory of Gender and Health. *Social Science and Medicine,* Vol.50, No.10, (May), pp. 1385-1401, ISSN 0277-9536

Craig, L. L. (1987). *Characteristics of Older Men and Their Ability to Comprehend Printed Health Education Materials.* Unpublished doctoral dissertation. University of Alabama at Birmingham, Birmingham

Davis, T. C.; Crouch, M. A.; Long, S. W.; Jackson, R. H.; Bates, P.; George, R. B. & Bairnsfather, L. E. (1991). Rapid Assessment of Literacy Levels of Adult Primary Care Patients. *Family Medicine.* Vol. 23, No.6, (August), pp. 433-435, ISSN 0742-3225

Davis, T. C.; Williams, M. V.; Marin, E.; Parker, R. M. & Glass, J. (2008). Health Literacy and Cancer Communication. *Cancer Journal for Clinicians,* Vol.52, No.3, (May-June), pp. 134-149, ISSN 0007-9235

Davison, J. & Degner, L. F. (1997). Empowerment of Men Newly Diagnosed with Prostate Cancer. *Cancer Nursing,* Vol.20, No.3, (June), pp. 187-196, ISSN 0162-220X

Derdiarian, A. (1987). Informational Needs of Recently Diagnosed Cancer Patients: A Theoretical Framework. Part I. *Cancer Nursing,* Vol.10, No.2, (April), pp. 107-115, ISSN 0162-220X.

Deslauriers, J.-P. & Deslauriers, J.-M. (2010). La Recherche Auprès des Hommes: Défis et Enjeux. [Research with Men: Challenges and Issues] In: *Regards Sur les Hommes et les Masculinités: Comprendre et Intervenir,* [Vision about Men and Masculinities: Understanding and Intervention], J.-M. Deslauriers, G. Tremblay, S. G. Dufault, D. Blanchette & J.-Y Desgagnés, 153-172, Les Presses de l'Université Laval, ISBN 978-2-7637-8954-5, Québec, Canada

Easton, P.; Entwistle, V. A. & Williams, B. (2010). Health in the 'Hidden Population' of People with Low Literacy: A Systematic Review of the Literature. *BMC Public Health,* Vol.10, (August), pp. 459-468, ISSN 1471-2458

Elder, K. T.; Wilshier, J. C.; McRoy, L.; Campbell, D.; Gary, L. C. & Safford, M. (2010). Men and Differences by Racial/Ethnic Group in Self Advocacy during the Medical Encounter. *Journal of Men's Health,* Vol.7, No.2, (June), pp. 135-144, ISSN 1875-6867

Feldman-Stewart, D.; Brennenstuhl, S.; Brundage, M. D. & Siemens, D. R. (2009). Overall Information Needs of Early-Stage Prostate Cancer Patients over a Decade: Highly Variable and Remarkably Stable. *Support Care Cancer,* Vol.17, No.4, (April), pp. 429-435, ISSN 1433-7339

Fieler, V. K.; Wlasowicz, G. S.; Mitchell, M. L.; Jones, L. S. & Johnson, J. E. (1996). Information Preferences of Patients Undergoing Radiation Therapy. *Oncology Nursing Forum,* Vol. 23, No.10. pp.1603-1608. ISSN 0190-535X

Francis, C. K. (1991). Hypertension, Cardiac Disease, and Compliance in Minority Patients. *The American Journal of Medecine.* Vol. 91, No.1A, (July), pp. 29S-36S, ISSN 0002-9343

Fujimura, J. (1996) *Crafting Science: A Sociohistory of the Quest for the Genetics of Cancer* Harvard University Press, ISBN 0 674 15553 0, Cambridge, United Kingdom

Fullwiley, D. (2007). The Molecularization of Race: Institutionalizing Human Difference in Pharmacogenetics Practice. *Science as Culture*, Vol.16, No.1, (March), pp. 1-30, ISSN 0950-5431

Gaster, B.; Edwards, K.; Trinidad, S. B.; Gallagher, T. H. & Braddock, C. H. (2010). Patient-Centred Discussions about Prostate Cancer Screening: A Real World Approach. *Annals of Internal Medicine,* Vol.123, No.10, (November), pp. 661-667, ISSN 1539-3704

Giddens, J. F. (2004). Nursing Management-Male Reproductive Problems. In: *Medical-Surgical Nursing: Assessment and Management of Clinical Problems*, S. M. Lewis, M. M. Heitkemper, & S. R. Dirksen, (6th Ed.), 1435-1462, Mosby, ISBN 9780323036900, St. Louis, Missouri, United States

Gil-Gómez, J. A.; Lloréns, R.; Alcañiz, M. & Colomer, C. (2011). Effectiveness of a Wii Balance Board-Based System (eBaViR) for Balance Rehabilitation: A Pilot Randomized Clinical Trial in Patients with Acquired Brain Injury. *Journal of Neuroengineering and Rehabilitation*, Vol.8, No.1, (May), pp. 30. Available from http://www.jneuroengrehab.com/content/8/1/30SSN 1743-0003

Gilmore, D. (1990). *Manhood in the Making: Cultural Concepts of Masculinity,* Yale University Press, ISBN 9780300050769, New Haven, United States

Golding, B. G. (2011). Social, Local, and Situated: Recent Findings about the Effectiveness of Older Men's Informal Learning in Community Contexts. *Adult Education Quarterly,* Vol.20, No.10, (May), pp. 1–18, ISSN 1552-3047

Gollop, C. J. (1997a). Health Information-Seeking Behavior and Older African American Women. *Bulletin of the Medical Library Association*, Vol.85, No.2, (April), pp. 141-146, ISSN 0025-7338

Gollop, C. J. (1997b). Where Have All the Nice Old Ladies Gone? Researching the Health Information-Seeking Behavior of Older African American Women. In: *Oral Narrative Research with Black Women,* K. M. Vaz (Ed.), 143-155, Sage, ISBN 9780803974296, Thousand Oaks, California, United States

Greene, M. G. & Adelman, R. D. (2003). Physician-Older Patient Communication about Cancer. *Patient Education Counselling,* Vol.50, No.1, (May), pp. 55-60, ISSN 0738-3991

Griffiths, M. & Leek, C. (1995). Patient Education Needs: Opinions of Oncology Nurses and Their Patients. *Oncology Nursing Forum,* Vol.22, No.1, (January-February), pp. 139-144, ISSN 0190-535X

Gwede, C. K. & McDermott, R. J. (2006). Prostate Cancer Screening Decision Making Under Controversy: Implications for Health Promotion Practice. *Health Promotion Practice,* Vol.7, No.1, (January), pp. 134-146, ISSN 1524-8399

Hack, T. F.; Degner, L. F. & Dyck, D. G. (1994). Relationship Between Preferences for Decisional Control and Illness Information among Women with Breast Cancer: A Quantitative and Qualitative Analysis. *Social Science & Medicine,* Vol.39, No.2, (July), pp. 279-289, ISSN 0277-9536

Health Canada (March 24, 1999). Literacy French- Profile. Available: http: //www.hc-sc.gv.ca/hppb/developpement-promotion/pubf/literacy-health/literacyfr2.htm

Hedgecoe, A. (2002). Reinventing diabetes: Classification, Division and the Geneticization of Disease. *New Genetics and Society*, Vol.21, No. (August), pp. 7-27, ISSN 1469-9915

Hogle, L. F. (2005). Enhancement Technologies and the Body. *Annual Review of Anthropology*, Vol.34, (October), pp. 695-716, ISSN 0084-6570

Houldin, A. D. & Wasserbauer, N. (1996). Psychosocial Needs of Older Cancer Patients: A Pilot Study. *MEDSURG Nursing*, Vol.5, No. 4, (August), pp. 253-256, ISSN 1092-0811

Illingworth, N.; Forbat, L.; Hubbard, G. & Kearney, N. (2010). The Importance of Relationships in the Experience of Cancer: A Re-working of the Policy Ideal of the Whole-Systems Approach. *European Journal of Oncology Nursing*, Vol.14, No.1, (February), pp. 23-28, ISSN 1532-2122

Jayadevappa, R.; Schwartz, S.; Chatre, S.; Wein, A. J. & Malkowicz, S. B. (2010). Satisfaction with Care: A Measure of Quality of Care in Prostate Cancer Patients. *Medical Decision Making*, Vol.30, No.2, (March-April), pp. 234-245, ISSN 1552-681X

Jensen, J. D.; King, A. J.; Davis, L. A. & Guntzviller, L. M. (2010). Utilization of Internet Technology by Low-Income Adults: The Role of Health Literacy, Health Numeracy, and Computer Assistance. *Journal of Aging and Health*, Vol.22, No.6, (September), pp. 804-826, ISSN 1552-6887

Jonsson, A.; Aus, G. & Bertero, C. (2009). Men's Experience of Their Life Situation when Diagnosed with Advanced Prostate Cancer. *European Journal of Oncology Nursing*, Vol.13, No.4, (September), pp. 268-273, ISSN 1532-2122

Jonnaert, P. (2009) *Créer des Conditions D'apprentissage: Un Cadre de Rréférence Socio-constructiviste pour une Formation Didactique des Enseignants*. [Create Conditions for Learning: A Socio-constructivist Framework for a Pedagogical Education of Teachers], De Boeck, ISBN 2804131548, Bruxelles, Belgium

Kaszap, M.; Viens, C.; Fortin, J. Ajar, D.; Ollivier, É. & Vandal, S. (2000). Rapport de Recherche. *Besoins D'éducation à la Santé Chez une Clientèle Âgée Peu Alphabétisée Atteinte de Maladies Cardio-vasculaires: Une Étude Exploratoire*. [Research Report. Health Education Needs of Low Literate Seniors Living with Cardiovascular Diseases: An Exploratory Study], Groupe de recherche Alpha-santé Éditeur, ISBN 2-98069 19-0-9, Québec, Canada

Kaszap, M.; Viens, C.; Ajar, D.; Ollivier, É.; Leclerc, L.-P. & Bah, Y. M. (2002). Rapport de Recherche. *Évaluation de L'applicabilité des Nouvelles Technologies de L'information et de la Communication dans le Domaine de L'éducation à la Santé des Adultes Peu Alphabétisés Atteints de Maladies Cardio-vasculaires*. [Research Report. Evaluation of the Applicability of New Information and Communication Technology for Health Education of Low Literate Seniors Living with Cardiovascular Diseases], Groupe de recherche Alpha-santé Éditeur, ISBN 2-9806919-1-7, Québec, Canada

Kaszap, M. (2006). Understanding Low Literate Elderly's Health Decisions by Recording Their Misconceptions and Metaphors. *Proceedings of the 12th Qualitative Health Conference*, p. 75, Edmonton, Alberta, Canada, April 2-5, 2006

Kaszap, M.; Drolet, M. & Gagné, I. (2008). Formation des Professionnels de la Santé et des Intervenants Communautaires à L'épistémologie de la Littératie en Santé des Personnes Âgées; Une Approche Socioconstructiviste Basée sur la Chronologie

Iconographique Thématique. [Education of Health Professionals and Community Workers According to the Epistemology of Seniors' Health Literacy: A Socioconstructivist Approach based on a Chronological, Iconography Theme], *Proceedings, 15th International Conference on Globalization and Education Towards A Knowledgeable Society*, Vol.1, pp. 447-448, Marrakech, Morocco, June 2-6, 2008

Kaszap, M. ; &Clerc, I. (2008). Réflections autour des concepts d'alphabétisme et de littératie. [Reflection on the concepts of alphabetization and literacy]. Rapport: Suites à donner au 2e Forum national de recherche en santé des communautes francophones en situation minoritaire, Unpublished manuscript. Ottawa, Canada, Novembre 22-24, 2007

Kaszap, M. & Drolet M. (December 2009) Rapport de Recherche. *L'animation Télévisuelle en Santé*. [The Tele-visual Animation in Health]. Available: http://www.ccl-cca.ca/CCL/Research/FundedResearch/201007Kaszap-FoodTV-2.html

Kaszap, M. & Zanchetta, M. S. (2009). La Littératie en Santé, Vécue dans la Simplicité mais Comprise à Travers la Complexité: Regard sur les Communautés Culturelles (Francophones, Minoritaires et Multiethniques) [Health Literacy, Lived in Simplicity but Understood Through Complexity: Issues of Cultural Communities (Francophone, Minority and Multiethnicity], In: *Les littératies multiples: lire au 21e siècle* [Multiple literacies: Reading in the 21st century], D. Masny (Ed.), 287-325, Les Presses de l'Université d'Ottawa, ISBN 978-2-7603-0702-5, Ottawa, Ontario, Canada

Kelly, D. (2009). Changed men: The Embodied Impact of Prostate Cancer. *Qualitative Health Research*, Vol.19, No.2, (February), pp. 151-163, ISSN 1049-7323

Kimmel, M. (1987). Rethinking Masculinity: New Directions in Research, In: *Changing men: new directions in research on men and masculinities*, M. Kimmel (Ed.), 9-24, Sage, ISBN 0803929978, Thousand Oaks, California, United States

Kimmel M. (1995). *Manhood in America: A Cultural History*, Free Press, ISBN 978-0-02-874067-6, New York, United States

Ko, N. Y.; Shiau, C. & Sheu, S. L. (1997). Informational Needs and Information-seeking Behaviors of Recently Diagnosed HIV Seropositive Gay Men. *Hu Li Za Zhi* (The Journal of Nursing), Vol.44, No.3, (June), pp. 32-40, ISSN 0047-262X.

Krist, A. H.; Woolf, S. H.; Johnson, R. E. & Kerns, J. W. (2007). Patient Education on Prostate Cancer Screening and Involvement in Decision Making. *Annals of Family Medicine*, Vol.5, No.2, (March-April), pp. 112-119, ISSN 1544-1717

Knight, S. J. & Latini, D. M. (2009). Sexual Side Effects and Prostate Cancer Treatment Decisions: Patient Information Needs and Preferences. *Cancer Journal*, Vol.15, No.1, (January-February), pp. 41-44, ISSN 1528-9117

Kruger, J.; Prohaska, T. R. & Furner, S. E. (2007). Preferences for Health Inquiry among Adults Aged 50 and Over. *Research on Aging*, Vol.29, No.4 (July), pp. 283-296, ISSN 1552-7573

Lallas, C. D. & Trabulsi, C. J. (2010). Laparascopic and Robotic Radical Prostatectomy. In: *Glenn's Urologic Surgery* (7th Ed.), S.D. Graham & T.E. Keane (Ed.), 867-880, Lippincott Williams & Wilkins, ISBN 0781791413, Philadelphia, Pennsylvania, United States

Lavery, J. F. & Clarke, V. A. (1999). Prostate Cancer: Patients' and Spouses' Coping and Marital Adjustment. *Psychology, Health & Medicine*, Vol.4, No.3 (August), pp. 289-302, ISSN 1354-8506

Lenoir, T. (2002a). Makeover: Writing the Body into the Posthuman Technoscape Part Two: Corporeal Axiomatics. *Configurations,* Vol.10, No.3 (September), pp. 373-385, ISSN 1063-1801

Lenoir, T. (2002b). Makeover: Writing the Body into the Posthuman Technoscape Part One: Embracing the Posthuman. *Configurations,* Vol.10, No.2 (April), pp. 203-220, ISSN 1063-1801

Lenoir, T. (2004). The Virtual Surgeon: New Practices for an Age of Medialization, In: *Data Made Flesh: Embodying Information*, R. Mitchell and P. Thurtle (Eds.), 137-153, Routledge, ISBN 9780415969055, New York, United States

Lenz, E. R. (1984). Information-seeking: A Component of Client Decisions and Health Behavior. *Advances in Nursing Science,* Vol.6, No.3, (April), pp. 59-72, ISSN 0161-9268

Lerman, N.; Oldenziel, R.; Mohun, A. (2003) (Eds.). *Gender and Technology: A Reader,* Johns Hopkins University Press, ISBN 0-8018-7259-6, Baltimore, Maryland, United States

Levasseur, M. & Carrier, A. (2010). Do Rehabilitation Professionals Need to Consider Their Clients' Health Literacy for Effective Practice? *Clinical Rehabilitation,* Vol.24, No.8, (August), pp. 756-765, ISSN 1477-0873

Lohan, M. (2007). How Might We Understand Men's Health Better? Integrating Explanations from Critical Studies on Men and Inequalities in Health. *Social Science and Medicine,* Vol.65, No.3 (August), pp. 493-504, ISSN 0277-9536

Mackert, M.; Love, B. & Whitten, P. (2009). Patient Education on Mobile Devices: An E-health Intervention for Low Health Literate Audiences. *Journal of Information Science*, Vol.35, No.1, (October), pp. 82–93, ISSN 1741-6485

Mahalik, J.; Burns S. & Syzdek, M. (2007). Masculinity and Perceived Normative Health Behaviors as Predictors of Men's Health Behaviors. *Social Science and Medicine,* Vol.64, No.11, (June), pp. 2201-2209, ISSN 0277-9536

Martinez, L. S.; Schwartz, J. S.; Freres, D.; Fraze, T. & Hornik, R. C. (2009). Patient-clinician Information Engagement Increases Treatment Decision Satisfaction among Cancer Patients Through Feeling of Being Informed. *Patient Education and Counseling,* Vol.77, No.3, (December), pp. 384-390, ISSN 1873-5134

Mayeaux, E. J.; Murphy, P. W.; Arnold, C.; Davis, T. C.; Jackson, R. H. & Sentell, T. (1996). Improving Patient Education for Patients with Low Literacy Skills. *American Family Physician.* Vol.53, No.1, (January), pp. 205-211, ISSN 0002-838X

Meischke, H. & Johnson, D. (1995). Women's Selection of Sources for Information on Breast Cancer Detection. *Health Values,* Vol.19, No.5 (December), pp. 30-38, ISSN 0147-0353

Mellstrom, U. (2004). Machines and Masculine Subjectivity: Technology as an Integral Part of Men's Life Experiences. *Men and Masculinities,* Vol.6, No.4 (April), pp. 368-382, ISSN 1097-184X

Miaskowski, C. (1999). Prostate Cancer. In: *Oncology Nursing: Assessment and Clinical Care,* C. Miaskowski & P. Buchsel (Eds.), 1471-1501, Mosby, ISBN 978-081-5169-90-1, St. Louis, Missouri, United States

Mishel, M. H. (1990). Reconceptualization of the Uncertainty in Illness Theory. *Image: Journal of Nursing Scholarship,* Vol.22, No.4, (December), pp. 256–262, ISSN 0743-5150

Mishel, M. H.; Belyea, M.; Germino, B.; Stewart, J. L.; Bailey, D. E. & Robertson, C. (2002). Helping Patients with Localized Prostate Carcinoma Manage Uncertainty and Treatment Side Effects: Nurse Delivered Psychoeducational Intervention Over the Telephone. *Cancer,* Vol.94, No.6, (March), pp. 1854–1866, ISSN 0008-543X

Monteiro, M. (2000). *"Tenham Piedade dos Homens!": Masculinidades em Mudança* ["Have Pity on Men!": ChangingMasculinities], FEME, ISBN 85-86913-06-5, Juiz de Fora, Brazil

Monteiro, M. (2001). Corpo e Masculinidade na Revista VIP Exame [Body and Masculinity in VIP Exame Magazine], *Cadernos Pagu,* No.16 (December), pp. 235-266, ISSN 0104-8333

Monteiro, M. (2011). *Dilemas do Humano: Reinventando o Corpo Numa Era (Bio)tecnologica* [Dilemmas of the Human: Reinventing the Body in a (Bio)technological Era]. Social Sciences, São Paulo: Annablume. (in press)

Monteiro, M. (2009). Molecular representations: Reflections on microarrays and prostate cancer. *Leonardo Electronic Almanac,* Vol.16, (May), pp. 1-12

Monteiro, M. & Keating, E. (2009). Managing Misunderstandings: The Role of Language in Interdisciplinary Scientific Collaboration. *Science Communication* Vol.31, No.1, (February), pp. 6-28, ISSN 1552-8545

Moon, P. J. (2011). Bereaved Elders: Transformative Learning in Late Life. *Adult Education Quarterly,* Vol.61, No.1 (February), pp. 22-39, ISSN 1552 3047

Morasso, G.; Alberisio, A.; Capelli, M.; Rossi, C.; Baracco, G. & Costantini, M. (1997). Illness Awareness in Cancer Patients: A Conceptual Framework and a Preliminary Classification Hypothesis. *Psycho-Oncology,* Vol.6, No. 3, (September), pp. 212-217, ISSN 1057 9249

Morrow, D. G.; Weiner, M.; Steinley, D.; Young, J. & Murray, M. D. (2007). Patients' Health Literacy and Experience with Instructions : Influence Preferences for Heart Failure Medication Instructions. *Journal of Aging & Health,* Vol.19, No.4 (August), pp. 575-593, ISSN 0898-2643

Mróz, L. W.; Chapman, G. E.; Oliffe, J. L. & Bottorff J. L. (2011). Men, Food, and Prostate Cancer: Gender Influences on Men's Diets. *American Journal of Men's Health,* Vol.5, No.2, (March), pp. 177-187, ISSN 1557-9891

Nanton, V.; Docherty, A.; Meystre, C. & Dale, J. (2009). Finding a Pathway: Information and Uncertainty along the Prostate Cancer Patient Journey. *British Journal of Health Psychology,* Vol.14, No.3 (September), pp. 437-458, ISSN 1359-107X

Oldfield, S. R. &Dreher, H. M. (2010). The Concept of Health Literacy within the Older Adult Population. *Holistic Nursing Practice,* Vol.24, No.4, (July-August), pp. 204–212, ISSN 1550-5138

Orel, N. O.; Spence, M. & Steele, J. (2005). Getting the Message Out to Older Adults: Effective HIV Health Education Risk Reduction Publications. *Journal of Applied Gerontology*, Vol.24, No.5, (November), pp. 490-508, ISSN 1552-4523

Paley, J.; Cheyne, H.; Dalgleish, L.; Duncan, E. A. S. & Niven, C. A. (2007). Nursing's Ways of Knowing and Dual Process of Theories of Cognition. *Journal of Advanced Nursing*, Vol.60, No.6, (December), pp. 692-701, ISSN 0309-2402

Peerson, A. & Saunders, M. (2009). Health Literacy Revisited: What Do We Mean and Why Does it Matter? *Health Promotion International*, Vol.24, No.3, (September), pp. 285-296. ISSN 1460-2245

Perlow, E. (2010). Accessibility: Global Gateway to Health Literacy. *Health Promotion Practice*, Vol.11, No.1, (January), pp. 123–131, ISSN 1524 8399

Picker Institute. *About.* Retrieved May 30, 2011, from http://pickerinstitute.org/about

Pierce, P. F. (1996). When the Patient Chooses: Describing Unaided decisions in Health Care. *Human Factors*, Vol.38, No.2 (June), pp. 278-287, ISSN 0018-7208

Prasauskas, R. & Spoo, L. (2006). Literally Improving Patient Outcomes. *Home Health Care Management Practice*, Vol.18, No.4, (June), pp. 270-271, ISSN 1552-6739

Prins, E.; Willson, B.; Kai, T. & Schafft, A. (2009). Social Interaction and Support among Women in Adult Education and Family Literacy. *Adult Education Quarterly*, Vol.59, No.4, (August), pp. 335-352, ISSN 0741-7136

Prout, A.; Hayes, L. & Gelder, L. (1999). Medicines and the Maintenance of Ordinariness in the Household Management of Childhood Asthma. *Sociology of Health & Illness* Vol. 21, No.2, (December), pp. 137–162, ISSN 0141–9889

Rajan, K. S. (2006). *Biocapital: The Constitution of Postgenomic Life*, Duke University Press, ISBN 0-8223-3720-7, Durham, North Carolina, United States

Roberts, N. J. & Partridge, M. R. (2011). Evaluation of a Paper and Electronic Pictorial COPD Action Plan. *Chronic Respiratory Disease*, Vol.8, No.1, (February), pp. 31–40, ISSN 1479-9731

Rootman, I.; Frankish, J. & Kaszap, M. (2007). Health Literacy in Canada, In: *Health Promotion in Canada*, M. O'Neill, A. Pederson, S. Dupere & I. Rootman (Eds.), 61-74, Canadian Scholars' Press, ISBN 1551303256, Toronto, Ontario, Canada

Saposnik, G.; Teasell, R.; Mamdani, M.; Hall, J.; McIlroy, W.; Cheung, D.; Thorpe, K. E.; Cohen, L. G. & Bayley M. (2010). Effectiveness of Virtual Reality Using Wii Gaming Technology in Stroke Rehabilitation: A Pilot Randomized Clinical Trial and Proof of Principle. *Stroke*, Vol.41, No.7, (July), pp. 1477-1484, ISSN 1524-4628

Scott, J. (1989). *Gender and the Politics of History*, Columbia University Press, ISBN 0-231-11857-0, New York, United States

Shaw, C. R.; Wilson, S. A. & O'Brien, M. E. (1994). Information Needs Prior to Breast Biopsy. *Clinical Nursing Research*, Vol.3, No.2 (May), pp. 119-131, ISSN 1054-7738

Shen, M. & Abate-Shen, C. (2010). Molecular Genetics of Prostate Cancer: New Prospects for Old Challenges. *Genes and Development*, Vol.24, No.18, (September), pp. 1967-2000, ISSN 1549-5477

Siegel, K. & Raveis, V. (1997). Perceptions of Access to HIV-related Information, Care, and Services among Infected Minority Men. *Qualitative Health Research*, Vol.7, No.1, (February), pp. 9-31, ISSN 1552-7557

Sinfield, P.; Baker, R.; Agarwal, S. & Tarrant, C. (2008). Patient-Centred Care: What Are the Experiences of Prostate Cancer Patients and Their Partners? *Patient Education and Counseling* Vol.73, No.1, (October), pp. 91–96, ISSN 0738-3991

Stacey, D.; Paquet, L. & Samant, R. (2010). Exploring Cancer Treatment Decision-making by Patients: A Descriptive Study. *Current Oncology,* Vol.17, No.4, (August), pp. 85-93, ISSN 1198-0052

Steinberg, D. L. (1997). *Bodies in Glass: Genetics, Eugenics, Embryoethics,* Manchester University Press, ISBN 978-0719046681, Manchester, Greater Manchester, United Kingdom

Taylor, J. S. (2005). Surfacing the Body Interior. *Annual Review of Anthropology,* Vol.34, No. (June), pp. 741-56, ISSN 0084-6570

Torres, M. I.; Marquez, D. X.; Carbone, E. T.; Stacciarini, J-M. R. & Foster, J. W. (2008). Culturally Responsive Health Promotion in Puerto Rican Communities: A Structuralist Approach. *Health Promotion Practice,* Vol.9, No.2 (April), pp. 149-158, ISSN 1524-8399.

Van Dijck, J. V. (2005). *The Transparent Body: A Cultural Analysis of Medical Imaging,* University of Washington Press, ISBN 0-295-98490-2, Seattle, Washington, United States

Walker, B. L.; Nail, L. M.; Larsen, L.; Magill, J. & Schwartz, A. (1996). Concerns, Affect, and Cognitive Disruption Following Completion of Radiation Treatment for Localized Breast or Prostate Cancer. *Oncology Nursing Forum,* Vol.23, No.8, (September), pp. 1181-1187, ISSN 0190-535X

Walker, L. G.; Köhler, C. R. D.; Heys, S. D. & Eremin, O. (1998). Psychosocial Aspect of Cancer in the Elderly. *European Journal of Surgical Oncology,Vol.*24, No.5, (October), pp. 375-378, ISSN 0748 7983

Wall, D. & Kristjanson L. (2005). Men, Culture and Hegemonic Masculinity: Understanding the Experience of Prostate Cancer. *Nursing Inquiry,* Vol.12, No.2 (June), pp. 87-97, ISSN 1320-7881

Wallerstein, N. & Bernstein, E. (1988). Empowerment Education: Freire's Ideas Adapted to Health Education. *Health Education & Behavior,* Vol.15, No.4, (December), pp. 379-394, ISSN 1552-6127

Wallington, S. F. (2008). The Internet as an Emerging Patient Education Tool Among African American Men With Prostate Cancer: An Exploratory Study. *American Journal of Men's Health,* Vol. 2, No.2 (June), pp. 106-121, ISSN 1557 9891

Weiss, B. D.; Hart, G.; McGee, D. L. & D'Estelle, S. (1992). Health Status of Illiterate Adults: Relation Between Literacy and Health Status Among Persons with Low Literacy Skills. *Journal of American Board Family Practice,* Vol. 5, No.3, (May-June), pp.257-264, ISSN 0893-8652

Weiss, B. D.; Blanchard, J. S.; McGee, D. L.; Hart, G.; Warren, B.; Burgoon, M. & Smith, K. J. (1994). Illiteracy Among Medicaid Recipients and its Relationship to Health Care Costs. *Journal of Health Care for the Poor and Underserved,* Vol. 5, No.2, (August), pp. 99-111, ISSN 1049-2089

Weiss, B. D. & Coyne, C. (1997). Communication with Patients Who Cannot Read. *The New England Journal of Medecine,* Vol. 337, No.4, (July), pp. 272-273, ISSN 1049-2089

Wilkin, H. A. & Ball-Rokeach, S. J. (2006). Reaching at Risk Groups: The Importance of Health Storytelling in Los Angeles Latino Media. *Journalism,* Vol.7, No.3 (August), pp. 299-320, ISSN 1741-3001

World Health Organization (2002). *Mainstreaming Gender Equity in Health: The Need to Move Forward- Madrid Statement.* Gender Mainstreaming Programme, WHO Regional Office for Europe. Copenhagen, Denmark World Health Organization. Available from http://www.euro.who.int/__data/assets/pdf_file/0008/76508/A75328.pdf

World Health Organization (January 1998). Division of Health Promotion, Education and Communications Health Education and Health Promotion Unit. *Health Promotion Glossary.* Geneva, Switzerland: World Health Organization. Available from http://www.who.int/hpr/NPH/docs/hp_glossary_en.pdf

Zanchetta, M.; Kaszap, M.; Mohamed, M.; Racine, L.; Maheu, C.; Masny, D.; Cèsar, I.; Maltais, C.; Sangwa-Lugoma, G.; Lussier, N. & Kinslikh, D. (2011). Lessons Learned from Francophone Families' Health Literacy: Linguistic Minority Status As a New Social Determinant of Health. Unpublished manuscript

Zanchetta, M.; Monteiro, M. S.; GorospeIV.; F. F.; Pilon, R. S. & Peña, A. (2010). Ideas of Masculinities in Latin America Countries and Their Influences on Immigrant Men's Attitudes toward Health, Prostate Cancer Prevention: An Analysis of Literature. *International Men's Health and People,* Vol.7, No.3, (October), pp. 259-269, ISSN 1875-6867.

Zanchetta, M. S.; Perreault, M.; Kaszap, M. & Viens, C. (2007). Patterns in Information Strategies Used by Older Men to Understand and Deal with Prostate-cancer-related Information: An Application of the Modélisation Qualitative Research Design. *International Journal of Nursing Studies,* Vol.44, No.6 (August), pp. 961-972, ISSN 0020-7489

Zanchetta, M. S.; Cognet, M.; Xenocostas, S.; Aoki, D. & Talbot, Y. (2007). Prostate Cancer among Canadian Men: A Transcultural Representation. *International Journal of Men's Health,* Vol.6, No.3, (September), pp. 224-258, ISSN 1532-6306

Zanchetta, M. S. & Moura, S. (2006). Self-determination and Information-seeking in End Stage of Cancer. *Clinical Journal of Oncology Nursing,* Vol.10, No.6, (December), pp. 803-807, ISSN 1092-1095

Zanchetta, M. S. (2005). Uncertainty and Health Information-seeking Behavior. *Online Brazilian Journal of Nursing,* Vol.4, No.2. Available from: www. uff.br/neape/obj402zanchetta.htm, ISSN 1676-4285

Zanchetta, M.; Cognet, M.; Xenocostas, S.; Talbot, Y.; Upshur, E. G. R.; Aoki, D. & Wildfong, D. (2004). *Family Values and Ethno-cultural Background Underlie Attitudes and Beliefs about Prostate Cancer: Time + Urgency+ Effectiveness…a Challenging Equation.* "Hospitals in a culturally diverse Europe" International conference on quality-assured health care and health promotion for migrants and ethnic minorities. December 9-11, Amsterdam, Netherlands. (Abstracts book, pp. 89-90). Available from: http: //www.mfh-eu.net/conf/results/poster2

Zanchetta, M. S. (2004). Understanding Functional Health Literacy in Experiences with Prostate Cancer: Older Men as Consumers of Health Information. *Online Brazilian*

Journal of Nursing, Vol.3, No.2, (July), ISSN 1676-4285. Available from http://www.uff.br/nepae/siteantigo/objn302zanchetta.htm

Zanchetta, M. S. (2002). *Older Men's Self-reported Levels of Functional Health Literacy and the Process of Constructing Strategies to Live and Deal with Prostate Cancer-related Information within Their Natural Environments: A Qualitative Model.* Unpublished PhD. Thesis, Université de Montréal. Publication number NQ75925

8

Future of Prostate Biopsy: Who will get it and How?

Tine Hajdinjak
Center UROL Maribor
Department of Surgery, General Hospital Murska Sobota
Medical Faculty, University of Maribor
Slovenia

1. Introduction

Prostate biopsy is a motor, driving force and entrance ticket for dealing with parade discipline in urology of recent years - prostate cancer. Therefore it receives a lot of attention and standard techniques are constantly challenged by new developments. Enormous amount of literature seem to have addressed all possible aspects regarding prostate biopsy. This chapter focuses less on historical overview but mainly on recent developments, controversies and questions.

Prostate cancer has already become leading cancer among males in developed world (Jemal et al., 2011), second reason for death due to cancer among men in US (Jemal et al., 2010) and third in Europe (Malvezzi et al., 2011). Future is looking even more serious - numbers are expected to rise much further, as recently predicted in Canadian forecast analysis (Quon et al, 2011). The authors claim expected estimates of increase in prostate cancer cases should not be limited only to aging of population, which is huge itself and is expected to cause 39% increase in prostate cancer cases. At least three further factors should be taken into account. First and most important is lowering of PSA threshold for biopsy. It seems the move of decreasing PSA cutoff from 4 to 2.5 is getting from university centers to every urologist's and generalist's office (this is especially important as they are the ones who pick and refer patients to urologists for biopsy). Increase in number of people, referred to biopsy for this reason is estimated to be much greater compared to aging of population and may increase prostate cancer incidence by 200%. If it will increase prostate cancer incidence by 200%, increase in number of biopsies should be disproportionally higher, as biopsies have lower yield for this new target population with PSA values between 2.5 and 4. PSA screening is creating at present a lot of debate, it is a very hot topic and there are very strong opponents and supporters. Introduction of formal screening would of course increase burden of cancer and burden of biopsy. It is at present unlikely to happen, probably because people who decide on health policies and their advisers do not meet, treat and care for people with advanced prostate cancer. But, call it case finding or however one prefers, a "non-formal" screening programs are actually already available in many health systems, not only in selected first adopters, like Tyrol in Austria (Oberaigner et al., 2006), but also for example in Slovenia, where every general practitioner has available extra funds for PSA measurement on all of his male patients, every two years. Extent of "non-formal" screening programs can be seen from well-known PLCO trial, where control, supposedly non-screened arm had 50% screening in comparison to intervention arm, supposedly "screened", where the rate was approximately 85% (Andriole et al., 2009). Some do not believe into usefulness of screening (Miettinen, 2010) and results of studies, which clearly show improved survival and necessity for screening, for example of European Randomized Trial of Screening for Prostate Cancer (Schröder et al., 2009). Despite those doubts, screening in one way or another is in fact increasingly taking place in every-day life. Further increase in screening is expected because recent analyzes of prostate screening studies seem to greatly reduce predicted numbers needed to screen and numbers needed to treat to save a life in prostate cancer and dispel previous doubts about usefulness of screening (Crawford et al., 2011) and treatment (Bill-Axelson et al., 2011).

Last reason for estimation of huge increase in prostate cancer cases expected in the next decade is stated (Quon et al., 2011) as "improved sensitivity of prostate biopsy". Will this really happen? This review will summarize some of the present developments in this field. If this is really the case, it may be at least one good sign, sign of relief: with improved biopsy specificity, number of repeat biopsies, which at present already represent significant burden and may also represent group of patients with higher risk for biopsy-related complications, may decrease.

Prostate biopsy aims to detect prostate cancer with as little problems and sequela as possible. Further, it aims to predict prognosis of detected cancer, therefore sampling must not only take any cancer, but representative cancer tissue samples from possibly all cancer focuses in the prostate. Third goal of modern prostate biopsy is to guide targeted therapy, which is expected to rise with increased number of lower stage cancers detected.

2. Selection of biopsy candidates

Only main criteria, which are in clinical use or are available and may be used in Europe in 2011 are included here and they are: 3 PSA's (total, free and -2proPSA), urine marker (PCA3), race, family history, previous biopsy technique and result, age and life expectancy.

There are markers, which were proposed and also used in the past, but are now outdated, like cPSA and other PSA's, not mentioned above. There are markers, which may become very useful in the future, but are at present not ready yet (for example SNP's and other genetic data or new urine markers, which may use advantage of being excreted and therefore no aggressive rectal prostate massage would be necessary (Pandha et al., 2011)).

Should we really biopsy all men with PSA above 2.5? Obviously we do not want to do that. It remains unresolved task, how should we select between those who would benefit from biopsy even earlier, at PSA 1, from those who do not need biopsy at PSA 10.

2.1 PSA's

Prostate specific antigen, during history of its discovery named with other names, for example semenogelase, is an androgen-regulated serine protease (EC 3.4.21.77), human tissue kallikrein 3 (Balk et al, 2003). Gene is located on 19q13.4. Mainly it is produced in secretory epithelial cells in prostate acini and ducts and secreted into lumen. Its function is in ejaculate liquefaction.

PSA is expressed in preproPSA form (17 aminoacid leading peptide), excreted into prostate lumen as proPSA (7 aminoacid propeptide on N-terminal) and activated by trypsine-like human kallikrein 2 (hK2), which is expressed on prostate secretory epithelial cells (Balk et.al, 2003). ProPSA can undergo cleavage at position -7, removing 7 aminoacid propeptide to form active PSA. ProPSA cleavage can also occur at positions -5 or -2. Those PSA isoforms are not catalytically active. Active PSA in part undergoes further degradation/internal cleavage by different proteases, thereby also forming inactive PSA. In seminal plasma approximately 30% of PSA is in active form. Remaining PSA represents different forms of inactive PSA. Some PSA (all forms) leaks to circulation and can be measured in serum. Active form of PSA in serum binds (complexes) to protease inhibitors, mostly to alpha1-antichymotrypsin (ACT). It represents main part of total serum PSA (70-90%) and can be measured as cPSA. Catalytically inactive PSA forms circulate freely in serum as they are not complexed to ACT or other inhibitors. This fraction represents main result of free PSA assay. Antibodies were also developed for measuring serum concentrations of specific PSA isoforms, for example [-5]pro PSA and [-2]proPSA. Assays which measure total PSA aim at detecting all isoforms, active (complexed) and inactive PSA.

As prostate cancer characteristic is disruption of basal cell layer and basement membrane, this allows increased amount of PSA and its isoforms to enter circulation (Balk et al, 2003). Free PSA fraction is decreased in serum of cancer patients. It is hypothesized there is relatively less free PSA in serum in cancer patients because more PSA enters circulation directly and complexes immediately to protease inhibitors. As there is less exposure of PSA to luminal and seminal fluid proteases, there is less chance for inactivating and producing inactive, free PSA. ProPSA isoforms are increased in serum of prostate cancer patients. Two hypotheses aim to explain this. One believes there is decreased cleavage of proPSA by hK2 in prostate cancer tissue (Balk et al., 2003). Other hypothesis believes proPSA isoforms are increased in cancer as a result of increased proPSA production from benign looking cancer associated areas in prostate gland (Makarov et al., 2009).

Higher serum PSA values were related to prostate cancer in 1980-ties. Hybritech, first commercial PSA measurement kit manufacturer, identified in a small study in 1986 in their sample 99% of tested men (different ages) had PSA below 4 and suggested this value as a cut-off. With this in hand, Catalona conducted a trial and published in 1991: 8% of tested men (mean age 68) had PSA values above 4, 22% of those with PSA between 4 and 10 had prostate cancer detected on sextant biopsy (and 67% among those with PSA above 10). Biopsy was performed using 18G needle. PSA was independent prognostic factor and positive DRE increased chance of positive biopsy (Catalona et al., 1991). 20 years later - we made a progress - now we do 12 core biopsies, use PSA cut-off 2.5 and use some other PSA derivatives to help in decisions. This modifies our outcomes a few percentages here and there, but main achievement, decrease in mortality due to prostate cancer, which was, after two decades of doubt, finally recently confirmed by a few large independent trials from both US and EU (see Introduction), was a result of a twenty years old approach, which is, with all its drawbacks and deficiencies, still valid and widely practiced around the world.

Inadequacy of PSA cut-off value of 4 was in depth explained by publication of results of control biopsies in prostate cancer prevention trial (Thompson et al., 2004). They found, among men in age range 62 to 91, median 69, 6.6% of cancers among those with PSA 0.5 or less and 12.5% among them with Gleason 7 or more (=0.8% of all men with median age 69 with PSA below 0.6 had important cancer). Among men with PSA of 1.1 to 2.0, cancer was found in 10% and 10% of those had Gleason 7 or more (=1% of all men with PSA between 1 and 2, median age 69, had Gleason 7 or higher prostate cancer). For PSA 2-3, the percentage of Gleason 7 or more among all tested was 4.6% and for PSA 3-4 it was 6.7%. Those numbers were found in a prescreened population and with sextant biopsy. Now it is believed those numbers are still accurate for overall cancer presence, but for Gleason 7 or higher cancers in general referral population, real numbers are about twice those estimates. Several thoughts follow from this data. One is related to high percentage of high grade cancers in population with median age 69 and relatively low PSA values. Once upon a time, it was suggested we should not measure PSA in men above 70. Should we now turn this completely around and biopsy all men with life expectancy of 10 yeas or more at the age of 70 irrespectively of their PSA? Or should we use other tests, like PSA isoforms derivatives?

Free PSA is measured to calculate fraction towards total PSA value, which is expressed as percentage. In PSA ranges between 4 and 10, with % free PSA below 10%, probability for biopsy detected prostate cancer in DRE negative patients was 56% and with % free PSA above 25% probability of cancer was only 8%. In PSA range between 2.5 and 4, with % free PSA below 10%, probability of cancer was 46% and with % free PSA above 20% probability of cancer was 8% (Catalona et al., 1998).

[-2]proPSA or p2PSA is new kid on the block, which is not yet universally available or accepted. It seems it will become next widely used PSA derivative, which is also used together with free PSA value (p2PSA/freePSA) or together with total and free PSA as value, calculated as p2PSA/freePSA times square root of total PSA and proprietary named by Beckman Coulter (Brea, California, USA) as PHI - prostate health index. Cut-off values for biopsy decisions using %p2PSA (p2PSA/free PSA) and PHI are not yet universally accepted and differ with regard to free PSA and total PSA calibration method (Hybritech or WHO), but it seems PHI values above 40 or 45 indicate high and below 21 low risk of prostate cancer. PHI of more than 48.5 was reported as 43% specific at 90% sensitive for detecting prostate cancer at initial prostate biopsy (Guazzoni et al., 2011). Another study reported PHI values above 34.2 to show increased probability for high risk disease (Isharwal et al., 2011). PHI was shown to indicate development of prostate cancer years before biopsy and correlated well with grade of future prostate cancer (Bektic et al., 2010). On negative side, using p2PSA compared to free PSA using ROC curves at area of high sensitivity (if we are to find cancer), increase in performance may seem marginal.

PSA density and different variants (PSA density of transitional zone etc), calculated from total PSA value and measurement of prostate volume using transrectal ultrasound, were in the past extensively evaluated. Drawback is variability of prostate volume measurements, need for this additional investigation and low sensitivity (Pepe et al., 2009). One example of cutoff value was density above 0.15 ng/ml PSA /ml prostate volume indicating higher risk of cancer. It may represent additional useful piece of information, also for example regarding prediction of disease course for patients on watchful waiting (Kotb et. al, 2011).

PSA velocity was in recent years proposed as another potentially helpful tool in picking cancers or high-risk cancers. Cutoff value of 0.35 ng/ml/year was proposed when total PSA values are less than 4. This may need adjustment for race (Tang et al., 2011). Although some doubts about value of PSA velocity in biopsy decisions were posed from analysis of PCPT trial data (Vickers et al., 2011), there are suggestions a lot of clinically important cancers in younger men may be detected by regularly and meticulously following and analyzing sequential PSA values (Bektic et al., 2011).

PSA values increase with age due to BPH. This became known early after PSA test introduction and "age-specific" PSA values were suggested. For Caucasian Americans, median, 75th and 95th percentiles of PSA were for age group 40-49 - 0.7, 1.0 and 2.1, for 50-59 age group 1.0, 1.6 and 3.6, for 60-69 age group 1.4, 2.5 and 4.3, for 70-79 decade 1.8, 3.5 and 5.8 (Morgan et al., 1996). One approach of integrating age specific PSA values in prostate biopsy decisions may be using as cutoff half of age-specific 95th percentile PSA value together with %free PSA below 18%, which was in part used in Innsbruck (Tyrol, Austria).

High increase of PSA with infection or any irritation of prostate is well known and sometimes antibiotic or anti-inflammatory treatment is suggested and repeat measurement. PSA decreases in high body-mass index-correction and decreased of cutoff values may be needed (Pater et al., 2011). Diseases (liver cirrhosis) and medications (NSAID's, thiazides and statins) may also decrease PSA values (Nieder et al., 2011). If using free PSA values as trigger for biopsy decisions, it may be important to note that use of herbal products, like Serenoa repens, may (artifically?) increase free PSA values.

2.2 Age and life expectancy

Risk of prostate cancer significantly increases with age. Age is significant independent predictor of high risk prostate cancer. Although we need age as a criterion (we do not start to think about prostate cancer before age of 40 or 35), it is clear age could not be the only factor which would preclude decisions about PSA measurement, digital rectal exam and biopsy. Age is only one parameter in estimation of life expectancy. Life expectancy, not age, is crucial factor in decisions regarding prostate cancer screening interventions. Age does increase probability of cancer and cancer related death and therefore higher age - for example 75 years or more (with additional criterion of more than 10 years life expectancy) means strong indication in-favor of PSA screening and prostate biopsy. It is true that not all men at age 75 or more have more than 10 years of life expectancy, but significant number have and for them, prostate cancer screening is most useful and fruit bearing (much higher yield compared to younger men). This thinking is in strong contrast to past belief (and even now supported by some outdated recommendations of non-urological organizations), when PSA testing was not recommended generally for all older men.

2.3 Digital rectal exam

Digital rectal exam remains important part of prostate evaluation (Gosselaar et al., 2008). Although still on occasion declined by a patient and despite hopes PSA or any other method would completely replace it (Schroder et al., 1998), one still finds from time to time a case, where PSA is low and DRE is suspicious. For such a patient, next year, when PSA has increased, may be (and cases were confirmed it was) too late. Although after many suspicious DRE's biopsy comes negative, we are more and more aware of the fact that prostate cancer may progress without PSA increase. DRE can estimate sphincter tone, in a way prepare patient for biopsy, if needed, on occasion register some other, non-urological pathology and appreciate prostate size, which may give different dimension compared to ultrasound impression. DRE is necessary for sampling prostate cells in post-massage urine - at present for PCA3 only, but in the future maybe also for other markers. DRE is necessary for clinical staging of prostate cancer. DRE is limited, it can not palpate whole gland, but at present it is here to stay (Yossepowitch, 2008).

2.4 PCA3

Comparison of mRNA expression patterns of prostate cancer and benign tissues identified significantly different expression of non-coding mRNA sequence, first called DD3 (Bussemakers et al., 1999) and later renamed PCA3. Technology (a variant of quantitative nucleic acid amplification test) was developed to identify very minute amounts of PCA3 mRNA from prostate cells shed in prostate urethra after prostatic massage and washed out immediately in first voided urine portion. Its estimated amount (number of copies) is normalized to estimated number of PSA mRNA copies in the same sample and multiplied by 1000, resulting in PCA3 score. Test is known as Progensa PCA3 Assay (Gen-Probe Inc, San Diego, USA). Higher PCA3 score values indicate greater risk of presence of prostate cancer. Values from approximately 4 to 125 can be obtained, 35 being most often suggested cut-off, which, according to package insert has 53% sensitivity and 74% specificity for detection of prostate cancer on subsequent biopsy. Other cut-off opinions are continuously evaluated (Auprich et al., 2011). Although PCA3 mRNA theoretically could be measured in urine also with standard molecular-medicine techniques, which first isolate mRNA from cells in the sample and then perform RT-PCR, is this, due to very small amounts of PCA3 mRNA, very difficult and inconsistent, therefore dedicated patented method from Gen-Probe which uses direct amplification and avoids isolation step, has become standard.

PCA3 use was suggested and marketed as help in biopsy decisions in previously negative prostate biopsies, in men with other risk factors (family history) and normal PSA values, in men with big prostates or other prostatic conditions where it is unclear whether high PSA is driven by cancer or other factor and in men on watchful waiting where high PCA3 score may indicate higher burden of disease.

Use of consecutive PCA3 tests for follow up of biopsy candidates or men on watchful waiting was questioned due to high variability of results, if test is repeated in the same individual with low risk disease (Shikanov et al., 2011).

Pre-biopsy PCA3 test results were evaluated together with PSA in relation to tumor characteristics in radical prostatectomy specimens (Vlaeminck-Guillem et al., 2011). It was found PCA3 score did not correlate with PSA and prostate volume. PCA3 score was also not related to Gleason score and pT stage. PCA3 did correlate with total tumor volume and index lesion volume. Further, multifocality was significantly correlated with PCA3. PCA3 expression can be identified on malignant and benign prostate tissue samples, only quantity varies (Quiles et al., 2011).

PCA3 test is, with many mentioned drawbacks and despite its high price, widely marketed and used in USA and EU. It seems sometimes may help in biopsy related decisions, but its role at present is still evolving.

2.5 Family history, race, previous biopsy result

Theoretically one may differentiate between familial (unpredictable clustering of disease in a family, slightly increased risk for offspring) and hereditary cancer (strong clustering pattern consistent with passage of a susceptibility gene via Mendelian inheritance) (Potter & Partin, 2000). Criteria for hereditary prostate cancer would be three or more first-degree relatives had prostate cancer, three successive generations had prostate cancer and where two relatives were affected at or before age 55. Despite identification of such families, their investigation has not resulted in such successful discoveries as in colon, ovary and breast cancers. In those classic hereditary cancers presence of a certain identifiable mutation with high probability predicts development of cancer in all affected offspring, which has resulted in formal screening programs for affected families and preventive surgery at early age. This is at present not known in prostate cancer.

Familial history of prostate cancer increases risk. In a meta-analysis brother with prostate cancer increases risk 3.3 times, father 2.2 times, two first-degree relatives 5 times (Zeegers et al., 2003).

It is accepted increased risk due to family history should result in earlier start of screening (at age 40 or 35). Some risk calculators do use family history information to modify risk estimation (increased risk for presence of cancer in first degree relatives, this means father, brother or son), which may influence biopsy decision, if based on calculated risk. But apart from this, it does not tell us anything - PSA and other cut-offs for decision about biopsy are the same as in men without family history. Also procedures for biopsy, treatment and also treatment outcomes are the same between familial, hereditary and sporadic prostate cancer. There is no known 100% risk situations, which would provoke preventive removal of prostate, as is known for breast cancer, although people sometimes do ask for this.

Recent research focused also on risk of prostate cancer in men whose family members have other forms of cancer. Men with first degree relative with breast cancer, who developed breast cancer at the age 35 or earlier, are at significantly increased risk of prostate cancer (5 to 18 times in case of BRCA mutation) (Dite et al., 2010). Other cancers in family may also increase risk of prostate cancer (Izmirlian et al., 2011).

Race is used in many prostate cancer risk calculators - African American race increases risk compared to Caucasians, Hispanic or Asian have decreased risk. But, the same as for family history, apart from earlier start of screening or a little different risk estimates from calculators, there are no other practical consequences of this fact at present.

Previous negative biopsy decreases risk of positive subsequent biopsy. There are, however, two findings, which differ: PIN (=HGPIN - high grade prostatic intraepithelial neoplasia, low grade PIN was abandoned) and ASAP (atypical small acinar proliferation). HGPIN is most probable precursor of prostate cancer. There are structurally benign ducts and acini with abnormal secretory cells with prominent nucleoli (Schoenfield et al., 2007). HGPIN is a histological entity in itself, it is not cancer. ASAP indicates finding of small focus of structure in a 2-dimensional view, which is not large enough to satisfy criteria for cancer. It may represent only specific cut of top of benign acinus or PIN. One may define different characteristics under ASAP category, like adenosis, intraductal hyperplasia... which have in common that pathologist can not say for certain, whether they represent cancer or not. As ASAP may represent cancer, is was identified as predictor of positive repeat biopsy. Identification of multiple HGPIN in a biopsy specimen was also identified as predictor of positive repeat biopsy (Akhavan et al., 2007). Therefore, ASAP and HGPIN require consideration about repeat biopsies. ASAP may require immediate scheduling for repeat biopsy. HGPIN requires careful follow up and in most cases other criteria (PSA increase) cause repeat biopsy sooner or later (for example in 1-2 years time).

2.6 Risk based strategies

Different nomograms were developed, which can predict risk of positive biopsy. They take into account risk for age, family history, race, PSA and free PSA, digital rectal exam and some also for body mass index and even new decision aids, for example PCA3 and PHI.

Nomograms have introduced new dimension in patient-physician pre-biopsy discussion. Need for individual's risk adjustment is illustrated by cardiology example. Do general practitioners and cardiologists decide whether one needs aspirin or statin on a single total cholesterol measurement (for example with result of 5.3 mmol/L, just above normal)? No. They measure HDL, LDL cholesterol, they ask for age, gender, blood pressure, smoking history. They consult nomograms and then decide whether statin drug is necessary (and reimbursed) or not. But urologists were dependent on a single PSA value? This has changed with risk calculators availability. Using single PSA cutoff value would be the same as claiming for a man, who runs marathon, has normal blood pressure, normal BMI, is a non-smoker, his parents lived till age 100 and has cholesterol of 5.3 mmol/L - to be at high risk for cardiac event because his cholesterol is elevated (above 5.2). Using single PSA value for biopsy decision would be the same as claiming for an overweight (BMI 30), sedentary man, heavy smoker, on three anti-hypertensive medications whose parents both died of cardiac event, because his cholesterol is 5.1 mmol/L (just normal) - not to be at risk for cardiac event. Everyone can clearly see ridiculosity, absurdity of such approach in cardiology - but we in urology use PSA as single dichotomous variable in our prostate biopsy decisions?! Risk calculators allow us to tell men with any PSA value their individual chances for biopsy outcome. Calculators report risk for high grade (Gleason 7 or more) and overall cancer probability. For example if calculator predicts 6% chance of significant prostate cancer (Gleason 7 or more) and 26% of overall cancer risk, we should tell patient his chance of being without cancer at present is approximately 74% (100-26), he has 6% chance of finding important high risk cancer and he has approximately 20% (26-6) chance biopsy would find cancer which may not be clinically important at present (but maybe in the future) and we would have to deal with this. If we explain this way, most men can and do take their own decision, whatever it is (to proceed with biopsy or continue PSA follow up).

Using risk calculators often surprises us with values one would not expect. For example use Sunnybroke Prostate risk calculator (see below) and take 75 years old healthy Caucasian male with PSA of 3.9, %free PSA 22%, IPSS 9, in a good health (for example upper 25% of his generation), no family history for prostate cancer and negative DRE. He has more than 15 years of life expectancy, 39% risk of prostate cancer and 20% risk of having at present high grade prostate cancer (Gleason 7 or more). 20% risk of high grade cancer and more than 15 years of life expectancy - would you suggest a biopsy?

At present (june 2011), one of the most modern (can take into account PCA3, p2PSA...) pre-biopsy nomograms is available from UT Health Science Center, San Antonio, head Ian Thompson (http://deb.uthscsa.edu/URORiskCalc/Pages/calcs.jsp). Opponents of his calculator state it has good estimation of overall cancer risk, but underestimates high risk cancers. Large urology collection of nomograms, also many pre-biopsy nomograms including estimation of biopsy risks, are available from Pierre Karakiewicz, Cancer Prognostics and Health Outcomes Unit from University of Montreal Health Centre, Canada (www.nomograms.org). Calculators derived from European Randomized study of Screening for Prostate Cancer (Fritz Schroeder) are available at SWOP Prostate Cancer Research Fundation: http://www.prostatecancer-riskcalculator.com/via.html. Useful, simple and modern (more accurate high risk cancers estimation) pre-biopsy nomogram is available from SunnyBrook Health Sciences Centre, Toronto: http://sunnybrook.ca/content/?page=OCC_prostateCalc.

Different nonograms, for example taking into account 3D biopsy approach (Sakura et al., 2011) are being developed and published constantly. Also, comparisons (Oliveira et al., 2011) and evaluations (Ngo et al., 2011) are permanently performed and published. When using nomograms, one should be aware of their limitations (Vickers & Cronin, 2010).

NCCN guidelines on prostate cancer early detection not require nomogram use, follow in part risk adapted approach, cover most "before biopsy" issues, are regularly updated and modern. They are available freely after registration from www.nccn.org.

3. Methods of biopsy

Prostate cancer was in the past diagnosed most often using histology from transurethral resection, which was performed for local complications of prostate cancer or merely BPH. As it became clear such diagnosis is most often too late, makes subsequent radical surgical treatment more difficult and as PSA become available, biopsy had become diagnostic method of choice. At first, it was finger guided, blind. With development of transrectal ultrasound (trus - transrectal ultrasound guided prostate biopsy) and coupling it to 18G needle, Pandora box of prostate cancer was opened.

3.1 Transrectal or transperineal approach?

Most prostate biopsies around the world are performed transrectally, as this naturally developed from transrectal finger guided approach, is cheaper, simpler, does not need any analgesia or anaesthesia (although it is highly recommended, see section 4.3). Transperineal approach does need at least local anaesthesia. On same occasions, like post surgical amputation of the rectum, if it is sutured, transperineal biopsy (or transgluteal) may be the only way. However, such biopsy is guided by US probe on the perineum or in the urethra or more often by CT or MRI, which is not the way transperineal biopsy is performed regularly. Regular transperineal biopsy is performed using probe in the rectum and needle is advanced through the skin above rectal opening. Transperineal approach has similarity with the way some treatments are performed (brachytherapy...). Treatment templates may be used for biopsy which may guide biopsy needle to a specific part of prostate, which is seen as potentially more effective and with better gain. Recently, stereotactic templates (even motorized and computer guided) have become available also for transrectal prostate sampling - mechanically assisted 3D TRUS guided biopsy system (Megwalu et al., 2008). Supporters of transperineal approach suggest transperineally apical and anterior parts of the prostate may be better accessed compared to transrectal approach. For those reasons, studies were designed to compare yields of transrectal versus transperineal biopsy approach in primary 12-core and saturation 20-core schemes (Hara et al., 2008; Abdollah et al., 2011). Those studies uniformly showed no difference in cancer yields. However, this has not convinced proponents of transperineal approach. In regions, where transperineal approach was used routinely and claimed to be better compared to transrectal (for example some parts of Italy), they are only lately discovering prostate biopsy with end-fire probe (Galosi et al., 2010). Due to technical development of ultrasound equipment, some manufacturers (also very respectful one), were using side-fire probe with needle "through-the-probe" technology. This was proved to be inferior (Chin et al., 2009) in comparison to end-fire biopsy approach (see below). Therefore comparison of perineal to side-fire transrectal approach is not appropriate. Combination of transrectal and transperineal approach has also been used and described, aiming at gaining best from both approaches and maximizing cancer detection rate (Kawakami et al., 2007).

Transrectal approach is recommended for routine primary and also saturation prostate biopsy. On rare occasions, where stereotactic guidance may be needed, decision on approach depends on availability of equipment. At present, equipment for transperineal stereotactic approach is more often available and more widespread, due to its use for brachytherapy (and different other new experimental approaches, such as cryotherapy or photodynamic therapy), compared to new and only limited availability of transrectal computer and motor guided tools for prostate biopsy. Therefore, transperineal biopsy may be method of choice in selected cases.

3.2 Transrectal ultrasound probe

After analogue ultrasound probes have settled to history, electronic probes prevailed. Rotating mechanical sector probes have not gained popularity in the past. Present standard is electronic multi-element transducer - array. They come in two configurations. Side-fire probes have longitudinal transducer and take biopsies in longitudinal sections – sagittal plane, while end-fire probes have curved array detector and allow biopsies to be taken also in transverse plane. In the past, Bruel and Kjaer and Kretz offered for prostate biopsy primarily side-fire probes and this was subjectively seen as better approach compared to end-fire probes (vaginal probes), used "secondarily" also for prostate biopsies. However, end-fire proponents build hypothesis better detection rate to be expected with end-fire sampling in transverse plane due to ability to direct needle more towards lateral part of the peripheral zone, where most tumors arise. This hypothesis was at first tested and confirmed for sextant biopsy in PSA range 4-10 (Paul et al., 2004). This issue was challenged again in 2009, hypothesising end-fire probe has more oblique angled trajectory allowing better peripheral sampling (Ching et al., 2009). To reach anterior gland and apex in longitudinal plane, side-fire probe should be turned a lot and moved in a way which often causes pain as moves point of entry of the needle below dentate line of the rectum. End-fire probe allows better manipulation and targeting desired areas of prostate. Hypothesis was confirmed in their study, finding significantly better detection rate overall in the end-fire group compared to side-fire group and better detection in side-fire group for biopsies with more than 8 cores (8-12, 13-19 and 20 and more) and all PSA ranges (below 2.5, 2.5-4, 4-10 and more than 10) (Ching et al., 2009)

Later, side-fire probes were often bi-planar, therefore allowing better orientation in the prostate, if one views it in two planes and offering choice between end-fire or side-fire biopsy guide. At present, interest has moved from purely end-fire or side-fire biopsy towards combined biopsy opinions and probe designs are now aiming further at 3-plane, 3D imaging and computer guidance... Biplanar probes have become standard equipment also because linear longitudinal array on the probe is necessary for transperineal prostate procedures guidance, while end-fire part is used for standard transrectal biopsy. Ideally, one should have the ability to use biplanar probe, but probably prefer end-fire setting for taking most biopsy cores.

As history is repeating and revealing again in many aspects of human life, new TargetScan device (Envisioneering Medical Technologies, St. Louis, MO, USA) uses mechanical sector probe with single rotating element, applying it in "side-fire" configuration, but with needle, which bends, thus overcoming drawbacks from side-fire systems (Taneja, 2006).

3.3 Biopsy needle

Form, length, thickness, shape of biopsy needle, as everything regarding prostate biopsy, is being constantly challenged. It seems at present thickness of the needle is settled to 18G, needles are side-notch, true-cut, straight with stroke length of 22 mm.

But it was not always so – aspiration biopsy (cytological biopsy) was around and well not so many years ago (Gustafsson et al., 1990). Length of the needle may not seem important at first sight, but for systematic sampling of all areas of big prostates, standard needle length may become limiting factor, as it may simply not be possible to advance needle from biopsy guide into the prostate enough to get sampling of all desired areas in a big or a bit differently formed prostate. For example, TargetScan (Envisoneering) declares needle movement of 2.2 cm (standard for most biopsy guns, but not all) and possibility of needle protruding 2 cm from tip of biopsy guide before firing - together 42 mm of needle penetration. This is a description of a dedicated "robotic" system. In every day life, where ultrasound system and needle guide are one thing, hospital's supply for needles another and hospital's selection of biopsy-guns third issue, this should be considered, measured and perhaps some longer needles acquired for bigger prostates. Many other variants of needle characteristics were evaluated. Regarding stroke length, 33 mm end-cut was proposed (Dogan et al., 2005) by some, others proposed 29 mm side-notch instead of 22 mm (Fink et al., 2005). It is obvious longer is better and at least 22 mm should be used instead of old 15 mm, which was used at introduction of now obsolete sextant biopsy scheme (Hodge et al., 1989). Also thickness of needle was questioned - 18G (1.27 mm) was compared to thinner needles (0.9 mm (20G), 0.8 mm and 0.7 mm(22G)) - this old study found 0.9 mm may be acceptable (Norberg et al., 1994) - however it is not used in practice today. More recent studies evaluated thickness of needles again - non-ferromagnetic titanium needles were evaluated for quality of yield in comparison to standard needles - 16G (1.65 mm) titanium needle was found to provide samples of good quality and better compared to 18G regular (Franiel et al., 2006). However, also for MRI guided puncture, commercially available product is 18G needle (TSK, Japan) with characteristics comparable to regular needles.

Until recently, only straight needles were in wide use. This creates problem with accessibility (see section 3.2). Recent machine for stereotactic trus biopsy Targetscan aims to overcome this problem with new pliable needle, which bends and allows good approach to most sites in the prostate in side-fire configuration.

3.4 Image guidance

In the beginning of transrectal prostate ultrasound era, large efforts were made attempting to recognize cancerous areas of prostate on gray ultrasound picture. Although hypoechoic lesions were identified as important (Terris et al., 1991) and we still lean toward specifically sampling hypoechoic areas as suspect in our every-day prostate biopsy work, we can not rely on them. After color doppler ultrasound was introduced, suspect areas were proposed to be the ones, which have higher or disorganized blood flow. Many studies have confirmed better sampling with the help of doppler or color flow imaging. However, presentation of subtly disorganized prostate vasculature and blood flow in potential cancer foci is very delicate and very dependent on sonographist, so only highly specialized individuals were and are able to put theory into practice. They are still trying to improve visualization of vasculature, either with ultrasound contrast or with other pharmacological agents, but other three presently available imaging techniques seem more promising as they may be more standardized and therefore easier for every urologist or radiologist, who, in a hurry and overwhelmed with other everyday work, perform mass of prostate biopsy burden: elastography, ANNA C-TRUS and HistoScanning.

3.4.1 Role of MRI

Magnetic resonance imaging with different modalities has established its role in prostate cancer imaging. Apart from T1 and T2 weighted images (Jager et al., 1996), which are not enough, multi-modal approach, like diffusion weighted imaging and dynamic contrast enhanced imaging was found necessary to identify tumor suspicious regions. Role of endorectal coil, although sometimes debated (for example for 3T may not be so important as for 1.5T), seems also well established (Comet-Batlle et al., 2003). Tumor suspicious regions are found in different proportions, depending on criteria and number of different imaging modalities applied and can reach up to 98% even in post-trus-negative biopsy setting. After tumor suspicious regions are identified, sampling is needed.

The easiest approach would be image fusion to trus picture, which is moving from development phase (Hu et al., 2010) and in some centers already represents routine practice (for example Heidelberg, Germany). Two systems are in development: transrectal Artemis - Eigen, Grass Valley, CA, USA (Natarajan et al., 2011) and transperineal BiopSee - MedCom, Darmstadt, Germany (Hadaschik et al., 2011). Incidental reports show identification and confirmation of cancer in patients with previously negative ANNA C-TURS biopsy, however, at present there are no studies which would compare any of the mentioned techniques and show individual strengths and indications.

Some researchers perform MRI examination with plastic simulator of endorectal probe in-situ to simulate deformation expected during trus biopsy setting (Ukimura et al., 2010). Others perform 3D ultrasound imaging and use electromagnetic positioning device to perform biopsies (Turkbey et al., 2011).

Straightforward use of MRI would be MRI guided biopsy of MRI identified suspicious regions of prostate. Although at present available only in few institutions, this may very soon become more widespread as technology, procedure and equipment seem more and more ready for prime time (Roethke et al., 2011). Two independent retrospective series, performed with 1.5T or 3T magnets, from Netherlands (Hambrock et al., 2010) and from Germany (Roethke et al., 2011), report 52% and 58% (of patients with tumour suspicious regions identified) of positive MRI-guided biopsies after previous negative trus guided prostate biopsies.

3.4.2 ANNA C-TRUS and HistoScanning

Idea about reflected ultrasound wave analysis, which should reveal more data than can be seen just with naked eye, is old. There were and are still experiments taking place in developing algorithms of data analysis. Most often prostate is evaluated with transrectal ultrasound before radical prostatectomy and pictures are saved. After radical prostatectomy, histological sections of prostate with known areas of cancer and benign tissue are correlated with saved ultrasound data. Aim is to allow identification of cancer regions on ultrasound before biopsy or surgery. There may be many usages - HistoScanning is evaluated for prediction of Gleason score, volume of cancer, number and localization of cancer foci, prediction of location of cancer focus in relation to neurovascular bundle and in relation to prostate borders - all those data may be useful not only for decision to proceed or postpone biopsy and to guide biopsy, but also for pre- and peri-operative or other treatment planning.

ANNA C-TRUS is a method, which analyzes typical transrectal ultrasound pictures of prostate in transversal plane (for example 5, on sections, where one normally takes biopsy cores). Pictures can be taken with any digital US scanner. Pictures are then sent, uncompressed (using either .tif, .bmp or .png format), using internet, to the provider. After analysis, suspect areas are marked on pictures and urologist repeats examination, this time taking samples from areas marked. All data available about this method seem at present still from the inventor and copyright holder of the technique, prof. Loch from Flensburg, they seem at present not independently evaluated. From author's report in 2010, it seems C-TRUS

ANNA technique detected 66 cancers, taking up to 6 cores in a series of 132 patients with previous negative prostate biopsy. Series included 62 patients with previous 1 negative biopsy, 41 with previous 2 negative biopsies, 18 with 3 negative biopsies, 6 with 4 negative biopsies and 5 with previous more negative biopsies (5-6) (Loch, 2010). This indicates 50% positive biopsy in a setting where lower numbers would be obviously expected, but data are not clear which part of the C-TRUS ANNA positive biopsies belongs to group of only one previous negative biopsy, some of them with only 6 cores, and which was percentage in a subgroup of patients with more negative biopsies. Method is commercially available from Fresenius Kabi Deutschland, Bad Homburg and costs in 2010 without tax (VAT) approximately 378 eur per use (one set of pictures analysis - one patient).

Prostatic HistoScanning was developed proprietary by company AMD, Waterloo, Belgium in cooperation with B/K ultrasound manufacturer. According to company's web site (accessed in April 2011), it is commercially available in EU and Canada and awaits FDA approval for US. First it was aimed as "triage test for men deemed to be at risk for prostate cancer and who wish to avoid prostate biopsy" (Braeckman et al., 2008). Later it seems they realized getting rid of biopsy is at present not attainable goal and they focused on improving sampling of the prostate at biopsy (Braeckman et al., 2008). It seems method was developed by comparing raw ultrasound data from prostates before biopsy to histological results of patients, positive for cancer, who underwent radical prostatectomy. In this way it seems development was similar to ANNA C-TRUS, each using own mathematical modeling for differentiation between benign and malign areas of prostate. However, AMD's HistoScann uses in a way "more straightforward" data, in a technical sense - but it needs specific B/K ultrasound machine and specific probe and is limited regarding other US manufacturer's data. In the community, availability of proper US machines for addition of HistoScann technology is limited. Advantage, compared to C-TRUS ANNA is in data analysis and processing in a "black box", which is for AMD's HistoScanning on site, while with C-TRUS ANNA one has to send data (over internet) to central facility and wait for analysis, therefore ultrasound prostate examination and biopsy can not be performed the same day, while HistoScann allows this. How often algorithms are changed and which are better, has not been evaluated yet although both systems are already commercially available in Europe and are, as such, competitors.

Some specific claims about HistoScanning were challenged in the letter to the editor of BJU (Aigner & Frauscher, 2009), objecting name of the method and questioning resolution and ability of ultrasound to detect small tumor foci. In response, authors admit some limitations of their method, specifically lower quality of signal and therefore potentially less reliable analysis in case of dense calcifications in the prostate or for analyzing anterior component of a very large prostate. They compare it with MRI claiming there is wider availability or US compared to MRI. It is at present not true - MRI is available in a lot of hospitals, endorectal coils are single use, however, specific B/K ultrasound machine with particular probe and motorized machine for rectal probe guiding and AMD's "black box" are not available and seem at present more costly compared to MRI examination. Advantage of all ultrasound approaches compared to MRI approaches lies in assumption of ultrasound picture to be easier for use in subsequent sample acquisition. With the expected development of programs for US - MRI picture fusion, this advantage of pure-ultrasound approach may disappear. Question which is better or are all those methods (MRI (T-2, DW and spectroscopy), elastography, C-TRUS ANNA and HistoScanning) comparable or perhaps they may supplement each other, will become important source of research endeavours in the future. HistoScanning manufacturer intends to use the technology also for other cancers, like ovary, thyroid and breast, which may be advantageous as prostate diagnosis may benefit from multidisciplinary team. On the other side, C-TRUS ANNA was developed by urologists for urologists, can be used in almost any setting (any digital ultrasound machine is good) and seems to have at present more peer reviewed data. HistoScanning is not aiming only towards prostate biopsy guidance, but also aims at other potentially useful predictions regarding prostate cancer and seems to have larger research base with groups from different countries (UK, Germany) who study its potential applications. Whether one or both techniques will stand the test of time and what role they will play remains open.

3.4.3 Elastography

Real time transrectal ultrasonoelastograpy of the prostate is aimed at discrimination between harder and softer areas of prostate tissue. MRI elastography technology was also developed (S. Li et al., 2011), but here only ultrasound is described. Back-scattered ultrasound waves are displaced with compression or decompression of tissue (approximately 2%), harder areas showing less displacement compared to softer (Salomon et al., 2008). Elastography is performed in real-time, at the time of biopsy - no previous transrectal ultrasound examination (as for C-TRUS ANNA) is necessary. By subjectively observing US elastography picture, operator aims at evaluating symmetry of stiffness, focal areas of hardness and persistence of stiffness with probe tilting, aiming at stiff nodule more than 5 mm in diameter and persistence of stiffness after probe tilting (Giurgiu et al., 2011). There are different scoring systems (Salomon et al., 2009), some focus on identifying smaller lesions and potentially showing increased sensitivity (Kamoi et al., 2008). Technique of elastography is still improving, better differentiation markers are being developed constantly (Zhang et al., 2011). Further, standardization of compression with idea of leaving this part to the machine is also in testing (Tsutsumi et al., 2010). Regarding companies which provide elastography equipment, most studies have been performed using Hitachi machine, which is commercially available for prostate applications and most tested, although other manufacturers also offer this technology. Among target-biopsy techniques elastograpy seems at present most widely spread as technology is also in use for breast cancer (primarily) and investment needed is only in US machine and probe, there are no per-investigation charges as for C-TRUS ANNA. Elastography procedure is also much simpler compared to MRI-US fusion. Another advantage of elastography is in its compatibility with power/color doppler techniques for image guidance, which can be performed simultaneously, therefore gaining from two sources. There are quite a few published studies describing experience with prostate elastograpy from different parts of the world. Study results are positive and seem to support claims that elastography improves cancer detection rate. One of the very appealing studies, from USA, analyzed help of elastograpy in biopsy of men with PSA values between 1.25 and 4 and free/total PSA ratio less than 18% (Aigner et al., 2010). They were able to detect 24% of cancers using 5 cores with elastography guidance compared to 5.1% cancers using 10 systematic biopsies. Another study, from Romania, used and compared in the same set of patients gray scale, doppler and elastograpyh data (Giurgiu et al., 2011). They found, in a series of 65 patients and 43% of them with identified cancer on biopsy, sensitivity of elastograpy to be 68% and specificity 62%. Particularly promising was elastography in a subgroup of older than 70 years, where sensitivity increased above 80% and lead authors to propose, if their results are further confirmed, in case of negative elastography and doppler, biopsy in this group and in relatively stable PSA, may be avoided.

On recent demonstration of C-TRUS ANNA and elastography at the occasion of EAU Congress in Vienna (march 2011), where both techniques were exposed to a patient with 4 previous negative biopsies and rising PSA, both techniques failed to find cancer in those two patients. This shows, as one can deduce from literature cited above: in approximately 50% of patients with suspicious characteristics (PSA) and previous negative biopsy, we are unable to find cancer at present. For how long? Will they develop cancer in the future? What is the right strategy to follow them? How they end? All those questions are important and need answers in future research.

3.4.4 Color, power doppler

Angiogenesis is important in development of cancer and increased vascularity was detected in tumors in general and in radical prostatectomy specimens, therefore use of ultrasound to detect those changes was proposed. Color doppler imaging estimates mean frequency shift of doppler signal to determine velocity and direction of flow. Power doppler shows total energy of the signal by integrating it, therefore resulting in sig`nal with homogenous background and more precise detection of smaller and low flow vessels (Remzi et al., 2004). Study of usefulness of power and color doppler for evaluation of hypoechoic lesions showed 80% sensitivity and 82% specificity for detecting prostate cancer (Cho et al., 2000). Standardized criteria for scoring different degrees and distributions of prostatic vascularity were developed and also subjective scales seem to work well (Mitterberger et al., 2010), however this points to high subjectivity of the method, which is its drawback.

Power doppler was used for evaluation of peripheral prostatic capsular vessels, parenchymal vessels and vessels anastomosing with extraprostatic vessels (Sauvain et al., 2003). Criteria for suspicion of cancer in this study were increase in number of intra-lesional vessels, disoriented vessels or verticalized vessels in peripheral gland, asymmetrical blood flow, mass effect on the intraprostatic perilesional vessels and vessels in peripheral margins. Analyzing all those criteria, they aimed at estimation of prostate cancer stage by dividing lesions into three groups: absent extracapsular involvement, undetermined extracapsular involvement and presumably present extracapsular involvement. In this series, 55.7% patients had cancer and sensitivity of power doppler ultrasound was claimed to be 92%, specificity 72% (compared to 88% and 58% for ultrasound only). Group with ultrasound estimated lack of extracapsular involvement had this found in final pathology in 11%, while group with ultrasound suspicious for extracapsular involvement had it confirmed in 87%. Authors (Sauvain et al., 2003) conclude power doppler ultrasound improves accuracy of ultrasound imaging in the diagnosis of cancer, can increase detection rate, optimize number of biopsy cores and also predict extracapsular invasion by identification of capsule perforating vessels.

When using ultrasound for evaluation of minor differences in prostate blood flow between cancerous and benign areas, many factors can interfere with the results - for example position of the patient - it was shown left decubitus position caused flow asymmetry resulting in more biopsies directed toward left side without improving detection rate (Halpern et al., 2002).

Different pharmaceutical interventions were proposed to increase difference between cancer and benign tissue: improved view with contrast agent, increased flow with phosphodiesterase inhibitor (vardenafil) (Morelli et al., 2011) or decreased flow with 5-alpha reductase inhibitor or combination of 5-alpha reductase inhibitor with contrast agent (Mitterberger et al., 2008).

Contrast enhanced transrectal prostate ultrasound was extensively evaluated in multiple research projects (Wink et al., 2008). Microbubbles act as additional reflectors in bloodstream and increase sensitivity of color and power doppler imaging. Newer techniques, for example harmonic imaging, were also tested. Use of ultrasound contrast agent is associated with only minimal side effects, like alterations in taste, flush or pain at the injection site. However, it costs additional money for contrast. It should be performed in 4 minutes after contrast injection (half life of bubbles). Further drawback is strong operator-dependence of the technique. Contrast enhanced ultrasound enables visualisation of prostate cancer (in up to 78% of cases), but sensitivity and specificity are not enough to avoid systematic biopsies. Targeted biopsies using this technique are claimed to allow lower number of cores per session without decrease in detection rate (Wink et al., 2008).

Use of 5-alpha reductase inhibitor was proposed in two staged approach: first color/power doppler evaluation of prostate is followed by 1-3 week of dutasteride and than reevaluation and biopsy guided to areas, where vascular signals have not decreased after treatment. Additional sextant systematic sample was also taken. Researchers claimed increased yield in targeted cores (20%) compared to sextant cores (8%) (Ives et al., 2005).

3.5 Biopsy schemes and number of cores

After finger guided biopsy strategies were replaced with ultrasound guided, it soon became clear (group around dr. Stamey, Stanford) 6 cores, taken in a systematic fashion, finds more cancer than aiming at hypo-echoic areas or randomly (Hodge et al., 1989). Standard approach, which hold for more than 10 years, was established: six cores were taken in parasagittal plane, one at the base, one mid-gland and one at apex. However, patients with negative biopsies and still suspicious for cancer, had repeat biopsies, which were almost as often positive as first biopsy - therefore it was obvious the system was not perfect. Aim should be - perform biopsy - if it is negative, then there is no cancer. Reality was - perform classic sextant scheme biopsy - if it is negative, then there is almost the same probability for cancer as before biopsy. So - search has begun for improvement of systematic biopsy scheme (mainly searching for optimal number of cores and location of cores) and this search has not settled yet. As this text aims at the future, not past, only some examples will be pointed out. Inadequacy of sextant scheme was proven many times, for example (Norberg et al., 1997) and also recent larger and longer retrospective data analyzes still turn to this question, for example regarding sextant biopsy's ability to predict unilateral disease (Mayes et al., 2011). First it became clear biopsies should be directed more laterally in the peripheral zone of the prostate (Eskew et al., 1997). Later, it seemed transitional zone inclusion may improve cancer detection, however this was abandoned for initial biopsy, because of inferior gain from transitional zone directed cores compared to more sampling toward far lateral mid-gland and anterior-apical areas. A lot of cancers are located on anterior horn of prostate. With repeat biopsy, of course, anterior transitional zone is also sampled (Chun et al., 2010). Innumerous analyzes have shown - more cores - more cancer. Prostate size has a role (Taneja, 2006). Nomogram was developed to optimize number of cores needed in relation to prostate size - so called Vienna nomogram (Remzi et al., 2005), as it is obvious higher number of cores gives better sampling and improves detection. Later, while some still questioned Vienna nomogram's usefulness (Lecuona & Heyns, 2010), it became obvious number of biopsy detected cancers is related to sampling density, which is a quotient between prostate size and number of cores taken. A lot of nomograms, which predict probability of positive prostate biopsy, take sampling density into account (Chun et al., 2007). Regarding number of cores, it went up from six at first to eight, later ten, later twelve (a lot of us still using this number at present for majority of patients for first biopsy), fifteen, eighteen... up to twenty-one (Guichard et al., 2007) core per biopsy session. This number seems to be highest present routine extended systematic biopsy scheme, simply because twenty-four or more cores is called saturation biopsy (Ahyai et al., 2010). Many have also argued they were unable to increase their cancer detection rate after increasing number of cores from for example 12 to 18. This underscores importance not only of number, but also direction of cores.

3.6 Free hand systematic biopsy, targeted biopsy, prostatic mapping or combination

Goal of prostate biopsy is not only to find "some" cancer in the prostate, as it was in the past. Now, it has not only to provide representative sample of DIL (dominant intraprostatic lesion), but also to show all "important" cancer areas in the prostate, describe precisely where they are and ensure other regions are cancer free. This is in contrast to efforts of targeted biopsies which claim they may reduce pain and burden of biopsy by reducing number of cores.

Prostate-mapping biopsy approaches, for example TargetScann, have different approach - they aim at precisely sampling predefined sections of prostate with larger number of cores. Electronic doppler ultrasound probes are becoming increasingly complex and sensitive to detect blood flow signals in the prostate to help guiding biopsy. TargetScan's device ultrasound probe is sector and at present can not be used for image-guided approaches, but seems to provide relatively reliable results regarding prostate mapping, which is very important for all targeted therapy approaches (Andriole et al., 2007). "Robotic" probes (ultrasound systems, which are just inserted into rectum by physician and then guided by pressing buttons, are being developed also by other manufacturers.

We have therefore a mix of partly competing, some probably complementary and some excluding technologies aiming at improving prostate cancer detection and staging. Which will find its way into every-day practice and to what extent, remains open. It seems at present repeat biopsy yield is about 20%-40% and targeted biopsy methods claim, in repeat, previously negative setting, yield of 50%. All those new approaches need evaluation and confirmation. One way may be showing significantly better performance of targeted or mapping approaches compared to prediction of nomograms for repeat biopsy setting (Chun et al., 2007).

Overall, it seems at present first biopsy should be 10-18 laterally directed cores (depending on prostate size, for prostates larger than 50 ml minimum 14). Targeted biopsy only, with less than 6 cores, may generally not be appropriate for the first biopsy, as it is far from 100% and we need to assess whole prostate.

For second and later biopsies, as targeted opinions are becoming more and more widespread and therefore accessible and are not untested technical glitches any more, we may in 2011 suggest any of the recently developed opinions, depending on local availability, as follows.

1. If no targeted approach is available and also there is lack of funds (for example for C-TRUS ANNA), transrectal saturation biopsy may be performed and probably it may be useful to perform MRI or choline PET-CT to help identifying suspicious areas.
2. If equipment and local expertise allow, any of the targeted biopsy methods (for example C-TRUS ANNA or others) should be used.
3. Stereotactic biopsy (TargetScan or transperineal) is definitely better opinion compared to free-hand saturation biopsy. Stereotactic approach may also be suggested after diagnosis, regarding watchful waiting or minimally invasive therapies planning.

4. Periprocedural considerations

Prostate biopsy is potentially dangerous and painful procedure. Preparation, informed consent with explanation of possible complications, administration of proper antibiotic prophylaxis, policy on anticoagulant and antiaggregation medications and pain management should be standardized and followed in every patient.

4.1 Enema and needle handling

Although bowel preparation with enema or clear fluids are not necessary before biopsy (Zaytoun et al., 2011) or no statistically significant increase in complication rate was identified with change of regimen (Ruddick et al., 2011), some still claim less septic complications with enema use (Kanjanawongdeengam et al., 2009) or even with the way enema is properly administrated (Huang et al., 2006). In the light of modern approaches to bowel surgery, extensive enemas really look outdated, but it is obvious rectum should be empty before biopsy and suppository in the evening or morning before biopsy seems very reasonable and appropriate. The future with development of resistant bacteria may even bring back old classical methods (cleaning rectum with povidone iodine enema or simply povidone iodine suppository), but at present this is not standard.

Question of role of re-inserting "dirty" needle. Most of us use one needle for the whole procedure (all cores). Some (Kisner in Maribor, Slovenia) have insisted on using sterilized needle with every core, others studied cleaning needle with povidone iodine solution during procedure (Koc et al., 2010). No decrease in complications was shown with those techniques.

4.2 Antibiotics

Most common causative organism for infectious complications following trus prostate biopsy is E.coli. Antibiotic prophylaxis is necessary and guidelines from European and American urological societies have been issued and regulate this question, although different antibiotic regimens are used in practice. Guidelines are freely accessible on web from the issuing societies (EAU and AUA) and provide also extensive lists of literature, which will therefore not be reviewed again here.

EAU guidelines (www.uroweb.org, 2010 edition) recommend antimicrobial prophylaxis, but admit choice of regimens remains debatable. They list studies which suggest single doses for low-risk patients and remark, prolonged course should be considered for high-risk patients. Expected patogens are Enterobacteriaceae and possibly also anaerobes. Recommended antibiotics are fluoroquinolons, TMP+SMX and metronidazole with question mark (no evidence).

AUA guidelines (www.auanet.org, 2008 edition, reviewed 2010) also confirm prophylaxis is indicated in all patients as randomized controlled trials have confirmed significantly lower rates of complications in antibiotic groups. They also claim single dose may be adequate.

A lot depends on local antibiotic resistance patterns. For example, if TMP+SMX regimen is not used even for non-complicated urinary tract infections in one area, one would not use it for prostate biopsy prophylaxis either. One can never predict for sure future development of antibiotic resistance. Therefore, constant vigilance is needed and monitoring rates of infectious complications is necessary. Special attention should focus on repeat biopsies and this setting may sometimes deserve different antibiotic scheme or previous culture and susceptibility analysis. Later may be performed in two ways - patients with catheters or other urinary tract insertions may be screened using urine culture (Bruyere et al., 2010), but all who need screening should have their stools sample cultured for resistant strains. Resistant strains do occur and may significantly contribute to complications (Liss et al., 2011). Due to high probability of E.coli resistance to quinolones in cases of patients returning to hospital after prostate biopsy with quinolone prophylaxis, it is wise to use another antibiotic before cultures are known (although it seems obvious, people do often get prescribed flouroquinolone again). If there is no or low risk for ESBL, cephalosporines (probably third generation) may be the best initial guess (Zaytoun et al., 2011).

Although single dose is claimed useful, in our and many other situations most patients can be considered not low risk regarding infectious risk classifications (more than 65 years of age, concomitant diseases, like diabetes and lower urinary tract symptoms, incomplete bladder emptying). Therefore typical scheme (as we use it and others, for example (Campos-Fernandes et al., 2009), uses ciprofloxacin 500 mg twice daily started before biopsy and continued for three days. It was shown to decrease rate of complications after biopsy (Schaeffer et al., 2007). As every single infectious complication, even most minor, requiring any health-service contact, even only consultation, is seen as a big problem and aim is to avoid any complication, there are many patients who probably benefit from short course and not single dose antibiotic and this may be further reason why urologists are reluctant in accepting single dose only approach.

Metronidazol is added in some centers routinely, but most do not use it at present. However, it might be useful for specific patients, with specific predisposing conditions and in combination with other antibiotics (for example cephalosporins, although subjective experience shows more complications with their use for this purpose), when flouroquinolone resistance or intolerance is present.

Instead of 1-2 hour prior to procedure fluoroquinolone orally, same use parenteral aminogylcoside (gentamicin or amikacin) or aminopenicilline with betalactamase inhibitor (co-amoxiclav) at the time of biopsy, which is followed by oral antibiotic (often fluoroquinolone, but also others) at home. This scheme is used in some centers and may be helpful when compliance with oral regimen prior to biopsy is questionable or for allergy and non-tolerance to quinolones or in areas with high resistance to quinolones (Kehinde et al., 2008). Combination of periprocedural oral dose of ciprofloxacine with iv dose of gentamicin may be method of choice for single dose regimens.

Additional important recent problem regarding fluoroquinolones was finding significantly different serum concentrations of active drug comparing different generic manufacturers (Kehinde et al., 2010). Apart from probable reason for higher complication rate, substandard antibiotics preparations also contribute to resistance development as longer courses are needed and as a consequence low concentrations of drug are present in the environment for longer time.

4.3 Pain control

Only 11% of urologists in US used local anesthesia to reduce pain during trus biopsy in 2002 (Davis et al. 2002). At the time, a strong appeal from one of the most distinguished opinion leaders favored local anesthesia (Soloway, 2003). Thereafter, guidelines (AUA, EAU, NCCN) all recommended or even mandated (AUA) local pain medication use during this procedure. Intrarectal application of eutectic cream or lidocaine jelly may decrease pain as some anesthetic agent may reach site of pain with diffusion, but it is variable and is considered not adequate. Pain during transrectal prostate biopsy is caused by two sources.

First source of pain is probe insertion and presence and movement of probe in the anal canal during biopsy. This can be ameliorated with slow and gentle dilation and local lidocaine jelly or EMLA cream, but other measures for relaxation of sphincter were also used with success and are available - local glyceryl trinitrate oinment or spray or local 2% diltiazem or 0,2% - 0,5% nifedipine oinment. Using gylceryl trinitrate oinment, headache was noted as side effect in 10% of patients - dose was 2 mg (McCabe et al., 2007). It remains open, whether lower dose of spray (0,4 mg/activation) would reach same effect with less side effects.

Second source of pain during trus biopsy is related to nerves in prostate capsule and neurovascular bundles. After a lot of research (for example (Scattoni et al., 2010)) it seems accepted injection of 2x 5 ml (each side) of 1% lidocaine most appropriately reduces pain. Site of injection may be at the base (basolateral periprostatic nerve plexus area, described also as prostate-vesicular junction injections) or at the apex. Debate where to inject sill continues. Quality control suggested for standard technique of periprostatic block, observation of hypoechoic nodule ("wheal") formation on the site of injection is needed. It was shown least pain (best effect) was observed, when hypoechoic nodule formed after injection on both sides (Obek et al., 2006). Regarding injectable agents, for potential lidocaine allergic patients, tramadol has significant local anesthetic properties and is universally available and it has also been studied in this setting (Seckiner et al., 2011).

Addition of oral medication, either for sedation or for additional pain relief may be also helpful in selected patients.

5. Complications

Generally, complications are: hematuria (13%-74%), hemospermia (30%), blood at stools (1%), pain (4%), nausea (up to 1%), fever (up to 1%), epididymitis (up to 1%), infection which needs hospitalization (0,3%). Most feared complication is sepsis.

Another important complication is bleeding. Patients can bleed from rectum, they can observe hematuria or hemospermia. Bleeding is most often self limiting and settle in a few days. Rarely significant issues (bladder tamponade or significant rectal bleeding) would occur. Such occasions would of course necessitate hospitalization or use of appropriate standard measurements for treatment. Bleeding may be more significant with anticoagulant treatment. Warfarin is stopped well before biopsy and patient is covered with low molecular weight heparin. Low dose acetylsalicylic acid (aspirin) may be continued, although some still recommend a drug holiday for a few days (till bleeding settles). There are no experience with newer antithrombotic drugs (for example dabigatran and other factor Xa inhibitors) and it is generally suggested to be avoided during prostate biopsy (changed to low-molecular weight heparin, the same as for warfarin). Clopidogrel should also be stopped, although there is a report claiming 15% of urologists to continue with both clopidogrel or warfarin (Brewster et al., 2010). This is not advisable, except aspirin and low molecular weight haparin, all other similarly working medications should be stopped before biopsy. Regarding clopidogrel, explicit agreement and consent between patient, his cardiologist and urologist may result in exception, but extreme caution is needed.

Immediate complications, like fainting, diaphoresis should be controlled by adequate local pain control. It is also not advisable for patients to be completely fasted.

Rate of complications increases with time. Most important and frequent seem infectious complications. Reasons for increasing rates of complications may be increasing numbers of cores per procedure or increased antibiotic resistance (Nam et al., 2010).

Long term complications of prostate biopsy would be development of pain syndromes or problems with erectile function, which was described recently (Klein et al., 2010). This reminds us that indefinitely repeating biopsies and increasing number of cores per biopsy may not be the best way forward. Selective, targeted approaches must be taken seriously, as prostate biopsy is not without its consequences.

6. Chemopreventive stategies

Inhibitors of 5-alpha reductase (5ARI), finasteride or dutasteride, may be used short term to decrease blood flow in the prostate before biopsy (as described at the end of section 3.4.4). Further, it is speculated their longer term use (6 months or more) may decrease proportion of benign prostate in a whole gland and in this way increase chances for prostate cancer detection on prostate biopsy. It may also reduce development of low grade cancer. One possible strategy for use of 5ARI inhibitors is prescription of drug after first or second negative biopsy and then regular follow up of PSA. PSA is expected to decrease. Trigger for repeat biopsy is any increase of PSA above nadir or if PSA value under 5ARI is above 40% of initial PSA value. Described approach was recently retrospectively evaluated in abstract form, using REDUCE data (Roobol et al., 2011). However, a proportion of prostate cancers do progress (for example on watchful waiting) without this fact reflecting in increase of PSA. Therefore a possibility of prostate cancer progression (in patients on 5ARI treatment or without) while PSA values would not increase is a serious concern and needs further research. We should always be aware, none of our methods is 100% successful.

7. Conclusion

Future of prostate biopsy will be interesting, a lot of new ideas and technologies are competing at present and it remains open which will, in the end, dominate the market and our every-day practice.

Although new targeted technologies, either ultrasound or magnetic resonance, may improve detection and sampling and reduce need for increasing number of cores and repeat biopsy sessions, none seem at present nearing 100% sensitivity or specificity. At present, approximately 50% positive biopsy rate is expected in repeat biopsy setting using either C-TRUS ANNA or MRI-guided or MRI-US picture fusion guided biopsy.

As burden of biopsies may increase dramatically in the near future (as explained above - (Quon et al., 2011)) further increases in complexity and technological demands may not be able to satisfy mass biopsy needs. Prostate biopsy is not very demanding procedure, potential harms and problems for patients do exist, but are not nearly as large as for different forms of prostate cancer treatments. Therefore, such a breakthrough as happened in the field of prostate surgery regarding robotic assisted prostatectomy, is not expected. Perhaps we may expect in the near future coexistence of many different biopsy opinions and methods, which are showing comparable results, the same situation as developed for surgical treatment of prostate cancer, where robotic, laparoscopic and open radical prostatectomies progressed to the level, where all show same good results (Eden et al., 2011). It seems present simple system - transrectal probe with 10-20 samples per session, with some additional help of ultrasound picture analysis and systematic sampling systems or not - is here to stay and will be main working horse for enormous number of prostate biopsies which are expected to be performed in the next decade. New markers (PCA3 and p2PSA) will complement PSA and free PSA in decisions about second and further repeat biopsies. At the same time different US and MRI methods, tailored to different patients needs, wishes and different predicted treatment modalities will be available to supplement basic approach when needed and will develop further.

8. References

Abdollah, F., Novara, G., Briganti, A., Scattoni, V., Raber, M., Roscigno, M., Suardi, N., et al. (2011). Trans-rectal Versus Trans-Perineal Saturation Rebiopsy of the Prostate: Is There a Difference in Cancer Detection Rate? *Urology*, *77*(4), 921-925.

Ahyai, S. A., Isbarn, H., Karakiewicz, P. I., Chun, F. K. H., Reichert, M., Walz, J., Steuber, T., et al. (2010). The presence of prostate cancer on saturation biopsy can be accurately predicted. *BJU Int*, *105*(5), 636-641.

Aigner, F., & Frauscher, F. (2009). RE: Computer-aided ultrasonography (HistoScanning): a novel technology for locating and characterizing prostate cancer. *BJU Int*, *103*(1), 115-116.

Aigner, F., Pallwein, L., Junker, D., Schafer, G., Mikuz, G., Pedross, F., Mitterberger, M. J., et al. (2010). Value of real-time elastography targeted biopsy for prostate cancer detection in men with prostate specific antigen 1.25 ng/ml or greater and 4.00 ng/ml or less. *J Urol*, *184*(3), 913-917.

Akhavan, A., Keith, J. D., Bastacky, S. I., Cai, C., Wang, Y., & Nelson, J. B. (2007). The proportion of cores with high-grade prostatic intraepithelial neoplasia on extended-pattern needle biopsy is significantly associated with prostate cancer on site-directed repeat biopsy. *BJU Int*, *99*(4), 765-769.

Andriole, G. L., Bullock, T. L., Belani, J. S., Traxel, E., Yan, Y., Bostwick, D. G., & Humphrey, P. A. (2007). Is There a Better Way to Biopsy the Prostate? Prospects for a Novel Transrectal Systematic Biopsy Approach. *Urology*, *70*(6, Supplement 1), S22-S26.

Andriole, G. L., Grubb, R. L., Buys, S. S., Chia, D., Church, T. R., Fouad, M. N., Gelmann, E. P., et al. (2009). Mortality Results from a Randomized Prostate-Cancer Screening Trial. *NEJM*, *360*(13), 1310-1319.

Auprich, M., van Poppel, H., Marberger, M., Stenzl, Arnulf, Mulders, P. F. A., Huland, Hartwig, Abbou, C.-C., et al. (2011). 2320 Initial and repeat prostate biopsy: comparative peerformance analysis of PSA, %FPSA, prostate volume and urinary PCA3 including development of novel PCA3 cut-off tresholds. *J Urol*, *185*(4, Supplement 1), e930.

Balk, S. P., Ko, Y.-J., & Bubley, G. J. (2003). Biology of Prostate-Specific Antigen. *JCO*, *21*(2), 383 -391.

Bektic, J., Darte, C., Skradski, V., Steiner, E., Schaefer, G., Bartsch, G., Horninger, W., et al. (2010). 985 Access [-2]proPSA and Beckman Coulter prostate health index (PHI) and early detection of aggressive prostate cancers. *Eur Urol Supplements, 9*(2), 309.

Bektic, J., Carroll, P. R., Cooperberg, M. R., Klocker, H., Steiner, E., Skradski, V., Horninger, W., et al. (2011). 747 The worst cancers send early PSA signals that would allow early detection if monitoring focused on increasing PSA. *Eur Urol Supplements, 10*(2), 238.

Bill-Axelson, A., Holmberg, Lars, Ruutu, M., Garmo, H., Stark, J. R., Busch, Christer, Nordling, S., et al. (2011). Radical Prostatectomy versus Watchful Waiting in Early Prostate Cancer. *NEJM, 364*(18), 1708-1717.

Braeckman, J., Autier, P., Garbar, C., Marichal, M. P., Soviany, C., Nir, R., Nir, D., et al. (2008). Computer-aided ultrasonography (HistoScanning): a novel technology for locating and characterizing prostate cancer. *BJU Int, 101*(3), 293-298.

Braeckman, J., Autier, P., Soviany, C., Nir, R., Nir, D., Michielsen, D., Treurnicht, K., et al. (2008). The accuracy of transrectal ultrasonography supplemented with computer-aided ultrasonography for detecting small prostate cancers. *BJU Int, 102*(11), 1560-1565.

Brewster, S., Turkeri, L., Brausi, M., Ravery, V., & Djavan, B. (2010). 5A prospective survey of current prostate biopsy practices among oncological urologists. *Can J Urol, 17*(2), 5071-5076.

Bruyere, F., d'Arcier, B. F., Boutin, J.-M., & Haillot, O. (2010). Is urine culture routinely necessary before prostate biopsy? *Prostate Cancer Prostatic Dis, 13*(3), 260-262.

Bussemakers, M. J., van Bokhoven, A., Verhaegh, G. W., Smit, F. P., Karthaus, H. F., Schalken, J.A., Debruyne, F. M., et al. (1999). DD3: a new prostate-specific gene, highly overexpressed in prostate cancer. *Cancer Res, 59*(23), 5975-5979.

Campos-Fernandes, J.-L., Bastien, L., Nicolaiew, N., Robert, G., Terry, S., Vacherot, F., Salomon, L., et al. (2009). Prostate cancer detection rate in patients with repeated extended 21-sample needle biopsy. *Eur Urol, 55*(3), 600-606.

Catalona, W. J., Partin, Alan W., Slawin, K. M., Brawer, M. K., Flanigan, R. C., Patel, A., Richie, J. P., et al. (1998). Use of the Percentage of Free Prostate-Specific Antigen to Enhance Differentiation of Prostate Cancer From Benign Prostatic Disease. *JAMA, 279*(19), 1542 -1547.

Catalona, W. J., Smith, D. S., Ratliff, T. L., Dodds, K. M., Coplen, D. E., Yuan, J. J. J., Petros, J. A., et al. (1991). Measurement of Prostate-Specific Antigen in Serum as a Screening Test for Prostate Cancer. *NEJM, 324*(17), 1156-1161.

Ching, C. B., Moussa, A. S., Li, J., Lane, B. R., Zippe, C., & Jones, J. S. (2009). Does transrectal ultrasound probe configuration really matter? End fire versus side fire probe prostate cancer detection rates. *J Urol, 181*(5), 2077-2082.

Cho, J. Y., Kim, S. H., & Lee, S. E. (2000). Peripheral hypoechoic lesions of the prostate: evaluation with color and power Doppler ultrasound. *Eur Urol, 37*(4), 443-448.

Chun, F. K.-H., Briganti, A., Graefen, Markus, Porter, C., Montorsi, F., Haese, A., Scattoni, V., et al. (2007). Development and external validation of an extended repeat biopsy nomogram. *J Urol, 177*(2), 510-515.

Chun, F. K.-H., Epstein, J. I., Ficarra, V., Freedland, S. J., Montironi, R., Montorsi, F., Shariat, S. F., et al. (2010). Optimizing performance and interpretation of prostate biopsy: a critical analysis of the literature. *Eur Urol, 58*(6), 851-864.

Comet-Batlle, J., Vilanova-Busquets, J. C., Saladie-Roig, J. M., Gelabert-Mas, A., & Barcelo-Vidal, C. (2003). The value of endorectal MRI in the early diagnosis of prostate cancer. *Eur Urol, 44*(2), 201-207.

Crawford, E. D., Grubb, R., Black, A., Andriole, G. L., Chen, M.-H., Izmirlian, G., Berg, C. D., et al. (2011). Comorbidity and mortality results from a randomized prostate cancer screening trial. *J Clin Oncol, 29*(4), 355-361.

Davis, M., Sofer, M., Kim, S. S., & Soloway, M. S. (2002). The procedure of transrectal ultrasound guided biopsy of the prostate: a survey of patient preparation and biopsy technique. *J Urol, 167*(2 Pt 1), 566-570.

Dite, G. S., Whittemore, A. S., Knight, J. A., John, E. M., Milne, R. L., Andrulis, I. L., Southey, M. C., et al. (2010). Increased cancer risks for relatives of very early-onset breast cancer cases with and without BRCA1 and BRCA2 mutations. *Br J Cancer, 103*(7), 1103-1108.

Dogan, H. S., Eskicorapci, S. Y., Ertoy-Baydar, D., Akdogan, B., Gunay, L. M., & Ozen, H. (2005). Can we obtain better specimens with an end-cutting prostatic biopsy device? *Eur Urol, 47*(3), 297-301.

Eden, C. G., Arora, A., & Hutton, A. (2011). Cancer Control, Continence, and Potency After Laparoscopic Radical Prostatectomy Beyond the Learning and Discovery Curves. *J Endourol.* 25(5), 815-819.

Eskew, L. A., Bare, R. L., & McCullough, D. L. (1997). Systematic 5 region prostate biopsy is superior to sextant method for diagnosing carcinoma of the prostate. *J Urol, 157*(1), 199-202.

Fink, K. G., Hutarew, G., Pytel, A., & Schmeller, N. T. (2005). Prostate biopsy outcome using 29 mm cutting length. *Urol Int, 75*(3), 209-212.

Franiel, T., Fritzsche, F., Staack, A., Rost, J., Hamm, B., & Beyersdorff, D. (2006). [Histopathologic quality of prostate core biopsy specimens: comparison of an MR-compatible biopsy needle and a ferromagnetic biopsy needle used for ultrasound-guided prostate biopsy]. *Rofo, 178*(12), 1212-1218.

Galosi, A. B., Tiroli, M., Cantoro, D., Conti, A., & Muzzonigro, G. (2010). Biopsy of the anterior prostate gland: technique with end-fire transrectal ultrasound. *Arch Ital Urol Androl, 82*(4), 248-252.

Giurgiu, C. R., Manea, C., Crisan, N., Bungardean, C., Coman, I., & Dudea, S. M. (2011). Real-time sonoelastography in the diagnosis of prostate cancer. *Med Ultrason, 13*(1), 5-9.

Gosselaar, C., Roobol, Monique J., Roemeling, S., & Schroder, Fritz H. (2008). The Role of the Digital Rectal Examination in Subsequent Screening Visits in the European Randomized Study of Screening for Prostate Cancer (ERSPC), Rotterdam. *Eur Urol, 54*(3), 581-588.

Guazzoni, G., Nava, L., Lazzeri, M., Scattoni, V., Lughezzani, G., Maccagnano, C., Dorigatti, F., et al. (2011). Prostate-Specific Antigen (PSA) Isoform p2PSA Significantly Improves the Prediction of Prostate Cancer at Initial Extended Prostate Biopsies in Patients with Total PSA Between 2.0 and 10 ng/ml: Results of a Prospective Study in a Clinical Setting. *Eur Urol, In Press,* doi: 10.1016/j.eururo.2011.03.052

Guichard, G., Larre, S., Gallina, A., Lazar, A., Faucon, H., Chemama, S., Allory, Y., et al. (2007). Extended 21-sample needle biopsy protocol for diagnosis of prostate cancer in 1000 consecutive patients. *Eur Urol,* 52(2), 430-435.

Gustafsson, O., Norming, U., Nyman, C. R., & Ohstrom, M. (1990). Complications following combined transrectal aspiration and core biopsy of the prostate. *Scand J Urol Nephrol, 24*(4), 249-251.

Hadaschik, B., Kuru, T., Tulea, C., Teber, D., Huber, J., Popeneciu, V., Pahernik, S., et al. (2011). 2304 Stereotactic prostate biopsy with pre-interventional MRI and live US fusion. *J Urol 185*(4, Supplement 1), e924.

Halpern, E. J., Frauscher, Ferdinand, Forsberg, F., Strup, S. E., Nazarian, L. N., O'Kane, P., & Gomella, L. G. (2002). High-frequency Doppler US of the prostate: effect of patient position. *Radiology, 222*(3), 634-639.

Hambrock, T., Somford, D. M., Hoeks, C., Bouwense, S. A. W., Huisman, H., Yakar, D., van Oort, I. M., et al. (2010). Magnetic resonance imaging guided prostate biopsy in men with repeat negative biopsies and increased prostate specific antigen. *J Urol, 183*(2), 520-527.

Hara, R., Jo, Y., Fujii, T., Kondo, N., Yokoyoma, T., Miyaji, Y., & Nagai, A. (2008). Optimal approach for prostate cancer detection as initial biopsy: prospective randomized study comparing transperineal versus transrectal systematic 12-core biopsy. *Urology, 71*(2), 191-195.

Hodge, K. K., McNeal, J. E., Terris, M. K., & Stamey, T. A. (1989). Random systematic versus directed ultrasound guided transrectal core biopsies of the prostate. *J Urol, 142*(1), 71-74.

Hu, Y., Ahmed, H. U., Taylor, Z., Allen, C., Emberton, M., Hawkes, D., & Barratt, D. (2010). MR to ultrasound registration for image-guided prostate interventions. *Medical Image Analysis, In Press,* doi: DOI: 10.1016/j.media.2010.11.003

Huang, Y.-C., Ho, D.-R., Wu, C.-F., Shee, J.-J., Lin, W.-Y., & Chen, C.-S. (2006). Modified bowel preparation to reduce infection after prostate biopsy. *Chang Gung Med J, 29*(4), 395-400.

Isharwal, S., Makarov, D. V., Sokoll, L. J., Landis, P., Marlow, C., Epstein, J. I., Partin, Alan W., et al. (2011). ProPSA and Diagnostic Biopsy Tissue DNA Content Combination Improves Accuracy to Predict Need for Prostate Cancer Treatment Among Men Enrolled in an Active Surveillance Program. *Urology, 77*(3), 763-763.

Ives, E. P., Gomella, L. G., & Halpern, E. J. (2005). Effect of dutasteride therapy on Doppler US evaluation of prostate: preliminary results. *Radiology, 237*(1), 197-201.

Izmirlian, G., Crawford, E. D., Grub III, R., Hsing, A., Kramer, B. S., Church, T. R., Riley, T. M., et al. (2011). 333 Family history of various cancers and the risk of incident prostate cancer in the PLCO trial. *J Urol 185*(4, Supplement 1), e134-e135.

Jager, G. J., Ruijter, E. T., van de Kaa, C. A., de la Rosette, J. J., Oosterhof, G. O., Thornbury, J. R., & Barentsz, J.O. (1996). Local staging of prostate cancer with endorectal MR imaging: correlation with histopathology. *Am J Roentgenol, 166*(4), 845-852.

Jemal, A., Siegel, R., Xu, J., & Ward, E. (2010). Cancer statistics, 2010. *CA Cancer J Clin, 60*(5), 277-300.

Jemal, A., Bray, F., Center, M. M., Ferlay, J., Ward, E., & Forman, D. (2011). Global cancer statistics. *CA Cancer J Clin, 61*(2), 69-90.

Kamoi, K., Okihara, K., Ochiai, A., Ukimura, O., Mizutani, Y., Kawauchi, A., & Miki, T. (2008). The utility of transrectal real-time elastography in the diagnosis of prostate cancer. *Ultrasound Med Biol, 34*(7), 1025-1032.

Kanjanawongdeengam, P., Viseshsindh, W., Santanirand, P., Prathombutr, P., & Nilkulwattana, S. (2009). Reduction in bacteremia rates after rectum sterilization before transrectal, ultrasound-guided prostate biopsy: a randomized controlled trial. *J Med Assoc Thai, 92*(12), 1621-1626.

Kawakami, S., Okuno, T., Yonese, J., Igari, T., Arai, G., Fujii, Y., Kageyama, Y., et al. (2007). Optimal sampling sites for repeat prostate biopsy: a recursive partitioning analysis of three-dimensional 26-core systematic biopsy. *Eur Urol, 51*(3), 675-682.

Kehinde, E. O., Sheikh, M., Anim, J., Al-Maghrebi, M., Hussein, A. Y., & John, J. S. (2008). Addition of single dose amikacin to prophylactic quinolones significantly reduces infectious complications of transrectal ultrasound guided biopsy of the prostate gland. *J Urol, 179*(4, Supplement 1), 717-718.

Kehinde, E., Abdel-Hamid, M., Philips, O., Sharaf, L., & Babu, A. (2010). 811 A comparative pharmacokinetic study of seven brands of ciprofloxacin in NZW rabbits using liquid chromatography mass spectrometry technique. *J Urol, 183*(4, Supplement 1), e316-e317.

Klein, T., Palisaar, R. J., Holz, A., Brock, M., Noldus, J., & Hinkel, A. (2010). The impact of prostate biopsy and periprostatic nerve block on erectile and voiding function: a prospective study. *J Urol, 184*(4), 1447-1452.

Koc, G., Un, S., Filiz, D. N., Akbay, K., & Yilmaz, Y. (2010). Does washing the biopsy needle with povidone-iodine have an effect on infection rates after transrectal prostate needle biopsy? *Urol Int, 85*(2), 147-151.

Kotb, A. F., Tanguay, S., Luz, M. A., Kassouf, W., & Aprikian, A. G. (2011). Relationship between initial PSA density with future PSA kinetics and repeat biopsies in men with prostate cancer on active surveillance. *Prostate Cancer Prostatic Dis, 14*(1), 53-57.

Lecuona, A., & Heyns, C. F. (2010). A prospective, randomized trial comparing the Vienna nomogram to an eight-core prostate biopsy protocol. *BJU Int. In Press.* doi: 10.1111/j.1465-410X.2010.09887.x.

Li, S., Chen, M., Wang, W., Zhao, W., Wang, J., Zhao, X., & Zhou, C. (2011). A feasibility study of MR elastography in the diagnosis of prostate cancer at 3.0T. *Acta Radiol, 52*(3), 354-358.

Liss, M. A., Chang, A., Santos, R., Nakama-Peeples, A., Peterson, E. M., Osann, K., Billimek, J., et al. (2011). Prevalence and Significance of Fluoroquinolone Resistant Escherichia coli in Patients Undergoing Transrectal Ultrasound Guided Prostate Needle Biopsy. *J Urol, 185*(4), 1283-1288.

Loch, T. (2010). [Core needle biopsy twice negative with rising PSA level. Does imaging help?]. *Urologe A, 49*(3), 369-375.

Makarov, D. V., Isharwal, S., Sokoll, L. J., Landis, P., Marlow, C., Epstein, J. I., Partin, Alan W., et al. (2009). Pro–Prostate-Specific Antigen Measurements in Serum and Tissue Are Associated with Treatment Necessity among Men Enrolled in Expectant Management for Prostate Cancer. *Clinical Cancer Research, 15*(23), 7316 -7321.

Malvezzi, M., Arfe, A., Bertuccio, P., Levi, F., La Vecchia, C., & Negri, E. (2011). European cancer mortality predictions for the year 2011. *Ann Oncol, 22*(4), 947-956.

Mayes, J. M., Mouraviev, V., Sun, L., Tsivian, M., Madden, J. F., & Polascik, T. J. (2011). Can the conventional sextant prostate biopsy accurately predict unilateral prostate cancer in low-risk, localized, prostate cancer? *Urol Oncol, 29*(2), 166-170.

McCabe, J. E., Hanchanale, V. S., Philip, J., & Javle, P. M. (2007). A randomized controlled trial of topical glyceryl trinitrate before transrectal ultrasonography-guided biopsy of the prostate. *BJU Int, 100*(3), 536-538.

Megwalu, I. I., Ferguson, G. G., Wei, J. T., Mouraviev, V., Polascik, T. J., Taneja, S., Black, L., et al. (2008). Evaluation of a novel precision template-guided biopsy system for detecting prostate cancer. *BJU Int, 102*(5), 546-550.

Miettinen, O. S. (2010). Screening for a cancer: thinking before rethinking. *Eur J Epidemiol, 25*(6), 365-374.

Mitterberger, M., Aigner, Friedrich, Pinggera, G. M., Steiner, Eberhard, Rehder, P., Ulmer, H., Halpern, E. J., et al. (2010). Contrast-enhanced colour Doppler-targeted prostate biopsy: correlation of a subjective blood-flow rating scale with the histopathological outcome of the biopsy. *BJU Int, 106*(9), 1315-1318.

Mitterberger, M., Pinggera, G., Horninger, Wolfgang, Strasser, H., Halpern, E., Pallwein, Leo, Gradl, J., et al. (2008). Dutasteride prior to contrast-enhanced colour Doppler ultrasound prostate biopsy increases prostate cancer detection. *Eur Urol, 53*(1), 112-117.

Morelli, G., Pagni, R., Mariani, C., Minervini, R., Morelli, A., Gori, F., Ferdeghini, E. M., et al. (2011). Results of Vardenafil Mediated Power Doppler Ultrasound, Contrast Enhanced Ultrasound and Systematic Random Biopsies to Detect Prostate Cancer. *J Urol*, 185(6): 2126-2131.

Morgan, T. O., Jacobsen, S. J., McCarthy, W. F., Jacobson, D. J., McLeod, D. G., & Moul, J. W. (1996). Age-Specific Reference Ranges for Serum Prostate-Specific Antigen in Black Men. *NEJM, 335*(5), 304-310.

Nam, R. K., Saskin, R., Lee, Y., Liu, Y., Law, C., Klotz, L. H., Loblaw, D. A., et al. (2010). Increasing hospital admission rates for urological complications after transrectal ultrasound guided prostate biopsy. *J Urol, 183*(3), 963-968.

Natarajan, S., Marks, L. S., Margolis, D. J. A., Huang, J., Macairan, M. L., Lieu, P., & Fenster, A. (2011). Clinical application of a 3D ultrasound-guided prostate biopsy system. *Urol Oncol, 29*(3), 334-342.

Ngo, T. C., Turnbull, B. B., Lavori, P. W., & Presti Jr., J. C. (2011). The Prostate Cancer Risk Calculator From the Prostate Cancer Prevention Trial Underestimates the Risk of High Grade Cancer in Contemporary Referral Patients. *J Urol, 185*(2), 483-488.

Nieder, C., Norum, J., & Geinitz, H. (2011). Impact of Common Medications on Serum Total Prostate-specific Antigen Levels and Risk Group Assignment in Patients with Prostate Cancer. *Anticancer Research, 31*(5), 1735 -1739.

Norberg, M., Busch, C., Stavinoha, J., Scardino, P.T., & Magnusson, A. (1994). Transrectal ultrasound-guided core biopsies of the prostate. A comparison between the standard 1.2-mm needle and three thinner needles. *Acta Radiol, 35*(5), 463-467.

Norberg, M., Egevad, L., Holmberg, L., Sparen, P., Norlen, B. J., & Busch, C. (1997). The sextant protocol for ultrasound-guided core biopsies of the prostate underestimates the presence of cancer. *Urology, 50*(4), 562-566.

Obek, C., Ozkan, B., Tunc, B., & Can, G. (2006). Hypoechoic space formation with periprostatic nerve block: myth or reality? *Urol Int, 76*(3), 236-239.

Oberaigner, W., Horninger, Wolfgang, Klocker, Helmut, Schonitzer, D., Stuhlinger, W., & Bartsch, Georg. (2006). Reduction of prostate cancer mortality in Tyrol, Austria, after introduction of prostate-specific antigen testing. *Am J Epidemiol, 164*(4), 376-384.

Oliveira, M., Marques, V., Carvalho, A. P., & Santos, A. (2011). Head-to-head comparison of two online nomograms for prostate biopsy outcome prediction. *BJU Int, 107*(11), 1780-1783.

Pandha, H., Ismail, M., Boxall, A., Bhatt, A., Langley, S., Hindley, R., & Morgan, R. (2011). 2326 Engrailed-2 (EN2): a urinary biomarker for the diagnosis of prostate cancer without DRE. *J Urol, 185*(4, Supplement 1), e932-e933.

Pater, L. E., Hart, K. W., Blonigen, B. J., Lindsell, C. J., & Barrett, W. L. (2011). Relationship Between Prostate-specific Antigen, Age, and Body Mass Index in a Prostate Cancer Screening Population. *American Journal of Clinical Oncology, In Press.*

Paul, R., Korzinek, C., Necknig, U., Niesel, T., Alschibaja, M., Leyh, H., & Hartung, R. (2004). Influence of transrectal ultrasound probe on prostate cancer detection in transrectal ultrasound-guided sextant biopsy of prostate. *Urology, 64*(3), 532-536.

Pepe, P., Candiano, G., Fraggetta, F., Galia, A., Grasso, G., Allegro, R., & Aragona, F. (2009). Is PSA density still useful in diagnosing prostate cancer? *Arch Ital Urol Androl , 81*(4), 199-202.

Potter, S. R., & Partin, A.W. (2000). Hereditary and familial prostate cancer: biologic aggressiveness and recurrence. *Rev Urol, 2*(1), 35-36.

Quiles, M. T., Arbos, M. A., de Torres, I. M., Blazquez, C., Bastaros, J. M., Placer, J., Doll, A., et al. (2011). 2321 Comparative analysis of prostate cancer antigen 3 mRNA expression in benign peripheral prostatic tissue, cancer and isolated or cancer-associated high grade prostatic intraepithelial neoplasia. *J Urol, 185*(4, Supplement 1), e930-e931.

Quon, H., Loblaw, A., & Nam, R. (2011). Dramatic increase in prostate cancer cases by 2021. *BJU Int. In Press.* doi: 10.1111/j.1464-410X.2011.10197.

Remzi, M., Dobrovits, M., Reissigl, A., Ravery, V., Waldert, Mattias. Wiunig, C., Fong, Y. K., et al. (2004). Can Power Doppler Enhanced Transrectal Ultrasound Guided Biopsy Improve Prostate Cancer Detection on First and Repeat Prostate Biopsy? *Eur Urol, 46*(4), 451-456.

Remzi, M., Fong, Y. K., Dobrovits, M., Anagnostou, T., Seitz, C., Waldert, Matthias, Harik, M., et al. (2005). The Vienna nomogram: validation of a novel biopsy strategy defining the optimal number of cores based on patient age and total prostate volume. *J Urol, 174*(4 Pt 1), 1256-1260.

Roethke, M., Anastasiadis, A. G., Lichy, M., Werner, M., Wagner, P., Kruck, S., Claussen, C. D., et al. (2011). MRI-guided prostate biopsy detects clinically significant cancer: analysis of a cohort of 100 patients after previous negative TRUS biopsy. *World J Urol. In Press* doi: 10.1007/s00345-011-0675-2.

Roobol, M.J., Van Leeuwen, P. J., & Schroder, F.H. (2011). 19 Combining screening and chemoprevention of prostate cancer. *Eur Urol Supplements, 10*(2), 34.

Ruddick, F., Sanders, P., Bicknell, S. G., & Crofts, P. (2011). Sepsis rates after ultrasound-guided prostate biopsy using a bowel preparation protocol in a community hospital. *J Ultrasound Med, 30*(2), 213-216.

Sakura, M., Kawakami, S., Ishioka, J., Fujii, Y., Yamamoto, S., Iwai, A., Numao, N., et al. (2011). A novel repeat biopsy nomogram based on three-dimensional extended biopsy. *Urology, 77*(4), 915-920.

Salomon, G., Graefen, M., Heinzer, H., Huland, H., Pallwein, L., Aigner, F., & Frauscher, F. (2009). [The value of real-time elastography in the diagnosis of prostate cancer]. *Urologe A, 48*(6), 628-636.

Salomon, Georg, Kollerman, J., Thederan, I., Chun, F. K. H., Budaus, L., Schlomm, T., Isbarn, H., et al. (2008). Evaluation of prostate cancer detection with ultrasound real-time elastography: a comparison with step section pathological analysis after radical prostatectomy. *Eur Urol, 54*(6), 1354-1362.

Sauvain, J. L., Palascak, P., Bourscheid, D., Chabi, C., Atassi, A., Bremon, J. M., & Palascak, R. (2003). Value of Power Doppler and 3D Vascular Sonography as a Method for Diagnosis and Staging of Prostate Cancer. *Eur Urol, 44*(1), 21-31.

Scattoni, V., Maccagnano, C., Zanni, G., Angiolilli, D., Raber, M., Roscigno, M., Rigatti, P., et al. (2010). Is extended and saturation biopsy necessary? *Int J Urol, 17*(5), 432-447.

Schaeffer, A. J., Montorsi, F., Scattoni, V., Perroncel, R., Song, J., Haverstock, D. C., & Pertel, P. E. (2007). Comparison of a 3-day with a 1-day regimen of an extended-release formulation of ciprofloxacin as antimicrobial prophylaxis for patients undergoing transrectal needle biopsy of the prostate. *BJU Int, 100*(1), 51-57.

Schoenfield, L., Jones, J. S., Zippe, C. D., Reuther, A. M., Klein, E., Zhou, M., & Magi-Galluzzi, C. (2007). The incidence of high-grade prostatic intraepithelial neoplasia and atypical glands suspicious for carcinoma on first-time saturation needle biopsy, and the subsequent risk of cancer. *BJU International, 99*(4), 770-774.

Schroder, F.H., van der Maas, P., Beemsterboer, P., Kruger, A. B., Hoedemaeker, R., Rietbergen, J., & Kranse, R. (1998). Evaluation of the digital rectal examination as a screening test for prostate cancer. Rotterdam section of the European Randomized Study of Screening for Prostate Cancer. *J Natl Cancer Inst, 90*(23), 1817-1823.

Schröder, F. H., Hugosson, J., Roobol, Monique J., Tammela, T. L. J., Ciatto, S., Nelen, V., Kwiatkowski, M., et al. (2009). Screening and Prostate-Cancer Mortality in a Randomized European Study. *NEJM, 360*(13), 1320-1328.

Seckiner, I., Sen, H., Erturhan, S., & Yagci, F. (2011). A Prospective, Randomized Controlled Study Comparing Lidocaine and Tramadol in Periprostatic Nerve Blockage for Transrectal Ultrasound-guided Prostate Biopsy. *Urology, In Press,* doi: 10.1016/j.urology.2011.03.010.

Shikanov, S., Jayram, G., McGuire, M. S., & Brendler, C. B. (2011). 2322 PCA3 variability in men with very low risk prostate cancer. *J Urol, 185*(4, Supplement 1), e931.

Soloway, M. S. (2003). Do unto others - why I would want anesthesia for my prostate biopsy. *Urology, 62*(6), 973-975.

Taneja, S. S. (2006). Prostate biopsy: targeting cancer for detection and therapy. *Rev Urol, 8*(4), 173-182.

Tang, P., Du, W., Xie, K., Fu, J., Chen, H., Yang, W., & Moul, J. W. (2011). Characteristics of baseline PSA and PSA velocity in young men without prostate cancer: Racial differences. *The Prostate, In Press.* doi:10.1002/pros.21418

Terris, M. K., Freiha, F. S., McNeal, J. E., & Stamey, T. A. (1991). Efficacy of transrectal ultrasound for identification of clinically undetected prostate cancer. *J Urol, 146*(1), 78-83.

Thompson, I. M., Pauler, D. K., Goodman, P. J., Tangen, C. M., Lucia, M. S., Parnes, H. L., Minasian, L. M., et al. (2004). Prevalence of Prostate Cancer among Men with a Prostate-Specific Antigen Level ≤4.0 ng per Milliliter. *NEJM, 350*(22), 2239-2246.

Tsutsumi, M., Miyagawa, T., Matsumura, T., Endo, T., Kandori, S., Shimokama, T., & Ishikawa, S. (2010). Real-time balloon inflation elastography for prostate cancer detection and initial evaluation of clinicopathologic analysis. *AJR Am J Roentgenol, 194*(6), 471-476.

Turkbey, B., Xu, S., Kruecker, J., Locklin, J., Pang, Y., Bernardo, M., Merino, M. J., et al. (2011). Documenting the location of prostate biopsies with image fusion. *BJU Int, 107*(1), 53-57.

Ukimura, O., Hirahara, N., Fujihara, A., Yamada, T., Iwata, T., Kamoi, K., Okihara, K., et al. (2010). Technique for a hybrid system of real-time transrectal ultrasound with preoperative magnetic resonance imaging in the guidance of targeted prostate biopsy. *Int J Urol, 17*(10), 890-893.

Vickers, A. J., & Cronin, A. M. (2010). Everything You Always Wanted to Know About Evaluating Prediction Models (But Were Too Afraid to Ask). *Urology, 76*(6), 1298-1301.

Vickers, A. J., Till, C., Tangen, C. M., Lilja, H., & Thompson, I. M. (2011). An Empirical Evaluation of Guidelines on Prostate-specific Antigen Velocity in Prostate Cancer Detection. *Journal of the National Cancer Institute, 103*(6), 462 -469.

Vlaeminck-Guillem, V., Devonec, M., Colombel, M., Rodriguez-Lafrasse, C., Decaussin-Petrucci, M., & Ruffion, A. (2011). Urinary PCA3 score predicts prostate cancer multifocality. *J Urol, 185*(4), 1234-1239.

Wink, M., Frauscher, Ferdinand, Cosgrove, D., Chapelon, J.-Y., Palwein, L., Mitterberger, M., Harvey, C., et al. (2008). Contrast-Enhanced Ultrasound and Prostate Cancer; A Multicentre European Research Coordination Project. *Eur Urol, 54*(5), 982-993.

Yossepowitch, O. (2008). Digital Rectal Examination Remains an Important Screening Tool for Prostate Cancer. *Eur Urol, 54*(3), 483-484.

Zaytoun, O. M., Anil, T., Moussa, A. S., Jianbo, L., Fareed, K., & Jones, J. S. (2011). Morbidity of prostate biopsy after simplified versus complex preparation protocols: assessment of risk factors. *Urology, 77*(4), 910-914.

Zaytoun, O. M., Vargo, E. H., Rajan, R., Berglund, R., Gordon, S., & Jones, J. S. (2011). Emergence of Fluoroquinolone-resistant Escherichia coli as Cause of Postprostate Biopsy Infection: Implications for Prophylaxis and Treatment. *Urology. In Press* doi: 10.1016/j.urology.2010.12.067.

Zeegers, M. P. A., Jellema, A., & Ostrer, H. (2003). Empiric risk of prostate carcinoma for relatives of patients with prostate carcinoma: a meta-analysis. *Cancer, 97*(8), 1894-1903.

Zhang, Y., Tang, J., Li, Y.-M., Fei, X., Lv, F.-Q., He, E.-H., Li, Q.-Y., et al. (2011). Differentiation of prostate cancer from benign lesions using strain index of transrectal real-time tissue elastography. *Eur J Radiol. In Press* doi: 10.1016/j.ejrad.2011.02.037.

9

Testosterone for the Treatment of Mammary and Prostate Cancers: Historical Perspectives and New Directions

Moshe Rogosnitzky and Rachel Danks
MedInsight Research Institute
Israel

1. Introduction

After lung cancer, breast cancer and prostate cancer are the two most common forms of cancer. Approximately 209,060 women were thought to have been diagnosed with breast cancer in the US in 2010, and 217,730 men with prostate cancer (National Cancer Institute, 2007). Furthermore, a total of 39,840 women and 32,050 men were expected to have died of breast or prostate cancer during this year (National Cancer Institute, 2007).

It has been known for some time that the sex hormones, estrogen and testosterone, play a major role in the etiology of breast and prostate cancer (Bonkhoff & Berges, 2009; Carruba, 2007; Dimitrakakis & Bondy, 2009; Folkerd & Dowsett, 2010; Ho, 2004; Mcleod, 2003; Meyer, 1955; Suzuki et al., 2010). However, determining their precise impact in these cancers has proved controversial, and theories of their involvement have been repeatedly revised with the emergence of new scientific evidence (Drewa & Chlosta, 2010; Jensen et al., 2010; Margo & Winn, 2006; Morgentaler, 2006). Because causation has often been assumed where in fact mere association exists, ineffective treatment strategies have frequently been adopted while potentially successful avenues have been neglected.

A key insight that was missing for many years was that testosterone and estrogen can be considered as two sides of a see-saw. In other words, manipulation of one has a direct effect upon the other (Ellem & Risbridger, 2010). This connection was realized with the discovery of aromatization (Santen et al., 2009), but unfortunately did not lead to the necessary re-examination of previous findings in the treatment of hormone-related cancers.

Despite enormous clinical and research efforts, hormonal treatments for advanced breast cancer and prostate cancer have not resulted in significant prolongation of survival over the last few decades. A comprehensive reassessment of prevailing hormonal treatment strategies and the scientific logic behind them is therefore long overdue.

The following chapter examines the role of testosterone and estrogen in breast and prostate cancer from an historical perspective, and suggests that a revised approach of combined therapies targeting multiple pathways in the hormonal cascade is required in order to lead to the meaningful hormonal manipulation of these cancers.

2. Estrogen and testosterone: a biological balancing act

Although people have been aware of the sex hormones since ancient times (Freeman et al., 2001), estrogen and testosterone were only isolated and fully characterized in the 1920s and

1930s. The structure of estrogen was the first to be determined when Adolf Butenandt and Edward Adelbert Doisy independently identified the chemical configuration in 1929 (Tata, 2005). Isolation of testosterone quickly followed in 1935 (David et al., 1935), and this was characterized and named once again by Butenandt (Butenandt & Hanisch, 1935).

New organic synthetic methods emerging during and after the 1930s created ready access to testosterone and estrogen and their derivatives, allowing a period of prolific research into the sex hormones in what has been termed 'The Golden Age of Steroid Chemistry' from the 1930s until the 1950s (Schwarz et al., 1999).

The studies conducted during this time began to reveal similarities between the androgens and estrogens, and it was speculated that it might be possible to convert the C19 androgens directly into C18 estrogens (Santen et al., 2009). Indeed, in 1934, the German-Jewish gynecologist Bernhard Zondek demonstrated remarkable early insight when he stated, '*the female hormone which is regularly present in the male organism represents a normal physiological product of the metabolism of the sex hormones, especially since – due to our present chemical knowledge – a conversion of the male hormone into the female one appears to be quite possible*' (Zondek et al., 1934). This speculation was further supported when the Austrian endocrinology pioneer Steinach and his colleague Kun showed enhanced estrogenic activity in the urine of men administered testosterone propionate (Steinach & Kun, 1937).

The crucial biochemical step in the conversion of testosterone to estradiol, the major estrogen present in humans, is the formation of an aromatic ring from the only unsaturated ring of testosterone (ring 'A', Figure 1). This process is known as 'aromatization'.

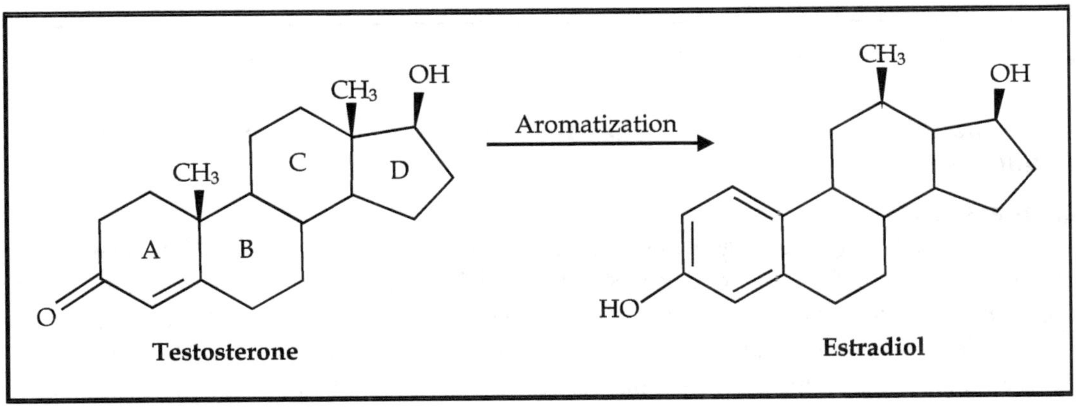

Fig. 1. Aromatization of testosterone to estradiol.

In 1955, a Swiss chemist named Meyer achieved this aromatization using bovine adrenal extracts (Meyer, 1955; Meyer et al., 1955). He recognized that this transformation was likely to be enzyme catalyzed, but the specific enzyme involved was not purified until the 1980s. The enzyme responsible for the aromatization of testosterone was ultimately found to be a member of the P450 cytochrome family of enzymes, and was named aromatase. Eventually, the full mechanism for the conversion of testosterone to estradiol was established (Figure 2).

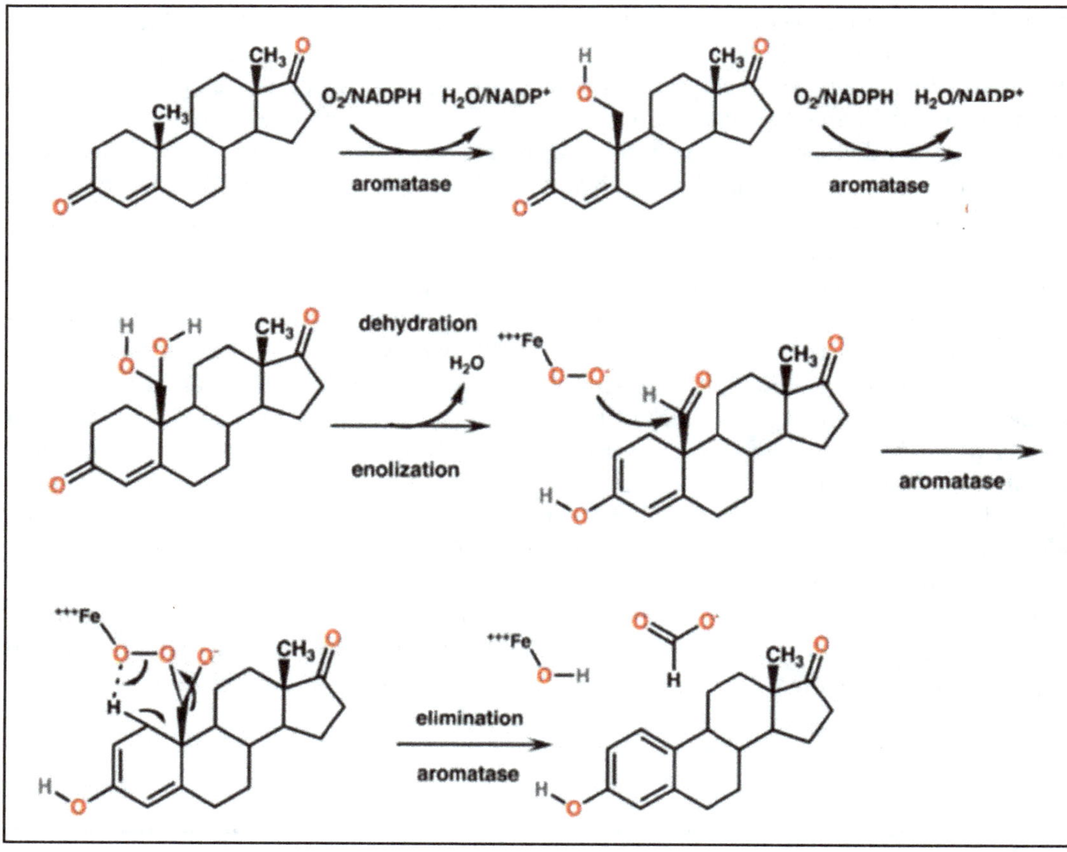

Fig. 2. Mechanism of action of aromatase in the conversion of testosterone to estradiol.

3. Hormonal manipulation in breast and prostate cancer: the controversy begins

3.1 Breast cancer

The first link between estrogen and breast cancer was observed in the late 1890s by a Scottish surgeon by the name of George Beatson (Mukherjee, 2011). Beatson had noticed that removal of the ovaries altered the capacity of cows to lactate, establishing for the first time a connection between breast and ovary. From this, he made the leap to speculate that removal of the ovaries in women with breast cancer may prove therapeutic. He successfully demonstrated the benefit of this intervention in a small group of his breast cancer patients when the tumors of three of his patients shrank dramatically following ovary removal (Beatson, 1896). Butenandt and Doisy's discovery of estrogen was still decades away and Beatson had no understanding of any mechanism for this effect. However, Beatson was convinced he had found a route to control breast cancer. When Beatson's experiments were repeated by others, around two thirds of breast cancer patients were found to benefit (Mukherjee, 2011). This was an important observation, the relevance of which would not become apparent for many years.

Despite its apparent success, removal of the ovaries was not considered a practical or viable treatment for breast cancer as it caused many side effects, including osteoporosis. The alternative was to suppress estrogen pharmacologically, and it was found that this could be achieved by administering testosterone (Mukherjee, 2011). Testosterone soon became an important and effective treatment for breast cancer, and was used extensively between the 1930s and 1960s (Fels, 1944; Goldenberg, 1964; Segaloff et al., 1951, 1964). However, when raised blood and urine levels of testosterone were found in breast cancer patients, testosterone was assumed to be the cause and not a simple associated factor, and successful testosterone therapy was abandoned (Malarkey et al., 1977; Secreto et al., 1983). Subsequent discovery of the confusion between total and free testosterone levels came too late redress the error (Vitola & Zeĭkate, 1976).

In 1968, an American chemist named Elwood Jensen made an important discovery when he identified the estrogen receptor (ER) in the breast, and began to look for the same receptor in breast cancer cells. He found that some breast cancers expressed high levels of the estrogen receptor (ER-positive tumors), while others expressed low levels (ER-negative tumors) (Mukherjee, 2011). This finally provided an explanation for why only a proportion of the early breast cancer patients investigated around 70 years earlier had responded to complete ovary removal. Only ER-positive tumors responded to the resulting estrogen deprivation.

Following this discovery, efforts were directed towards strategies to block the estrogen receptor in breast cancer. The first nonsteroidal antiestrogen developed, MER-25, was only weakly active in large doses and caused severe central nervous system side effects (Gajdos & Jordan, 2002). However, an alternative was soon found, although through an indirect route. Tamoxifen (Figure 3) was originally developed in an attempt to create an estrogen stimulator which would be effective as a female contraceptive drug. However, tamoxifen was very quickly shown to induce ovulation in women instead, acting as a fertility agent rather than a contraceptive (Klopper & Hall, 1971). Instead of stimulating estrogen, tamoxifen was acting as an estrogen antagonist, turning off the estrogen signal in many tissues. As an estrogen antagonist was thought to have no possible clinical benefit, clinical development of tamoxifen was very nearly abandoned.

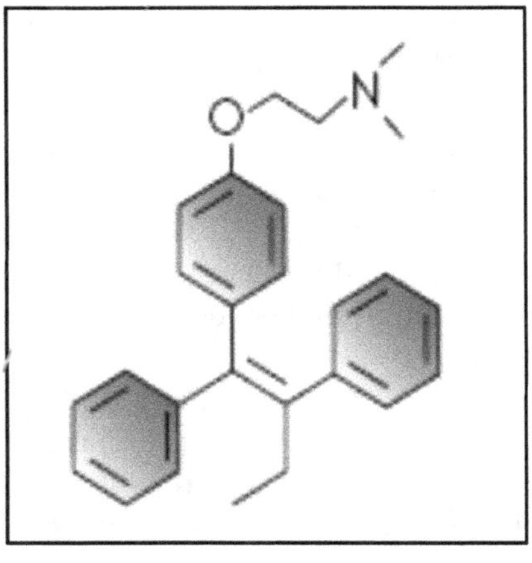

Fig. 3. Chemical structure of tamoxifen.

However, one chemist at ICI where tamoxifen had first been synthesized saw a possible connection between fertility drugs and cancer. Arthur Walpole had been intimately involved in the development of tamoxifen and knew of previous experiments of the sex hormones in prostate and breast cancer. Walpole wondered whether an estrogen antagonist could have a role in ER-positive breast cancer (Furr & Jordan, 1984). Unlike MER-25, tamoxifen is a selective estrogen receptor modulator (SERM), which means it is a partial antagonist effective in only a number of sites, and has relatively low toxicity (Cole et al., 1971; Furr & Jordan, 1984). Tamoxifen therefore appeared to have the attributes of a potential chemotherapeutic candidate for breast cancer.

In collaboration with an oncologist from Manchester, a clinical trial of tamoxifen in 46 women with breast cancer was quickly designed. The results were astonishing. An almost immediate response was observed in ten patients in the trial, with tumors visibly shrinking in the breast, reductions in lung metastases, and a dramatic reduction in bone pain.

Tamoxifen was quickly discovered to improve survival of ER-positive breast cancer patients (Early Breast Cancer Trialists' Collaborative Group, 1998) and soon became a standard adjunctive therapy (Lerner & Jordan, 1990). Tamoxifen held the dominant position for treatment of ER-positive breast cancer for nearly three decades, although numerous other SERMs were also developed (Gajdos & Jordan, 2002). The reduction in the number of deaths from breast cancer in the Western world over recent decades can largely be attributed to tamoxifen therapy (Gajdos & Jordan, 2002; Gradishar, 2010; Hackshaw et al., 2011).

For many years, tamoxifen was considered to act exclusively through its anti-estrogen activity. However, recent evidence has emerged to suggest that its benefit in breast cancer may be due to the up-regulation of androgen receptors (Labrie et al., 2003; Somboonporn & Davis, 2004; Wierman et al., 2006; Zhou et al., 2000). Thus tamoxifen therapy represents an indirect return to the testosterone therapy which was abandoned during the 1950s.

To complete the circle, a review of studies of androgen therapy has recently suggested testosterone itself has a protective effect against breast cancer (Dimitrakakis & Bondy, 2009), while the role of estrogen in the development of breast cancer is now firmly established (Ekmektzoglou et al., 2009; Rana et al., 2010; Sonne-Hansen & Lykkesfeldt, 2005; Thijssen & Blankenstein, 1989).

3.2 Prostate cancer

Just as female hormones were known to control the growth of breast tissue, so it was speculated around the same time that the androgens were responsible for the control of prostate growth. In the 1920s and 1930s, experiments conducted by the urologist Charles Huggins working at the University of Chicago showed that surgical removal of dog testicles led to a dramatic reduction in prostate size, an effect that could be ameliorated by injecting purified exogenous testosterone (Mukherjee, 2011). Soon, Huggins and his colleague, Hodges, published a paper reporting that reducing testosterone levels through castration or estrogen therapy achieved regression of metastatic prostate cancer, while administration of exogenous testosterone resulted in growth of prostate cancer (Huggins & Hodges, 1941). This paper marked the beginning of the long association of testosterone with increased prostate cancer risk and progression, establishing the enduring perception of testosterone as 'food for a hungry cancer' (Morgentaler, 2006). From this time onwards, the presence of prostate cancer, or any prior history of prostate cancer, became an absolute contraindication for use of testosterone therapy.

In an attempt to achieve medical, rather than surgical, castration, estrogens began to be routinely administered to prostate cancer patients in an attempt to halt the production of testosterone. The first results with diethylstilbestrol (DES), a xenoestrogen, appeared extremely encouraging. Patients with aggressive prostate cancer treated with estrogen derivatives responded rapidly and markedly (Mukherjee, 2011).

Estrogen therapy was soon hailed as the salvation for prostate cancer. The reduced side effects achieved were considered particularly important as the current pharmaceutical model of cancer management involved increasingly aggressive cytotoxic drugs which took patients to the very limits of their tolerance. Although patients frequently relapsed, remission could often be achieved for several months. It seemed that prostate cancer would finally be beaten by hormonal manipulation through estrogen therapy.

Over time, new methods for restricting testosterone levels became common place, notably novel phytoestrogens (Castle & Thrasher, 2002; Morrissey & Watson, 2003) and synthetic estrogens (Kim et al., 2002). Yet decades of estrogen-based therapies and testosterone deprivation have failed to make a significant impact on survival and have resulted in significant toxicities.

Despite numerous studies investigating the proposed link between testosterone and prostate cancer, no direct correlation has in fact been found (Jannini et al., 2011; Morgentaler, 2006). Equally, low testosterone levels have not conclusively been linked with the absence of prostate cancer (Jannini et al., 2011; Morgentaler, 2006). For example, prostate biopsies in a study of hypogonadal men revealed prostate cancer in 14.3% of men (Morgentaler et al., 1996), comparable with the 15.2% found in the placebo arm of the Prostate Cancer Prevention Trial (Thompson et al., 2004). Of even greater concern, neither prostate specific antigen (PSA), prostate volume, nor cancer progression has been found to increase with increasing testosterone levels in men with untreated prostate cancer (Morgentaler et al., 2011). Interestingly, evidence is even emerging to show that patients with a lower serum testosterone level may have a higher risk of prostate cancer than patients with high serum testosterone (Shin et al., 2010).

Recent scrutiny of the seminal work conducted by Huggins and Hodges has revealed some fundamental flaws and methodological failings (Morgentaler, 2006). Perhaps the most damning criticism of the causative link between testosterone and prostate cancer comes from the observation that prostate cancer rates are lowest during the late teens and early 20s when testosterone levels are highest, and highest in old age when testosterone levels are at their lowest (Figure 4). If testosterone truly was a cause of prostate cancer, the reverse relationship would be expected.

Not only does it appear that testosterone should be exonerated from its role in causing prostate cancer, but evidence is emerging to suggest that it may actually be beneficial in managing the condition (Gardiner et al., 2009; Dorff & Vogelzang, 2011; Algarté-Génin et al., 2004). For example, two preliminary phase I studies have shown that high-dose exogenous testosterone therapy can safely be administered in patients with castrate-resistant metastatic prostate cancer (Szmulewitz et al., 2009; Morris et al., 2009). Some response in terms of PSA reduction was noted in these trials, but neither study was designed to investigate efficacy of this regimen. A larger, randomized trial is under way to further characterize efficacy and impact on quality of life measures more fully.

To complete the absolute reversal of the conventional dogma regarding the role of estrogen and testosterone in prostate cancer, there is also now considerable evidence to suggest that estrogens, once used to treat prostate cancer, actually contribute to the genesis of the disease (Bonkhoff & Berges, 2009; Carruba, 2007; Jensen et al., 2010; Prins & Korach, 2008; M Singh et al., 2008; P Singh et al., 2008; Wibowo et al., 2011)

In summary, after decades of research and contradictory claims it now seems that, contrary to the received wisdom, estrogen is a causative factor in breast and prostate cancer while

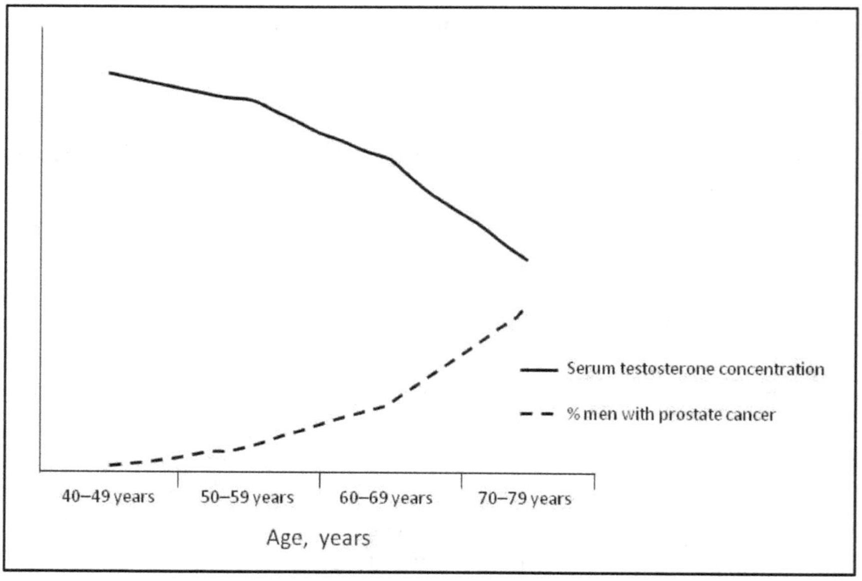

Fig. 4. Prostate cancer prevalence and testosterone levels with ageing. pCA: prostate cancer, T: testosterone. Reproduced from Morgentaler, 2006 with permission.

	Prostate cancer	Breast cancer
Estrogen	Causative	Causative
Testosterone	Protective	Protective

Table 1. Current understanding of the relationship between estrogen/testosterone and prostate/breast cancer.

testosterone actually offers protection against the conditions (Table 1). The concept of aromatization is the key to understanding the conflicting findings.

3.3 The importance of aromatization

From the earliest studies of the sex hormones, it was widely believed that estrogen was only formed in the ovaries and testosterone in the testes. However, research conducted during the 1970s demonstrated that aromatase was abundant in the adipose tissue of both men and women, demonstrating that the peripheral tissue is the major source of estrogen synthesis in men and postmenopausal women (Grodin et al., 1973; MacDonald et al., 1967; Santen et al., 2009).

The close connection between estrogen and testosterone in both men and women presented the possibility of fine-tuning the balance of the two hormones in the body. Scientists began to recognize the therapeutic potential of targeting aromatase to control the biosynthesis of estrogen, and started to develop selective aromatase inhibitors for therapeutic purposes (Barone et al., 1979; Santen et al., 2009; Thompson & Siiteri 1973, 1974).

Research conducted over recent years suggests that aromatase expression and activity in the breast and prostate may be up-regulated at the tumour site, resulting in an altered local hormonal environment and an increased estrogen/testosterone ratio (Ellem & Risbridger,

2010). This is thought to lead to proliferation of the tumor cells in both breast and prostate cancer through a positive feedback loop, established via paracrine and autocrine mechanisms leading to the continuing growth and development of the tumors (Simpson et al., 1997). Further research has suggested that estrogens are capable of inducing prostatic inflammation (Bianco et al., 2006), and this is likely to establish a cycle of increased aromatase, local estrogen activity and subsequently greater inflammation.

Development of inhibitors of the aromatase enzyme therefore represents a logical strategy for the management of hormonally-derived tumors. Aromatase inhibitors are currently used with great effect in the endocrine therapy of ER-positive breast cancer in postmenopausal women to counteract the local estrogens produced in the tumor and surrounding tissue which act as a stimulant for growth (Eisen et al., 2008; Ghosh et al., 2009). Their potential in male breast cancer is also being investigated and shows early promise (Doyen et al., 2010).

Aromatase inhibitors have advanced considerably since the first generation of agents was developed (Table 2). Third-generation aromatase inhibitors now used routinely (Bhatnagar, 2007).

Type	Generic	Dose	Selected brand names
First generation (non-selective)	Aminoglutethimide	250 mg	Cytadren®, Orimeten®
	Testolactone	50 mg	Fudestrin®, Teslac®
Second generation (selective)	Formestane	250 mg	Lentaron®
	Fadrozole	1 mg	Afema®
Third generation (selective)	Exemestane	25 mg	Aromasin®
	Anastrozole	1 mg	Arimidex®
	Letrozole	2.5 mg	Femara®
	Vorozole	2.5 mg	Rivizor®

Table 2. Aromatase inhibitors.

4. Applying current knowledge in future directions

After more than a century of research and controversy surrounding the hormonal treatment of breast and prostate cancer, some conclusions can finally be drawn. First, excessive estrogen levels can be implicated in both breast and prostate cancer, while testosterone appears to offer a protective effect. Second, aromatase inhibitors reduce the conversion of testosterone to estrogen, thus lowering levels of estrogen and increasing testosterone activity. Third, the SERM tamoxifen blocks estrogen activity and both directly and indirectly increases testosterone activity by up-regulating androgen receptors.

In view of these findings, the most rational approach to treatment of breast and prostate cancer would be to administer a combination of three drugs - tamoxifen, an aromatase inhibitor and testosterone. The combination of these three drugs would allow patients to greatly benefit from their synergistic effects in maintaining a desirable hormonal balance in the following way:

1. **Aromatase inhibitor** would allow both endogenous and exogenous testosterone levels to be maintained and estrogen levels to be reduced;

2. **Tamoxifen** would allow upregulation of androgen receptors and downregulation of estrogen receptors, thereby both increasing testosterone's action and ensuring further suppression of estrogen activity;
3. **Exogenous testosterone** in the presence of the aromatase inhibitor would allow increased testosterone levels whilst halting its aromatization to estrogen.

These effects are summarized in Figure 5.

	Increases testosterone	Decreases estrogen

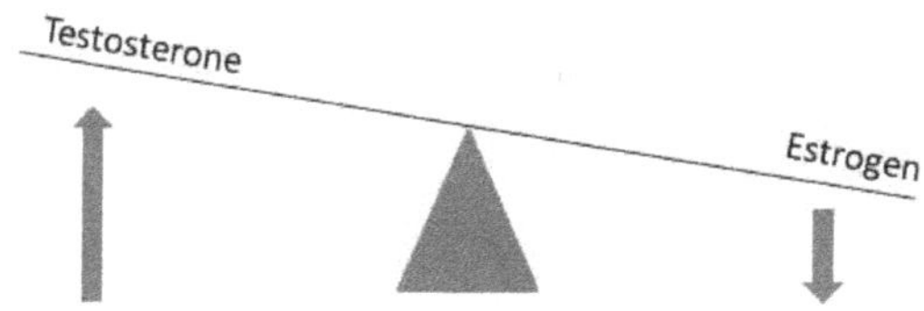

Exogenous testosterone	• Increases testosterone without aromatization	• No increase in estrogen
Aromatase inhibitor	• Prevents conversion to estrogen	• Prevents conversion to estrogen
Tamoxifen	• Upregulates androgen receptors	• Downregulates estrogen receptors

Fig. 5. Rationale for the combination of exogenous testosterone, an aromatase inhibitor, and tamoxifen for the treatment of breast or prostate cancer through elevation of testosterone and reduction of estrogen levels.

Considerable research efforts continue to be devoted to the development of new SERMs to improve upon tamoxifen (Clarke & Khosla, 2009; Silverman 2010). However, the now off-patent tamoxifen confers a significant advantage over newer drugs in being inexpensive and well-tolerated with a known side-effect profile. As well as an established role in the treatment and chemoprevention of hormone-related breast cancer, tamoxifen is also cardioprotective and increases bone mineral density, and appears to have other beneficial physiological effects (M Singh et al., 2008). Although usually prescribed at 20 mg daily, studies have revealed that tamoxifen may be as effective, and perhaps even more effective, at one-tenth the dose (Tormey et al., 1983). This is highly desirable as the risks associated with high dose tamoxifen include thrombo-embolism and uterine cancer.

Testosterone has been safely used for decades and its use does not require any regulatory approval. When used in combination with other drugs, it may have beneficial effects at much lower doses than usual. Ideally it would be possible to use at physiologic doses that would mean customizing the dose to each patient's individual requirement. This could be determined with comprehensive individual hormonal assessments.

There have been several clinical trials in the past 30 years demonstrating superior effects of combining a synthetic androgen with tamoxifen in treating advanced breast cancer over using tamoxifen alone (Ingle et al., 1991; Swain et al., 1988; Tormey et al., 1983), as well as preliminary research into thecombination of tamoxifen with an aromatase inhibitor (Coombes et al., 1982).

Combination therapy has been a common practice in the treatment of cancer for many years, and new combinations continue to be investigated (Lin et al., 2010). It is proposed here that hormonal therapy could also be used in combination in order to take advantage of the combined benefits of the drugs discussed above.

5. Conclusion

Despite considerable research, treatments for advanced breast cancer and prostate cancer have not resulted in significant prolongation of survival over recent years. A comprehensive reassessment of prevailing treatment strategies and the scientific logic behind them is long overdue.

New evidence discovered in the last few years concerning the role and interaction of tamoxifen, testosterone, and estrogen in these cancers is compelling. In the light of this new evidence a rigorous reinvestigation of the science and logic behind existing and long-abandoned therapies is now called for.

We propose that combination treatment with tamoxifen, an aromatase inhibitor, and testosterone may offer substantial survival benefits among patients with breast or prostate cancer. A formal investigation may reveal a significant benefit of this combination of treatments and provide an additional and effective treatment option for the improved management of patients with some of the most prevalent forms of cancer.

6. References

National Cancer Institute. (2007). United States Cancer Statistics (USCS): 1999-2007, In *Incidence and Mortality Web-based ReportExternal Web Site Policy.* 28.02.2011, Available from: http://seer.cancer.gov/csr/1975_2007/results_single/sect_01_table.01.pdf

Early Breast Cancer Trialists' Collaborative Group. (1998). Tamoxifen for early breast cancer: an overview of the randomised trials. *Lancet*, Vol.351, No.9114, pp. 1451-1467

Algarté-Génin, M.; Cussenot, O. & Costa, P. (2004). Prevention of prostate cancer by androgens: experimental paradox or clinical reality. *European Urology*, Vol.46, No.3, pp. 285-294

Barone, R.; Shamonki, I.; Siiteri, P. & Judd, H. (1979). Inhibition of peripheral aromatization of androstenedione to estrone in postmenopausal women with breast cancer using delta 1-testololactone. *The Journal of Clinical Endocrinology and Metabolism*, Vol.49, No.5, pp. 672-676.

Beatson, G. (1896). On the treatment of inoperable cases of carcinoma of hemamma. Suggestions for a new method of treatment with illustrative cases. *Lancet II*, 104-107

Bhatnagar, A. (2007). The early days of letrozole. *Breast Cancer Research and Treatment*, Vol.105, Suppl 1, pp. 3-5

Bianco, J.; McPherson, S.; Wang, H.; Prins, G. & Risbridger, G. (2006). Transient neonatal estrogen exposure to estrogen-deficient mice (aromatase knockout) reduces prostate weight and induces inflammation in late life. *The American Journal of Pathology*, Vol.168, No.6, pp. 1869-1878

Bonkhoff, H. & Berges, R. (2009). The evolving role of oestrogens and their receptors in the development and progression of prostate cancer. *European Urology*, Vol.55, No. 3, pp. 533-542

Butenandt, A. & Hanisch, G. (1935). Umwandlung des Dehydroandrosterons in Androstendiol und Testosterone; ein Weg zur Darstellung des Testosterons aus Cholestrin [About Testosterone. Conversion of Dehydro-androsterons into androstendiol and testosterone; a way for the structure assignment of testosterone from cholestrol]. *Hoppe Seylers Z Physiol Chem*, Vol.237, No. 2, pp. 89

Carruba, G. (2007). Estrogen and prostate cancer: an eclipsed truth in an androgen-dominated scenario. *Journal of Cellular Biochemistry*, Vol.102, No. 4, pp. 899-911

Castle, E. & Thrasher, J. (2002). The role of soy phytoestrogens in prostate cancer. *The Urologic Clinics of North America*, Vol.29, No.1, pp. 71-81

Clarke, B. & Khosla, S. (2009). New selective estrogen and androgen receptor modulators. *Current Opinion in Rheumatology*, Vol.21, No.4, pp. 374-379

Cole, M.; Jones, C. & Todd, I. (1971). A new anti-oestrogenic agent in late breast cancer. An early clinical appraisal of ICI46474. *British Journal of Cancer*, Vol.25, No.2, pp. 270-275

Coombes, R.; Powles, T.; Rees, L.; Ratcliffe, W.; Nash, A.; Henk, M.; Ford, H.; Gazet, J. & Neville, A. (1982). Tamoxifen, aminoglutethimide and danazol: effect of therapy on hormones in post-menopausal patients with breast cancer. *British Journal of Cancer*, Vol.46, No.1, pp. 30-34

David, K.; Dingemanse, E.; Freud, J. & Laqueur, E. (1935). Über krystallinisches mannliches Hormon aus Hoden (Testosteron) wirksamer als aus harn oder aus Cholesterin bereitetes Androsteron [On crystalline male hormone from testicles (testosterone) effective as from urine or from cholesterol]. *Hoppe Seylers Z Physiol Chem*, Vol.233, pp. 281

Dimitrakakis, C. & Bondy, C. (2009). Androgens and the breast. *Breast Cancer Research: BCR*, Vol.11, No.5, pp. 212

Dorff, T. & Vogelzang, N. (2011). Use of Testosterone Replacement Therapy in Patients with Prostate Cancer. *Current Urology Reports* (March 2).

Doyen, J.; Italiano, A.; Largillier, R.; Ferrero, J-M.; Fontana, X. & Thyss, A. (2010). Aromatase inhibition in male breast cancer patients: biological and clinical implications. *Annals of Oncology: Official Journal of the European Society for Medical Oncology*, Vol.21, No.6, pp. 1243-1245

Drewa, T. & Chłosta, P. (2010). Testosterone supplementation and prostate cancer, controversies still exist. *Acta Poloniae Pharmaceutica* Vol.67, No.5, pp. 543-546

Eisen, A.; Trudeau, M.; Shelley, W.; Messersmith, H. & Pritchard, K. (2008). Aromatase inhibitors in adjuvant therapy for hormone receptor positive breast cancer: a systematic review. *Cancer Treatment Reviews*, Vol.34, No.2, pp. 157-174

Ekmektzoglou, K.; Xanthos, T.; German, V. & Zografos, G. (2009). Breast cancer: from the earliest times through to the end of the 20th century. *European Journal of Obstetrics, Gynecology, and Reproductive Biology*, Vol.145, No.1, pp. 3-8

Ellem, S. & Risbridger, G. (2010). Aromatase and regulating the estrogen:androgen ratio in the prostate gland. *The Journal of Steroid Biochemistry and Molecular Biology*, Vol.118, No.4, pp. 246-251

Fels, E. (1944). Treatment of breast cancer with testosterone propionate.A preliminary report. *J Clin Endocrinol* 4: 121-125.

Folkerd, E. & Dowsett, M. (2010). Influence of sex hormones on cancer progression. *Journal of Clinical Oncology: Official Journal of the American Society of Clinical Oncology*, Vol.28, No.26, pp. 4038-4044

Freeman, E.; Bloom, D. & Mcguire, E. (2001). A brief history of testosterone. *The Journal of Urology*, Vol.165, No.2, pp. 371-373

Furr, B. & Jordan, V. (1984). The pharmacology and clinical uses of tamoxifen. *Pharmacology & Therapeutics*, Vol.25, No. 2, pp. 127-205

Gajdos, C. & Jordan V. (2002). Selective estrogen receptor modulators as a new therapeutic drug group: concept to reality in a decade. *Clinical Breast Cancer*, Vol.2, No.4, pp. 272-281

Gardiner, R.; Sweeney, C. & Tilley, W. (2009). Testosterone therapy in castrate-resistant prostate cancer: a possible new approach. *European Urology*, Vol.56, No.2, pp. 245-246

Ghosh, D.; Griswold, J.; Erman, M. & Pangborn, W. (2009). Structural basis for androgen specificity and oestrogen synthesis in human aromatase. *Nature*,Vol.457, No.7226, pp. 219-223

Goldenberg, I. (1964). Testosterone propionate therapy in breast cancer. *The Journal of the American Medical Association*, Vol.188, pp. 1069-1072

Gradishar, W. (2010). Adjuvant endocrine therapy for early breast cancer: the story so far. *Cancer Investigation*, Vol.28, No.4, pp. 433-442

Grodin, J.; Siiteri, P. & MacDonald, P. (1973). Source of estrogen production in postmenopausal women. *The Journal of Clinical Endocrinology and Metabolism*, Vol.36, No.2, pp. 207-214

Hackshaw, A.; Roughton, M.; Forsyth, S.; Monson, K.; Reczko, K.; Sainsbury, R. & Baum, M. (2011). Long-Term Benefits of 5 Years of Tamoxifen: 10-Year Follow-Up of a Large Randomized Trial in Women at Least 50 Years of Age With Early Breast Cancer. *Journal of Clinical Oncology*, doi:10.1200/JCO.2010.32.2933. http://www.ncbi.nlm.nih.gov/pubmed/21422412.

Ho, S-M. (2004). Estrogens and anti-estrogens: key mediators of prostate carcinogenesis and new therapeutic candidates. *Journal of Cellular Biochemistry*, Vol.91, No.3, pp. 491-503

Huggins, C. & Hodges, C. (1941). Studies on prostatic cancer, I: the effect of castration, of estrogen and of androgen injection on serum phosphatases in metastatic carcinoma of the prostate. *Cancer Res*, Vol.1, pp. 293-7

Ingle, J.; Twito, D.; Schaid, D.; Cullinan, S.; Krook, J.; Mailliard, J.; Tschetter, L.; Long, H.; Gerstner, J. & Windschitl, H. (1991). Combination hormonal therapy with tamoxifen plus fluoxymesterone versus tamoxifen alone in postmenopausal women with metastatic breast cancer. An updated analysis. *Cancer*, Vol.67, No.4, pp. 886-891

Jannini, E.; Gravina, G.; Mortengaler, A.; Morales. A.; Incrocci, L. & Hellstrom, W. (2011). Is testosterone a friend or a foe of the prostate? *The Journal of Sexual Medicine*, Vol.8, No.4, pp. 946-955

Jensen, E.; Jacobson, H.; Walf, A. & Frye, C. (2010). Estrogen action: a historic perspective on the implications of considering alternative approaches. *Physiology & Behavior*, Vol.99, No. 2, pp. 151-162

Kim, I.; Kim, B-C.; Seong, D.; Lee, D.; Seo, J-M.; Hong, Y.; Kim, H-T.; Morton, R. & Kim, S-J. (2002). Raloxifene, a mixed estrogen agonist/antagonist, induces apoptosis in androgen-independent human prostate cancer cell lines. *Cancer Research*, Vol.62, No.18, pp. 5365-5369

Klopper, A. & Hall, M. (1971). New Synthetic Agent for the Induction of Ovulation: Preliminary Trials in Women. *BMJ*, Vol.1, pp. 152-154

Labrie, F.; Luu-The, V.; Labrie, C.; Belanger, A.; Simard, J.; Lin, S-X. & Pelletier, G. (2003). Endocrine and Intracrine Sources of Androgens in Women: Inhibition of Breast Cancer and Other Roles of Androgens and Their Precursor Dehydroepiandrosterone. *Endocrinology Reviews*, Vol.24, No.2, pp. 152-182

Lerner, L. & Jordan, V. (1990). Development of antiestrogens and their use in breast cancer: eighth Cain memorial award lecture. *Cancer Research*, Vol.50, No.14, pp. 4177-4189

Lin, S-X.; Chen, J.; Mazumdar, M.; Poirier, D.; Wang, C.; Azzi, A. & Zhou, M. (2010). Molecular therapy of breast cancer: progress and future directions. *Nature Reviews. Endocrinology*, Vol.6, No.9, pp. 485-493

MacDonald, P.; Rombaut, R. & Siiteri, P. (1967). Plasma precursors of estrogen. I. Extent of conversion of plasma delta-4-androstenedione to estrone in normal males and nonpregnant normal, castrate and adrenalectomized females. *The Journal of Clinical Endocrinology and Metabolism*, Vol.27, No.8, pp. 1103-1111

Malarkey, W.; Schroeder, L.; Stevens, V.; James, A. & Lanese, R. (1977). Twenty-four-hour preoperative endocrine profiles in women with benign and malignant breast disease. *Cancer Research*, Vol.37, No.12, pp. 4655-4659

Margo, K.; & Winn, R. (2006). Testosterone treatments: why, when, and how? *American Family Physician*, Vol.73, No.9, pp. 1591-1598

Mcleod, D. (2003). Hormonal therapy: historical perspective to future directions. *Urology*, Vol.61, No.2, pp. 3-7

Meyer, A. (1955). Conversion of 19-hydroxy-delta 4-androstene-3,17-dione to estrone by endocrine tissue. *Biochimica Et Biophysica Acta*, Vol.17, No.3, pp. 441-442

Meyer, A.; Hayano, M.; Lindberg, M.; Gut, M. & Rodgers, O. (1955). The conversion of delta 4-androstene-3,17-dione-4-C14 and dehydroepiandrosterone by bovine adrenal homogenate preparations. *Acta Endocrinologica*, Vol.18, No.2, pp. 148-168

Morgentaler, A.; Bruning, C. & DeWolf, W. (1996). Occult prostate cancer in men with low serum testosterone levels. *The Journal of the American Medical Association*, Vol.276, No.23, pp. 1904-1906

Morgentaler, A. (2006). Testosterone and prostate cancer: an historical perspective on a modern myth. *European Urology*, Vol.50, No.5, pp. 935-939

Morgentaler, A.; Lipshultz, L.; Bennett, R.; Sweeney, M.; Avila, D & Khera, M. (2011). Testosterone Therapy in Men With Untreated Prostate Cancer. *The Journal of Urology*. doi:10.1016/j.juro.2010.11.084. http://www.ncbi.nlm.nih.gov/pubmed/21334649.

Morris, M.; Huang, D.; Kelly, W.; Slovin, S.; Stephenson, R.; Eicher, C.; Delacruz, A.; Curley, T.; Schwartz, L. & Scher, H. (2009). Phase 1 trial of high-dose exogenous testosterone in patients with castration-resistant metastatic prostate cancer. *European Urology*, Vol.56, No. 2, pp. 237-244

Morrissey, C. & Watson, W. (2003). Phytoestrogens and prostate cancer. *Current Drug Targets*, Vol.4, No.3, pp. 231-241

Mukherjee, S. (2011). *The emperor of all maladies. A biography of cancer* (1st ed). HarperCollins Publishers. ISBN 978-0-00-725091-2, London, UK

Prins, G. & Korach, K. (2008). The role of estrogens and estrogen receptors in normal prostate growth and disease. *Steroids*, Vol.73, No.3, pp. 233-244

Rana, A.; Rangasamy, V. & Mishra, R. (2010). How estrogen fuels breast cancer. *Future Oncology*, Vol.6, No.9, pp. 1369-1371

Santen, R.; Brodie, H.; Simpson, E.; Siiteri, P. & Brodie, A. (2009). History of Aromatase: Saga of an Important Biological Mediator and Therapeutic Target. *Endocrinology Review* Vol.30,No.4, pp. 343-375

Schwarz, S.; Onken, D. & Schubert, A. (1999). The steroid story of Jenapharm: From the late 1940s to the early 1970s. *Steroids*, Vol.64, No.7, pp. 439-445

Secreto, G.; Recchione, C.; Grignolio, E. & Cavalleri, A. (1983). Increased urinary androgen excretion is a hormonal abnormality detectable before the clinical onset of breast cancer. *Cancer Detection and Prevention*, Vol.6, No.4, pp. 435-438

Segaloff, A.; Gordon, D.; Horwitt, B.; Schlosser, J. & Murison, P. (1951). Hormonal therapy in cancer of the breast. I. The effect of testosterone propionate therapy on clinical course and hormonal excretion. *Cancer*, Vol.4, No.2, pp. 319-323

Segaloff, A.; Weeth, J.; Cuningham, M. & Meyer, K. (1964). Hormonal therapy in cancer of the breast. 23. Effect of 7-alpha-methyl-19-nortestosterone acetate and testosterone propionate on clinical course and hormonal excretion. *Cancer*, Vol.17, pp. 1248-1253

Shin, B.; Hwang, E.; Im, C.; Kim, S-O.; Jung, S.; Kang, T.; Kwon, D.; Park, K. & Ryu, S. (2010). Is a decreased serum testosterone level a risk factor for prostate cancer? A cohort study of korean men. *Korean Journal of Urology*, Vol.51, No.12, pp. 819-823

Silverman, S. (2010). New selective estrogen receptor modulators (SERMs) in development. *Current Osteoporosis Reports*, Vol.8, No.3, pp. 151-153

Simpson, E.; Zhao, Y.; Agarwal, V.; Michael, M.; Bulun, S.; Hinshelwood, M. & Graham-Lorence, S. (1997). Aromatase expression in health and disease. *Recent Progress in Hormone Research*, Vol.52: 185-213

Singh, M.; Martin-Hirsch, P. & Martin, F. (2008). The multiple applications of tamoxifen: an example pointing to SERM modulation being the aspirin of the 21st century. *Medical Science Monitor: International Medical Journal of Experimental and Clinical Research*, Vol.14, No.9, pp. RA144-148

Singh, P.; Matanhelia, S. & Martin, F. (2008). A potential paradox in prostate adenocarcinoma progression: oestrogen as the initiating driver. *European Journal of* Cancer, Vol.44, No.7, pp. 928-936

Somboonporn, W. & Davis, S. (2004). Testosterone Effects on the Breast: Implications for Testosterone Therapy for Women. *Endocrinology Review*, Vol.25, No.3, pp. 374-388

Sonne-Hansen, K. & Lykkesfeldt, A. (2005). Endogenous aromatization of testosterone results in growth stimulation of the human MCF-7 breast cancer cell line. *The Journal of Steroid Biochemistry and Molecular Biology*,Vol.93, No.1, pp. 25-34

Steinach, E. & Kun, H. (1937). Transformation of male sex hormones into a substance with the action of a female hormone. *Lancet* Vol.133, pp. 845

Suzuki, T.; Miki, Y.; Takagi, K.; Hirakawa, H.; Moriya, T.; Ohuchi, N. & Sasano, H. (2010). Androgens in human breast carcinoma. *Medical Molecular Morphology* Vol.43, No.2, pp. 75-81

Swain, S.; Steinberg, S.; Bagley, C. & Lippman, M. (1988). Tamoxifen and fluoxymesterone versus tamoxifen and danazol in metastatic breast cancer-a randomized study. *Breast Cancer Research and Treatment*, Vol.12, No.1, pp. 51-57

Szmulewitz, R.; Mohile, S.; Posadas, E.; Kunnavakkam, R.; Karrison, T.; Manchen, E. & Stadler, W. (2009). A randomized phase 1 study of testosterone replacement for patients with low-risk castration-resistant prostate cancer. *European Urology* Vol.56, No.1, pp. 97-103

Tata, J. (2005). One hundred years of hormones. *EMBO reports*, Vol.6, No.6, pp. 490-496

Thijssen, J. & Blankenstein, M. (1989). Endogenous oestrogens and androgens in normal and malignant endometrial and mammary tissues. *European Journal of Cancer & Clinical Oncology*, Vol.25, No.12, pp. 1953-1959

Thompson, E. & Siiteri, P. (1973). Studies on the aromatization of C-19 androgens. *Annals of the New York Academy of Sciences*, Vol.212, pp. 378-391

Thompson, E. & Siiteri, P. (1974). The involvement of human placental microsomal cytochrome P-450 in aromatization. *The Journal of Biological Chemistry*, Vol.249, No.17, pp. 5373-5378

Thompson, I.; Pauler, D.; Goodman, P.; Tangen, C.; Lucia, M.; Parnes, H. & Minasian, L. (2004). Prevalence of prostate cancer among men with a prostate-specific antigen level < or =4.0 ng per milliliter. *The New England Journal of Medicine*, Vol.350, No.22, pp. 2239-2246

Tormey, D.; Lippman, M.; Edwards, B. & Cassidy, J. (1983). Evaluation of tamoxifen doses with and without fluoxymesterone in advanced breast cancer. *Annals of Internal Medicine*, Vol.98, No.2, pp. 139-144

Vitola, G. & Zeĭkate, G. (1976). Blood levels of testosterone and dihydrotestosterone in breast cancer. *Voprosy Onkologii* Vol.22, No.8, pp. 26-30

Wibowo, E.; Schellhammer, P. & Wassersug, R. (2011). Role of estrogen in normal male function: clinical implications for patients with prostate cancer on androgen deprivation therapy. *The Journal of Urology*, Vol.185, No.1, pp. 17-23

Wierman, M.; Basson, R.; Davis, S.; Khosla, S.; Miller, K.; Rosner, W. & Santoro, N. (2006). Androgen Therapy in Women: An Endocrine Society Clinical Practice Guideline. *J Clin Endocrinol Metab*, Vol.91, No.10, pp. 3697-3710

Zhou, J.; Ng, S.; Adesanya-Famuiya, O.; Anderson, K. & Bondy, C. (2000). Testosterone inhibits estrogen-induced mammary epithelial proliferation and suppresses estrogen receptor expression. *FASEB J.* Vol.14, pp. 1725-1730

Zondek, B. (1934). Oestrogenic hormone in the urine of the stallion. *Nature*, 133, pp. 494

10

Monenin Induced Oxidative Stress Reduces Prostate Cancer Cell Migration and Cancer Stem Cell Population

Kirsi Ketola[1], Anu Vuoristo[2], Matej Orešič[2], Olli Kallioniemi[3] and Kristiina Iljin[1]

[1]Medical Biotechnology, VTT Technical Research Centre of Finland and University of Turku, Turku,
[2]VTT Technical Research Centre of Finland, Espoo,
[3]Institute for Molecular Medicine, Finland (FIMM), University of Helsinki,
Finland

1. Introduction

Prostate cancer is the most common malignancy and second leading cause of cancer related death in males in developed countries (Jemal et al. 2011). Patients with localized and metastatic prostate cancer are treated with anti-androgens. Although prostate cancer cell proliferation is initially blocked or slowed down with anti-androgen therapy, eventually castration-resistant disease develops (Sharifi, Gulley & Dahut 2010). Therapeutic options for castration-resistant prostate cancer are limited and treatment responses to currently existing therapies are often unsatisfactory (Bracarda et al. 2011). For example, the cytotoxic therapy often causes severe toxicity and eventually leads also to the development of chemo-resistance (Tannock et al. 2004, Berthold et al. 2008, Bracarda et al. 2011). Thus, there is an urgent need for novel agents to block the proliferation and to inhibit the progression of the primary prostate cancer cells to the advanced stage as well as to target advanced and metastatic prostate cancer. Therefore, understanding of disease progression and drug resistance mechanisms may provide valuable insights into the development of novel treatment options to improve the survival of prostate cancer patients.

We have recently performed a high-throughput cell-based screening of 4,910 known drugs and drug-like molecules in four prostate cancer cell models and two non-tumorigenic prostate epithelial cell lines to identify prostate cancer cell growth selective inhibitors (Iljin et al. 2009). Only four compounds, antibiotic ionophore monensin, aldehyde dehydrogenase (ALDH) inhibitor disulfiram, histone deacetylase inhibitor trichostatin A and fungicide thiram inhibited selectively cancer cell growth at nanomolar concentrations. The mechanistic studies indicated that monensin and disulfiram inhibited prostate cancer cell growth by inducing oxidative stress (Iljin et al. 2009, Ketola et al. 2010). In contrast to disulfiram, monensin induced apoptosis, reduced androgen receptor signalling and showed a synergistic anti-proliferative effect with anti-androgens in prostate cancer cells. Moreover, monensin increased the amount of reactive oxygen species (ROS) and induced an oxidative stress signature in prostate cancer cells (VCaP and LNCaP), but not in the non-malignant prostate epithelial cells (RWPE-1, EP156T) (Ketola et al. 2010). Furthermore, antioxidant vitamin C partially rescued the monensin induced growth inhibition, indicating that oxidative stress plays a key role in the antineoplastic effect of monensin in cultured prostate cancer cells (Ketola et al. 2010).

Oxidative stress occurs in the cell when redox regulation is imbalanced. Redox balance depends on the level of intracellular free radicals and reactive oxygen species as well as on the antioxidative capacity of the cell. Figure 1 illustrates the connection between the malignant progression and increase in intracellular ROS (Fig. 1).

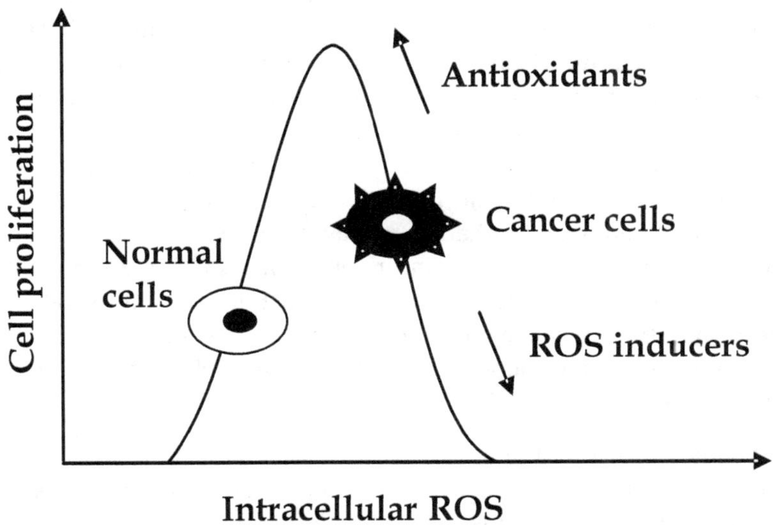

Fig. 1. The balance between cell proliferation and intracellular reactive oxygen species (ROS). The malignant progression and the effects of ROS inducers and antioxidants depend on the intracellular levels of ROS. In cancer cells, intracellular ROS levels are higher than in normal cells making them more vulnerable to agents inducing ROS. Figure idea adapted from Gupte & Mumper 2009.

Cancer cells benefit from the increased mutation rate induced via oxidative stress (Shibutani, Takeshita & Grollman 1991). Therefore, cancer cells need also an active antioxidative mechanism to be able to survive under high oxidative stress. The oxidative stress level is elevated in prostate cancer cells compared to non-malignant prostate epithelial cells (Khandrika et al. 2009, Yossepowitch et al. 2007, Kumar et al. 2008). Many oncogenes are known to protect cells from oxidative stress e.g. androgen receptor (AR), ERG and MYC are known to have antioxidative properties in cancer cells (Pinthus et al. 2007, Tam et al. 2003, Benassi et al. 2006, Swanson et al. 2011, DeNicola et al. 2011). Monensin may sensitize prostate cancer cells to oxidative stress via reducing the expression of these genes (Ketola et al. 2010). In addition, many other anti-neoplastic agents such as vinblastine, cisplatin, mitomycin C, doxorubicin, camptothecin, inostamycin, neocarzinostatin, etoposide, arsenic trioxide and nonsteroidal anti-inflammatory drugs are known to mediate their apoptotic effect by inducing oxidative stress (Fang, Nakamura & Iyer 2007, Rigas, Sun 2008, Sun et al. 2011). The increased sensitivity to oxidative stress combined with dependency on anti-oxidative system may provide a way to selectivity inhibit cancer cell proliferation (Iljin et al. 2009, Ketola et al. 2010).

Recently, redox control including antioxidative defence mechanisms and ROS-scavenging systems has been identified as an important regulator of cancer stem cell potential, metastasis and chemoresistance (Kobayashi, Suda 2011b, Cairns, Harris & Mak 2011, Pani, Galeotti & Chiarugi 2010). Aldehyde dehydrogenase activity is widely used as a marker for cancer stem cells and its activity has been shown to correlate with poor outcome in several cancers such as in prostate cancer (Davydov, Dobaeva & Bozhkov 2004, Burger et al. 2009, Li et al. 2010, Yu et al. 2011, Zhang et al. 2009a). Aldehyde dehydrogenases are detoxifying enzymes that are responsible for the oxidation of intracellular aldehydes (Duester 2000, Magni et al. 1996, Sophos, Vasiliou 2003, Yoshida et al. 1998). Moreover, ALDH oxidize retinol to retinoic acid (vitamin A) known to reduce oxidative stress whereas retinoic acid depletion induces oxidative stress and mitochondrial dysfunction (Ahlemeyer, Krieglstein 1998, Ahlemeyer et al. 2001, Chiu, Fischman & Hammerling 2008, Duester 2000, Chute et al. 2006). Thus, ALDH increases the antioxidative capacity in cells and protects cells from oxidative stress induction. Moreover, the inhibition of ALDH activity has recently been linked to reduced chemotherapy and radiation resistance in cancer stem cells (Croker, Allan 2011). These results suggest that not only cancer cells, but also cancer stem cells could be targeted by oxidative stress induction and/or reduction of antioxidative capacity. Interestingly, the results from mechanistic studies of prostate cancer selective compounds indicated that both disulfiram and monensin reduced the ALDH activity in prostate cancer cells (Iljin et al. 2009, Ketola et al., 2010).

In this study, we explored further the molecular mechanism of monensin induced growth inhibition in cultured prostate cancer cells. Cancer pathway reporter assays and steroid profiling was performed to get insights into altered signalling and metabolite levels in monensin exposed prostate cancer cells. Since monensin reduces ALDH activity, the putative effect on cancer stem cells was evaluated. Furthermore, we studied the effect of monensin on prostate cancer cell differentiation and motility.

2. Materials and methods

2.1 Cells

VCaP prostate carcinoma cells (TMPRSS2-ERG positive, received from Drs. Adrie van Bokhoven, University of Colorado Health Sciences Center, Denver, Colorado and Kenneth Pienta, University of Michigan, Michigan) were grown in Dulbecco's Modified Eagle's Medium (Korenchuk et al. 2001b, Korenchuk et al. 2001a). LNCaP prostate carcinoma cells (received from Dr. Marco Cecchini, University of Bern, Bern, Switzerland) were grown in T-Medium (Invitrogen). PC-3 prostate carcinoma cells were purchased from American Type Culture Collection (LGC Promochem AB) and grown according to provider's instructions. All cells were cultured in appropriate growth media described above including 10% fetal bovine serum (FBS), 2 mM L-glutamine, 100 U/ml penicillin, and 100 μg/ml streptomycin in an incubator with a humidified atmosphere of 95% air and 5% CO_2 at 37°C.

2.2 Compounds

Monensin was purchased from Sigma-Aldrich and diluted in ethanol.

2.3 Cancer 10-pathway reporter array

Cancer 10-pathway Reporter Luciferase Kit (Wnt (TCF/LEF), Notch (RBP-Jκ), p53/DNA damage, TGF-β (SMAD2/3/4), Cell cycle/pRb-E2F (E2F/DP1), NF-κB, Myc/Max, Hypoxia (HIF1A), MAPK/ERK (Elk-1/SRF) and MAPK/JNK (AP-1) was used to study the monensin modulated signalling (SABiosciences, Frederick, MD). The assay was performed according to manufacturer's instructions. In brief, inducible transcription factor responsive firefly luciferase reporters with constitutively expressing Renilla construct transcription factor reporters were plated onto 96-well plates with transfection reagent (siLentFect, Bio-Rad Laboratories), followed by addition of cells and incubation for 24 hours. A mixture of non-inducible firefly luciferase reporter and constitutively expressing Renilla construct was used as the negative control. After 24 hours of transfection, monensin (100 nM) and control treatment were added onto the cells and plates were incubated for 18 hours. The Dual-LuciferaseReporter (DLR™) Assay System (Promega) was utilized in quantitation of reporters and results according to the manufactorer's instructions. The change in the activity of each signalling pathway was determined by comparing the normalized luciferase activity of the reporters in monensin or solvent exposed cells.

2.4 Wound healing assay

The effect of monensin (10 nM, 100 nM and 1 μM) on prostate cancer cell migration was studied using a scratch wound assay. PC-3 cells were plated on 96-well plates (Essen ImageLock, Essen Instruments, UK) and a wound was scratched with wound scratcher (Essen Instruments). Compounds and appropriate controls were added immediately after wound scratching and wound confluence was monitored with Incucyte Live-Cell Imaging System and software (Essen Instruments). Wound closure was calculated for every hour for 24 hours by comparing the mean relative wound density of three biological replicates in each experiment.

2.5 Cell viability assay

Cell viability was determined with CellTiter-Glo (CTG) cell viability assay (Promega, Madison, WI) according to the manufacturer's instructions. Briefly, 2,000 cells per well were plated in 35 μl of their respective growth media and left to attach overnight. Monensin (100 nM) was added to the cells and incubated for 12 or 24 hours. CTG reagent was added and the signals were quantified using Envision Multilabel Plate Reader (Perkin-Elmer, Massachusetts, MA).

2.6 RNA extraction and quantitative real-time PCR

VCaP cells were exposed to monensin for 6 hours, total RNA was extracted and quantitative real-time PCR was done as previously described (Ketola et al. 2010). TaqMan gene expression probes and primers from the Universal Probe Library (Roche Diagnostics, Espoo, Finland) were used to study E-cadherin (5′-cccgggacaacgtttattac-3′ and 5′-gctggctcaagtcaaagtcc-3′) and β-actin (5´-ccaaccgcgagaagatga -3´ and 5´-ccagaggcgtacagggatag -3´) mRNA expression. Three replicate samples were studied.

2.7 Fluorescence-Activated Cell Sorting analysis (FACS)

VCaP and LNCaP cells were exposed to monensin (1 µM) for 6 hours, samples were fixed with 2% paraformaldehyde, and stained with CD44 (FITC-conjugated mouse monoclonal anti-human, BD Pharmingen™ 555478) and CD24 (PE-conjugated rat monoclonal anti-human, Abcam ab25281) antibodies for 45 minutes at 4°C in the dark. Cells were washed and the fluorescence intensity was measured using Accuri C6 Flow Cytometer.

2.8 Immuofluorescence staining

For immunofluorescence stainings, VCaP cells were grown on cover slip slides and exposed to monensin for 6 hours. Cells were fixed with 4 % paraformaldehyde in PBS, permeabilized with 0.2% Triton X-100 in PBS for 15 min, and blocked with 2 % BSA/PBS for 30 min. Cells were stained with E-cadherin antibody (1:100 dilution, polyclonal rabbit anti-human, Cell Signaling Technology, MA, USA) and Alexa-conjugated polyclonal donkey anti-rabbit antibody was used for secondary staining (1:300 dilution, Invitrogen, Molecular Probes, Carlsbad, CA). Cell nuclei were stained with DAPI present in Vectashield mounting medium (Vector Labs) and images were taken with Zeiss Axiovert 200M Microscope with the spinning disc confocal unit Yokogawa CSU22 and a Zeiss Plan-Neofluar 63× oil/1.4 NA objective. Z-stacks with 1 airy unit optical slices were acquired with a step size of 0.5 µm between slices, and the maximum intensity projections were created with SlideBook 4.2.0.7 software (Intelligent Imaging Innovations Inc., CO, USA).

2.9 Statistical analyses

Stars in the figures indicate the significance of the experiments calculated using Student's t-test (*$P<0.05$, **$P<0.01$, *** $P<0.001$).

2.10 Steroid quantification

VCaP cells ($1x10^7$ cells) were exposed to 1 µM monensin for 6 hours, harvested and counted. An internal standard (labeled C16:0) and chloroform:methanol (2:5) mixture were added, the samples were homogenized with Retsch system (5 min, 20 Hz), centrifuged and the supernatants were collected and evaporated. MOX (25 µl, TS-45950, Thermo Scientific, Helsinki, Finland) was added and the mixture was incubated at 45°C for 60 minutes. Next, 100 µl of MSTFA with 1% trimethylchlorosilane (Fluka, St. Louis, MO) was added and the mixture was incubated at 70°C for 60 minutes. Injection standard was added to the mixture before gas chromatography-mass spectrometry analysis (GC-MS, Agilent 6890 gas chromatograph (GC) combined with Agilent 5973 mass selective detector (MSD)). The injector (injection volume 1 µl with pulsed splitless injection) and MSD temperatures were 230°C (MS Source) and 150°C (MS Quad). The analyses were performed on Supelco 38499-02C capillary column. Selective ion monitoring using specific masses for each target analyte was used in the detection. The following steroids were quantified: 7-ketocholesterol, aldosterone, progesterone, pregnenolone, estrone, 17B-estradiol, 4B-hydroxycholesterol,

25-hydroxycholesterol, 5a,6a-epoxycholesterol (Mono-TMS), dihydrotestosterone and testosterone (the standards were from Steraloids, Newport, RI)).

3. Results

3.1 Monensin reduces NF-κB pathway activity in prostate cancer cells

Here, we studied the effect of monensin exposure on the activities of ten cancer signalling pathways using Cancer pathway Reporter Array in prostate cancer cells. Inducible transcription factor responsive firefly luciferase reporters were transfected to VCaP and LNCaP cells with constitutively active Renilla reporters and incubated for 24 hours. Monensin (100 nM) or solvent control was added onto the transfected cells for 18 hours followed by measure of luciferase activities. The results are presented in Fig. 2. Comparison of the basal pathway activities in VCaP prostate cancer cells indicated that NF-κB was

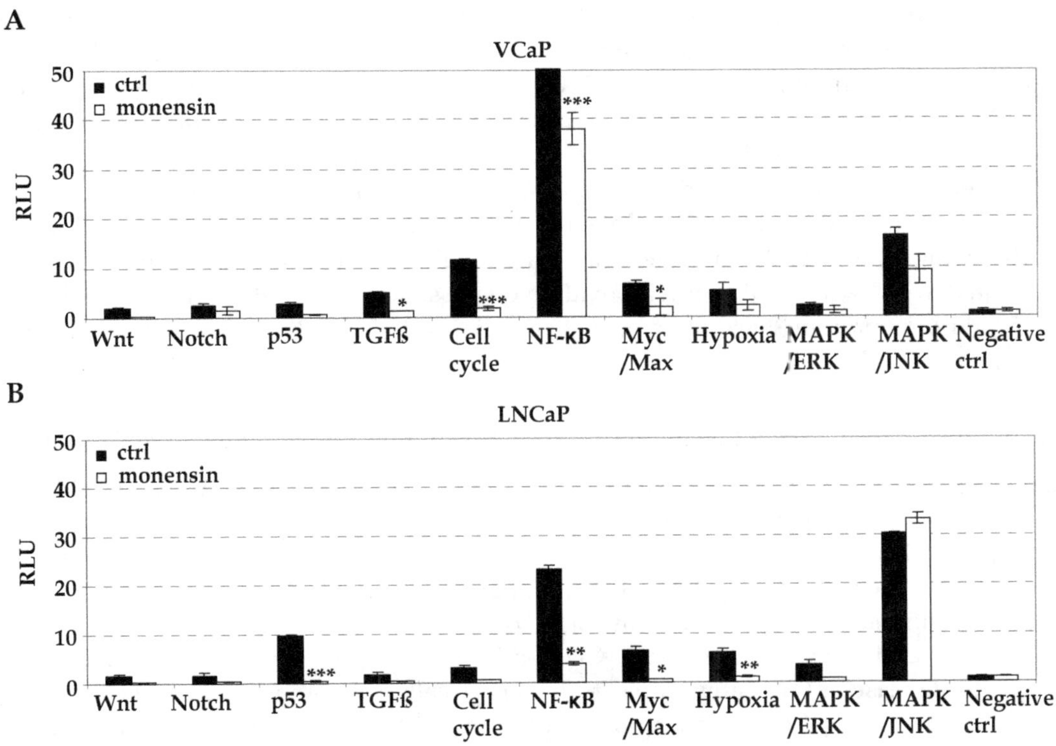

Fig. 2. Cancer pathway activities in VCaP and LNCaP prostate cancer cells. A) VCaP and B) LNCaP cells were exposed to ethanol or 100 nM monensin for 24 hours and pathway activities were measured as described in the text. Results with negative control measuring the background firefly luciferase activity (non-inducible firefly luciferase reporter and constitutively expressing Renilla construct) are indicated and used to determine the basal pathway activities in VCaP and LNCaP cells. The y-axis was set to 50 to allow direct comparison of relative luciferase units (RLU) in VCaP and LNCaP cells, although the basal NK-κB activity in VCaP cells extended RLU 324. Statistical significance of monensin induced changes are shown for the active pathways *P<0.05, **P<0.01, ***P<0.001.

clearly the most active pathway (fold change FC > 300, compared to the negative control). In addition, TGF-ß (FC = 5), cell cycle (FC = 12), Myc/Max (FC = 7) and hypoxia (FC = 5) were active in VCaP cells. In LNCaP cells, MAPK/JNK was the most active pathway (FC = 30 compared to the negative control), followed by NF-κB (FC = 23), p53 (FC = 10), Myc/Max (FC = 7) and hypoxia (FC = 6). Interestingly, NF-κB pathway was 14 times more active in TMPRSS2-ERG fusion positive VCaP cells than in ERG negative LNCaP cells. These results are in agreement with previous data indicating that ERG induces NF-κB activity in prostate cells *in vitro* and *in vivo* (Wang et al. 2010). The results with p53 pathway are also in accordance with the previous literature since VCaP cells are known to have an inactivating mutation in p53 (Trp-248) whereas LNCaP cells express the active form, supporting further the overall functionality of the assay (van Bokhoven et al. 2003).

Monensin exposure inhibited NF-κB activity in both VCaP (by 88%) and LNCaP (by 83%) cells. NF-κB is a transcription factor that regulates various cellular processes such as cellular antioxidant defence capacity (Gloire, Legrand-Poels & Piette 2006). These results suggest that monensin induced oxidative stress may result from reduced NF-κB signalling. In addition, monensin reduced TGF-ß (by 75%), cell cycle (by 85%) and Myc/Max (by 71%) activities in VCaP cells and p53 (by 94%), hypoxia (by 82%) and Myc/Max (by 90%) activities in LNCaP cells. The reduced Myc/Max signalling is supported by reduced MYC mRNA expression seen in monensin exposed VCaP and LNCaP cells (Ketola et al. 2010). Taken together, monensin reduced the activities of multiple signalling pathways such as NF-κB, TGF-ß, hypoxia and Myc/Max, all associated with cancer cell survival, oxidative stress, stem cell potential and metastasis (Jones, Pu & Kyprianou 2009, Blum et al. 2009, Mimeault, M. & Batra, S.K. 2011, Benassi et al. 2006, Koh et al. 2010).

3.2 Monensin reduces the cancer stem cell population in prostate cancer cell cultures

Monensin exposure reduced the activities of multiple pathways maintaining antioxidative capacity and promoting the growth and survival of cancer stem cells such as NF-κB, HIF1A, MYC and ALDH, in cultured prostate cancer cells. Therefore, the effect of monensin on prostate cancer stem cell population was studied. Prostate cancer stem cells can be identified by high expression of CD44 and low expression of CD24 antigens (Klarmann et al. 2009). Interestingly, CD44 cell surface glycoprotein has recently been shown to increase antioxidative capacity in cancer cells, indicating that cancer initiating cells could be targeted by impairing oxidative stress defence mechanisms (Ishimoto et al. 2011). Thus, we analyzed the effect of monensin exposure to the fraction of $CD44^{+}/CD24^{-}$ cells in cultured prostate cancer cells. VCaP and LNCaP cells exposed to monensin (1 μM) for 6 hours were stained with CD44 and CD24 recognizing antibodies and the samples were analyzed using FACS. The results showed that monensin reduced the fraction of $CD44^{+}/CD24^{-}$ cells in both VCaP (from 3 to 1.3%) and LNCaP (3.1 to 2.6%) cells (Fig. 3). In agreement with these results, genome-wide gene expression analysis indicated that monensin decreased CD44 (by 20%) and induced CD24 (by 30%) mRNAs compared to the levels in ethanol control at 6-hour time point (Ketola et al. 2010). Taken together, these results indicate that monensin reduces the fraction of cancer stem cells in prostate cancer cell cultures.

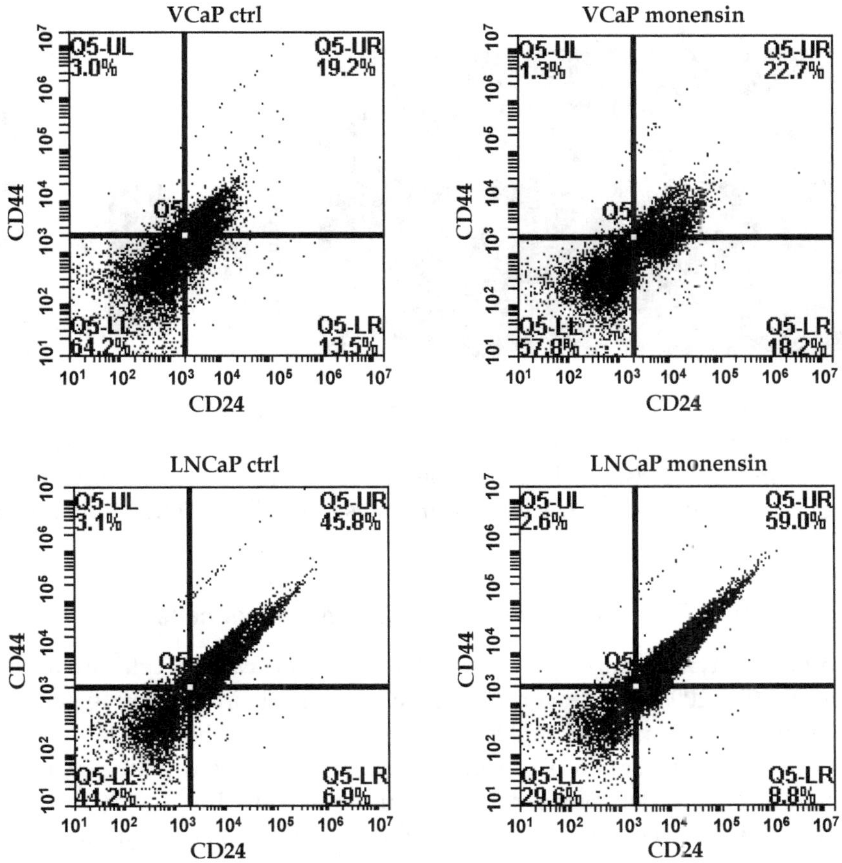

Fig. 3. FACS analysis of CD44 and CD24 immunostained VCaP and LNCaP prostate cancer cells. Monensin reduces the fraction of CD44+/CD24- cells in cultured prostate cancer cells. VCaP and LNCaP cells were stained with CD44 and CD24 antibodies in response to six hour monensin or ethanol exposure. Representative images from one out of four replicates are shown.

3.3 Monensin induces cell differentiation in prostate cancer cells

Cancer stem cells have been hypothesized to arise intrinsically through oncogenic transformation of normal tissue stem or progenitor cells in the early stage of the tumorigenesis or through induction of epithelial-to-mesenchymal transition (EMT) at later stages (Chaffer, Weinberg 2011). The expression of E-cadherin is considered as a marker of epithelial differentiation and it is lost during EMT. Interestingly, ERG knock-down in VCaP cells has been shown to induce E-cadherin expression (Gupta et al. 2010). Moreover, our previous results indicated that monensin reduced ERG expression in VCaP cells (Ketola et al. 2010). Thus, to study whether monensin affects prostate cancer cell differentiation, E-cadherin expression was analysed in monensin exposed VCaP cells. The results from immunochemical staining and quantitative RT-PCR showed that monensin induced E-cadherin expression in VCaP cells (Fig. 4A and B), indicating that monensin promotes cell differentiation in cultured prostate cancer cells.

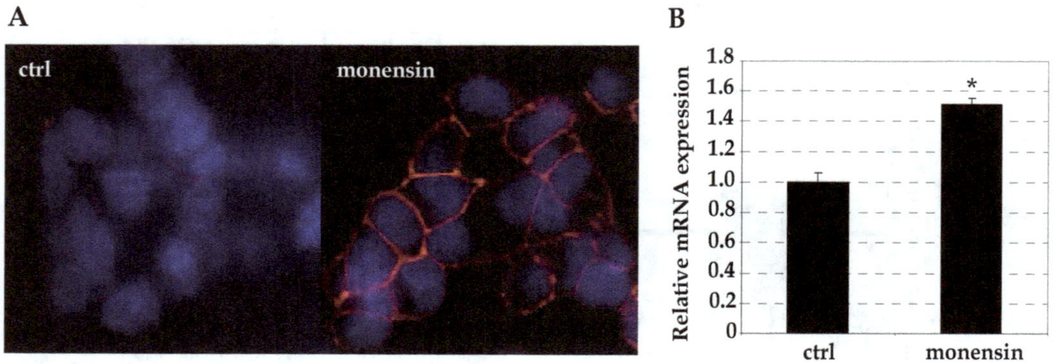

Fig. 4. Monensin induces E-cadherin expression in VCaP prostate cancer cells. A) Immunofluorescence staining of E-cadherin (red) in response to 1 μM monensin or ethanol (ctrl) for 6-hour in VCaP cells. Nuclei are stained with DAPI (blue). B) Relative mRNA expression of E-cadherin in response to 1 μM monensin or ethanol (ctrl) exposure for 6-hour in VCaP cells.

3.4 Monensin reduces migration in cultured prostate cancer cells

Epithelial-to-mesenchymal transition is a perquisite for cancer cell migration (Baum, Settleman & Quinlan 2008). Moreover, in addition to the role in promoting cancer stem cell growth and survival, NF-κB and ALDH activities as well as high CD44 and low CD24 expressions are known to enhance prostate cancer cell migration (van den Hoogen et al. 2010, Klarmann et al. 2009). Since monensin induced cell differentiation, the effect of monensin exposure on prostate cancer cell migration was studied. VCaP and LNCaP cells do not migrate and therefore PC-3 prostate cancer cells were used as a model in migration assay. The results are presented in Fig. 5. Interestingly, already at 10 nM concentration, monensin significantly reduced cell migration. The anti-migratorial effect was stronger at higher concentrations (100 nM and 1 μM) (Fig. 5A). Thus, monensin was able to reduce cell migration at nanomolar concentrations in PC-3 cells although the same concentrations did not significantly decrease cell viability in these cells even at 24 hour time point (Fig. 5B). Pictures showing the decrease in wound closure in monensin exposed PC-3 cells in comparison to control are shown at 12 and 24 hour time points in Fig. 5C.

3.5 Monensin increases oxidative stress inducing steroids as well as reduces the level of androgen precursor and antioxidative steroid

Our previous results indicated that monensin induced oxidative stress and altered the expression of genes involved in cholesterol and steroid biosynthesis (Ketola et al. 2010). Moreover, monensin reduced androgen receptor (AR) signalling and showed synergistic growth inhibitory effects with anti-androgens in prostate cancer cells. To validate the monensin induced changes in cellular steroid levels, steroid profiling was performed in VCaP prostate cancer cells. Cells were exposed to ethanol or monensin (1 μM) for six hours and steroid profiles were studied using gas chromatocraphy - mass spectrometry (GC-MS). The results presented as a heat-map in Fig. 6 show that the most prominent changes in response to monensin exposure were the induction of 7-ketocholesterol and aldosterone

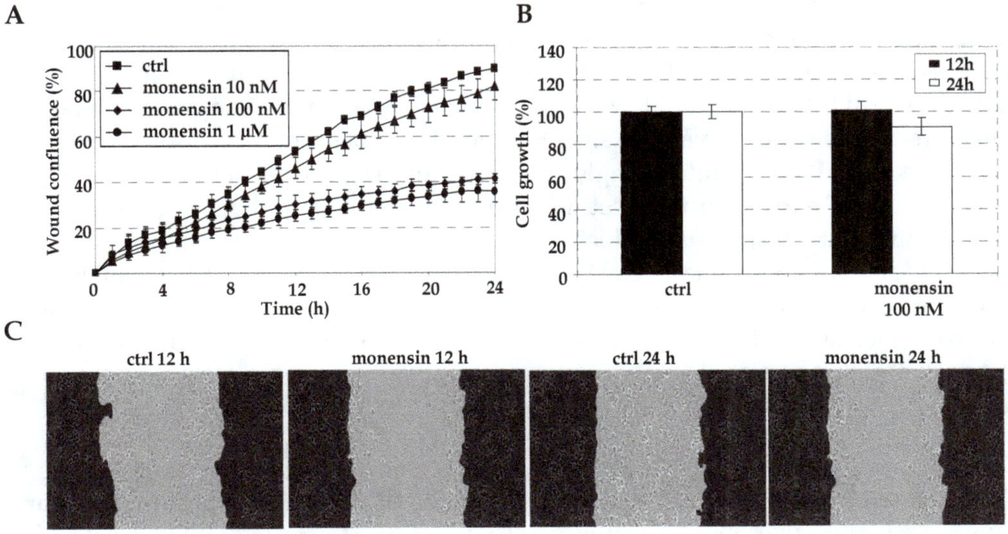

Fig. 5. The effect of monensin exposure on PC-3 prostate cancer cell migration. A) Relative wound confluency in response to monensin (10 nM, 100 nM and 1 µM) or control (ethanol) was monitored for 24 hours. B) Results from cell viability assay in response to monensin exposure (100 nM) for 12 and 24 hours in PC-3 cells. C) Pictures of scratch-wounded wells in response to 100 nM monensin or ethanol exposure at 12- and 24-hour time points. The wound margin in the beginning of the experiment is coloured in dark grey.

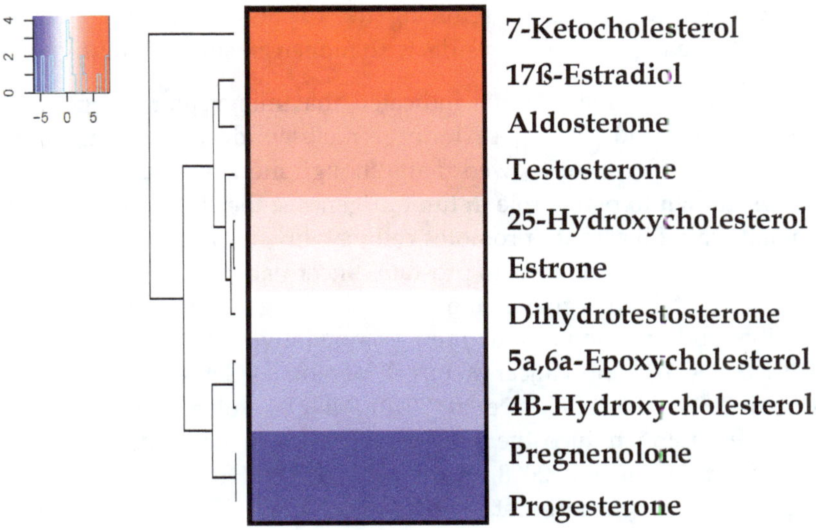

Fig. 6. Steroid profiling heat-map of monensin exposed VCaP prostate cancer cells. The cells were exposed to monensin (1 µM) for 6 hours and the steroid profile was measured with gas chromatography-mass spectrometry (GC-MS). The levels of individual steroids in monensin exposed cells were compared to ethanol exposed samples (presented as fold change, red: induction, blue: reduction).

levels as well as decrease in progesterone and pregnenolone levels. Aldosterone and 7-ketocholesterol are known oxidative stress inducers whereas progesterone has antioxidant properties (Leonarduzzi et al., 2006, Gramajo et al., 2010, Lee et al., 2009, Calo et al., 2010, Queisser et al., 2011, Ozacmak et al., 2009). Moreover, progesterone and pregnenolone are androgen precursors which have been suggested to play a major role in prostate cancer cell survival (Locke et al. 2008). Interestingly, progesterone has also been shown to promote mammary stem cell expansion (Joshi et al. 2010). The steroid profiling validates also the previous Connectivity Map results which indicated that monensin has opposite effects to progesterone and pregnenolone (Ketola et al. 2010). Taken together, monensin induced alterations in cellular steroid profile indicated that monensin induced oxidative stress results from increased aldosterone and 7-ketocholesterol levels as well as decreased progesterone and pregnenolone levels.

4. Conclusion

In this study, we explored the molecular consequences of monensin exposure in cultured prostate cancer cells. Our previous study indicated that monensin inhibited selectively prostate cancer cell viability at nanomolar concentrations by inducing oxidative stress. Cancer cells are constantly under pro-oxidative state (Szatrowski, Nathan 1991, Toyokuni et al. 1995). Long-term oxidative stress stimulates cell growth and proliferation, contributes to metastatic process and promotes cancer cell invasiveness and migration (Mori, Shibanuma & Nose 2004, Sung et al. 2006). Therefore, cancer cells need strong antioxidant mechanisms to survive and profit from these oxidative stress induced changes. Interfering redox balance has been suggested as a potential mean to selectively target cancer cells for example by increasing the cellular ROS level or reducing the expression of antioxidative enzymes (Pelicano, Carney & Huang 2004). Our results with monensin support this hypothesis.

Our previous Connectivity Map results indicated that monensin has agonistic effects to NF-κB inactivator and oxidative stress inducer niclosamide supporting monensin as a potent NF-κB inhibitor. Here, we showed that although monensin reduced the activities of several pathways known to play a role in tumourigenesis, the strongest reduction was seen in NF κB signalling. NF-κB activity promotes cell viability, tumorigenesis and metastasis as well as correlates with poor prognosis in prostate cancer patients (Blum et al. 2009, Sarkar et al. 2008). Importantly, NF-κB regulates the expression of genes responsible for antioxidant defence capacity and its inhibition induces oxidative stress as well as reduces tumourigenesis, metastasis and cancer stem cell potential (Gloire, Legrand-Poels & Piette 2006, Sarkar et al. 2008, Gluschnaider et al. 2010). NF-κB inhibitors are known to decrease AR signalling *in vitro* and reduce the growth of androgen deprivation-resistant prostate cancer xenografts *in vivo* (Jin et al. 2008, Zhang et al. 2009b). However, at present no specific NF-κB inhibitors have reached the stage of clinical trials for prostate cancer treatment (Mahon et al. 2011). Our results support NF-κB as the main mediator of monensin induced oxidative stress, which may also contribute to the reduced androgen signalling and induction of apoptosis in monensin exposed prostate cancer cells.

Recently, cancer stem cell targeting has raised a lot of interest as a prominent way to target cancer drug resistance and metastasic growth (Mimeault, Batra 2011, Clayton, Mousa 2011). In comparison to cancer cells, ROS levels in cancer stem cells are lower due to controlled redox balance system such as high ALDH and CD44 expression protecting cancer stem cells from oxidative stress (Kobayashi, Suda 2011a, Croker, Allan 2011, Ishimoto et al. 2011). Interestingly, NF-κB inhibition induces apoptosis in prostate cancer stem cells and thus NF-κB is considered as an attractive chemotherapeutic target also against cancer stem cells (Jin et al. 2008, Birnie et al. 2008). Since monensin reduced ALDH and NF-κB activities, we studied the fraction of $CD44^{+}/CD24^{-}$ cells in prostate cancer cell cultures in response to monensin exposure. The results confirmed that monensin reduced the amount of prostate cancer stem cells. Moreover, monensin induced epithelial cell differentiation and reduced motility in cultured prostate cancer cells, suggesting that monensin inhibits prostate tumorigenesis by multiple ways. Cancer stem cell inhibitor and cell differentiation inducer salinomycin shares a similar structure as monensin, supporting the functional similarities between these two compounds (Gupta et al. 2009).

Steroidogenic enzymes as well as stem cell markers are induced in castration-resistant prostate cancer both *in vitro* and *in vivo* (Blum et al. 2009, Pfeiffer et al. 2011). Several studies have shown that steroidogenesis is inhibited by ROS (Tsai et al. 2003, Stocco, Wells & Clark 1993, Kodaman, Aten & Behrman 1994, Lee et al. 2009, Abidi et al. 2008). Our previous results indicated that monensin reduced androgen receptor signalling. Here, we showed that monensin increases the levels of oxidative stress inducing steroids, 7-ketocholesterol and aldosterone, and reduces androgen precursor and antioxidative steroid progesterone in cultured prostate cancer cells. Interestingly, 7-ketocholesterol is a ligand for aryl hydrocarbon receptor (AhR) and acts as AhR antagonist (Savouret et al. 2001). AhR expression is elevated in malignant prostate cells and its signalling is activated in prostate cancer stem cells (Blum et al. 2009, Gluschnaider et al. 2010). AhR pathway increases the expression of ALDH proteins and protects cells against oxidative stress and foreign chemicals (Lindros et al. 1998, Vrzal, Ulrichova & Dvorak 2004, Nebert et al. 2000, Kohle, Bock 2007). Interestingly, AhR binds to NF-κB, induces MYC activation and reduces E-cadherin expression in breast cancer cells (Kim et al. 2000, Dietrich, Kaina 2010). Moreover, AhR can form a complex with androgen receptor and protect prostate cancer cells during androgen ablation (Ohtake, Fujii-Kuriyama & Kato 2009, Gluschnaider et al. 2010). Thus, our results indicate that monensin induced oxidative stress is potentially transmitted via reduced AhR signalling. This hypothesis is further supported by our previous gene expression results indicating that although AhR itself was not altered, the expression of AhR target gene mRNAs were decreased in response to monensin exposure (Ketola et al. 2010).

Taken together, we hypothesize that monensin induced anti-neoplastic effects result mainly due to increase in oxidative stress. The overview figure 7 illustrates the various changes occurring in prostate cancer cells in response to monensin exposure. The cancer selectiveness could be explained by increased intracellular ROS due to reduced antioxidative capacity sensitizing prostate cancer cells to oxidative stress. Since normal prostate epithelial cells are not under intensive oxidative stress and therefore, are less dependent on the function of antioxidative genes, they are not as sensitive to monensin exposure as cancer cells. In conclusion, our results support the idea that impairing the redox control, which has a crucial role in cancer cells enabling survival in high intracellular ROS, is a potent way to target prostate cancer cells.

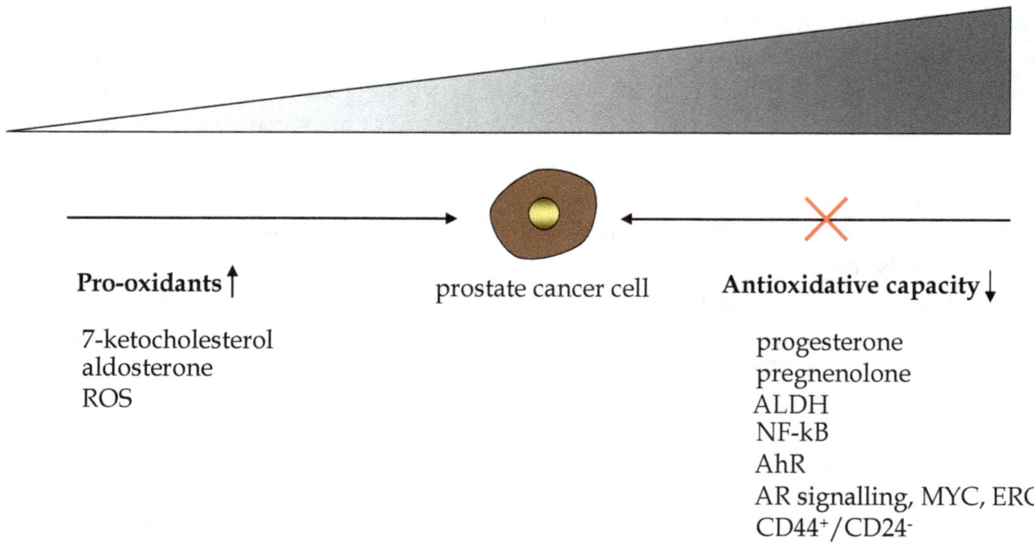

Fig. 7. Overview of monensin induced changes in prostate cancer cells. The figure idea adapted from Cairns, R.A., Harris, I.S. & Mak, T.W. 2011.

5. Acknowledgement

We thank Mika Hilvo, Tuulia Hyötyläinen, Anna-Liisa Ruskeepää (VTT Technical Research Centre of Finland, Espoo, Finland) for their contribution in steroid profiling part of this study.

6. References

Abidi, P., Zhang, H., Zaidi, S.M., Shen, W.J., Leers-Sucheta, S., Cortez, Y., Han, J. & Azhar, S. 2008, "Oxidative stress-induced inhibition of adrenal steroidogenesis requires participation of p38 mitogen-activated protein kinase signaling pathway", *The Journal of endocrinology,* vol. 198, no. 1, pp. 193-207.

Ahlemeyer, B., Bauerbach, E., Plath, M., Steuber, M., Heers, C., Tegtmeier, F. & Krieglstein, J. 2001, "Retinoic acid reduces apoptosis and oxidative stress by preservation of SOD protein level", *Free radical biology & medicine,* vol. 30, no. 10, pp. 1067-1077.

Ahlemeyer, B. & Krieglstein, J. 1998, "Retinoic acid reduces staurosporine-induced apoptotic damage in chick embryonic neurons by suppressing reactive oxygen species production", *Neuroscience letters,* vol. 246, no. 2, pp. 93-96.

Baum, B., Settleman, J. & Quinlan, M.P. 2008, "Transitions between epithelial and mesenchymal states in development and disease", *Seminars in cell & developmental biology,* vol. 19, no. 3, pp. 294-308.

Benassi, B., Fanciulli, M., Fiorentino, F., Porrello, A., Chiorino, G., Loda, M., Zupi, G. & Biroccio, A. 2006, "c-Myc phosphorylation is required for cellular response to oxidative stress", *Molecular cell,* vol. 21, no. 4, pp. 509-519.

Berthold, D.R., Pond, G.R., Soban, F., de Wit, R., Eisenberger, M. & Tannock, I.F. 2008, "Docetaxel plus prednisone or mitoxantrone plus prednisone for advanced prostate cancer: updated survival in the TAX 327 study", *Journal of clinical oncology : official journal of the American Society of Clinical Oncology,* vol. 26, no. 2, pp. 242-245.

Birnie, R., Bryce, S.D., Roome, C., Dussupt, V., Droop, A., Lang, S.H., Berry, P.A., Hyde, C.F., Lewis, J.L., Stower, M.J., Maitland, N.J. & Collins, A.T. 2008, "Gene expression profiling of human prostate cancer stem cells reveals a pro-inflammatory phenotype and the importance of extracellular matrix interactions", *Genome biology,* vol. 9, no. 5, pp. R83.

Blum, R., Gupta, R., Burger, P.E., Ontiveros, C.S., Salm, S.N., Xiong, X., Kamb, A., Wesche, H., Marshall, L., Cutler, G., Wang, X., Zavadil, J., Moscatelli, D. & Wilson, E.L. 2009, "Molecular signatures of prostate stem cells reveal novel signaling pathways and provide insights into prostate cancer", *PloS one,* vol. 4, no. 5, pp. e5722.

Bracarda, S., Logothetis, C., Sternberg, C.N. & Oudard, S. 2011, "Current and emerging treatment modalities for metastatic castration-resistant prostate cancer", *BJU international,* vol. 107 Suppl 2, pp. 13-20.

Burger, P.E., Gupta, R., Xiong, X., Ontiveros, C.S., Salm, S.N., Moscatelli, D. & Wilson, E.L. 2009, "High aldehyde dehydrogenase activity: a novel functional marker of murine prostate stem/progenitor cells", *Stem cells (Dayton, Ohio),* vol. 27, no. 9, pp. 2220-2228.

Cairns, R.A., Harris, I.S. & Mak, T.W. 2011, "Regulation of cancer cell metabolism", *Nature reviews.Cancer,* vol. 11, no. 2, pp. 85-95.

Chaffer, C.L. & Weinberg, R.A. 2011, "A perspective on cancer cell metastasis", *Science (New York, N.Y.),* vol. 331, no. 6024, pp. 1559-1564.

Chiu, H.J., Fischman, D.A. & Hammerling, U. 2008, "Vitamin A depletion causes oxidative stress, mitochondrial dysfunction, and PARP-1-dependent energy deprivation", *The FASEB journal : official publication of the Federation of American Societies for Experimental Biology,* vol. 22, no. 11, pp. 3878-3887.

Chute, J.P., Muramoto, G.G., Whitesides, J., Colvin, M., Safi, R., Chao, N.J. & McDonnell, D.P. 2006, "Inhibition of aldehyde dehydrogenase and retinoid signaling induces the expansion of human hematopoietic stem cells", *Proceedings of the National Academy of Sciences of the United States of America,* vol. 103, no. 31, pp. 11707-11712.

Clayton, S. & Mousa, S.A. 2011, "Therapeutics formulated to target cancer stem cells: Is it in our future?", *Cancer cell international,* vol. 11, pp. 7.

Croker, A.K. & Allan, A.L. 2011, "Inhibition of aldehyde dehydrogenase (ALDH) activity reduces chemotherapy and radiation resistance of stem-like ALDH(hi)CD44 (+) human breast cancer cells", *Breast cancer research and treatment,* .

Dakhova, O., Ozen, M., Creighton, C.J., Li, R., Ayala, G., Rowley, D. & Ittmann, M. 2009, "Global gene expression analysis of reactive stroma in prostate cancer", *Clinical cancer research : an official journal of the American Association for Cancer Research,* vol. 15, no. 12, pp. 3979-3989.

Davydov, V.V., Dobaeva, N.M. & Bozhkov, A.I. 2004, "Possible role of alteration of aldehyde's scavenger enzymes during aging", *Experimental gerontology,* vol. 39, no. 1, pp. 11-16.

DeNicola, G.M., Karreth, F.A., Humpton, T.J., Gopinathan, A., Wei, C., Frese, K., Mangal, D., Yu, K.H., Yeo, C.J., Calhoun, E.S., Scrimieri, F., Winter, J.M., Hruban, R.H., Iacobuzio-Donahue, C., Kern, S.E., Blair, I.A. & Tuveson, D.A. 2011, "Oncogene-induced Nrf2 transcription promotes ROS detoxification and tumorigenesis", *Nature,* vol. 475, no. 7354, pp. 106-109.

Dietrich, C. & Kaina, B. 2010, "The aryl hydrocarbon receptor (AhR) in the regulation of cell-cell contact and tumor growth", *Carcinogenesis,* vol. 31, no. 8, pp. 1319-1328.

Duester, G. 2000, "Families of retinoid dehydrogenases regulating vitamin A function: production of visual pigment and retinoic acid", *European journal of biochemistry / FEBS,* vol. 267, no. 14, pp. 4315-4324.

Fang, J., Nakamura, H. & Iyer, A.K. 2007, "Tumor-targeted induction of oxystress for cancer therapy", *Journal of drug targeting,* vol. 15, no. 7-8, pp. 475-486.

Gloire, G., Legrand-Poels, S. & Piette, J. 2006, "NF-kappaB activation by reactive oxygen species: fifteen years later", *Biochemical pharmacology,* vol. 72, no. 11, pp. 1493-1505.

Gluschnaider, U., Hidas, G., Cojocaru, G., Yutkin, V., Ben-Neriah, Y. & Pikarsky, E. 2010, "beta-TrCP inhibition reduces prostate cancer cell growth via upregulation of the aryl hydrocarbon receptor", *PloS one,* vol. 5, no. 2, pp. e9060.

Gupta, P.B., Onder, T.T., Jiang, G., Tao, K., Kuperwasser, C., Weinberg, R.A. & Lander, E.S. 2009, "Identification of selective inhibitors of cancer stem cells by high-throughput screening", *Cell,* vol. 138, no. 4, pp. 645-659.

Gupta, S., Iljin, K., Sara, H., Mpindi, J.P., Mirtti, T., Vainio, P., Rantala, J., Alanen, K., Nees, M. & Kallioniemi, O. 2010, "FZD4 as a mediator of ERG oncogene-induced WNT signaling and epithelial-to-mesenchymal transition in human prostate cancer cells", *Cancer research,* vol. 70, no. 17, pp. 6735-6745.

Gupte, A. & Mumper, R.J. 2009, "Elevated copper and oxidative stress in cancer cells as a target for cancer treatment", *Cancer treatment reviews,* vol. 35, no. 1, pp. 32-46.

Iljin, K., Ketola, K., Vainio, P., Halonen, P., Kohonen, P., Fey, V., Grafstrom, R.C., Perala, M. & Kallioniemi, O. 2009, "High-throughput cell-based screening of 4910 known drugs and drug-like small molecules identifies disulfiram as an inhibitor of prostate cancer cell growth", *Clinical cancer research : an official journal of the American Association for Cancer Research,* vol. 15, no. 19, pp. 6070-6078.

Ishimoto, T., Nagano, O., Yae, T., Tamada, M., Motohara, T., Oshima, H., Oshima, M., Ikeda, T., Asaba, R., Yagi, H., Masuko, T., Shimizu, T., Ishikawa, T., Kai, K., Takahashi, E., Imamura, Y., Baba, Y., Ohmura, M., Suematsu, M., Baba, H. & Saya, H. 2011, "CD44 variant regulates redox status in cancer cells by stabilizing the xCT subunit of system xc(-) and thereby promotes tumor growth", *Cancer cell,* vol. 19, no. 3, pp. 387-400.

Jemal, A., Bray, F., Center, M.M., Ferlay, J., Ward, E. & Forman, D. 2011, "Global cancer statistics", *CA: a cancer journal for clinicians,* vol. 61, no. 2, pp. 69-90.

Jin, R.J., Lho, Y., Connelly, L., Wang, Y., Yu, X., Saint Jean, L., Case, T.C., Ellwood-Yen, K., Sawyers, C.L., Bhowmick, N.A., Blackwell, T.S., Yull, F.E. & Matusik, R.J. 2008, "The nuclear factor-kappaB pathway controls the progression of prostate cancer to androgen-independent growth", *Cancer research,* vol. 68, no. 16, pp. 6762-6769.

Jones, E., Pu, H. & Kyprianou, N. 2009, "Targeting TGF-beta in prostate cancer: therapeutic possibilities during tumor progression", *Expert opinion on therapeutic targets,* vol. 13, no. 2, pp. 227-234.

Joshi, P.A., Jackson, H.W., Beristain, A.G., Di Grappa, M.A., Mote, P.A., Clarke, C.L., Stingl, J., Waterhouse, P.D. & Khokha, R. 2010, "Progesterone induces adult mammary stem cell expansion", *Nature,* vol. 465, no. 7299, pp. 803-807.

Ketola, K., Vainio, P., Fey, V., Kallioniemi, O. & Iljin, K. 2010, "Monensin is a potent inducer of oxidative stress and inhibitor of androgen signaling leading to apoptosis in prostate cancer cells", *Molecular cancer therapeutics,* vol. 9, no. 12, pp. 3175-3185.

Khandrika, L., Kumar, B., Koul, S., Maroni, P. & Koul, H.K. 2009, "Oxidative stress in prostate cancer", *Cancer letters,* vol. 282, no. 2, pp. 125-136.

Kim, D.W., Gazourian, L., Quadri, S.A., Romieu-Mourez, R., Sherr, D.H. & Sonenshein, G.E. 2000, "The RelA NF-kappaB subunit and the aryl hydrocarbon receptor (AhR) cooperate to transactivate the c-myc promoter in mammary cells", *Oncogene,* vol. 19, no. 48, pp. 5498-5506.

Klarmann, G.J., Hurt, E.M., Mathews, L.A., Zhang, X., Duhagon, M.A., Mistree, T., Thomas, S.B. & Farrar, W.L. 2009, "Invasive prostate cancer cells are tumor initiating cells that have a stem cell-like genomic signature", *Clinical & experimental metastasis,* vol. 26, no. 5, pp. 433-446.

Kobayashi, C.I. & Suda, T. 2011a, "Regulation of reactive oxygen species in stem cells and cancer stem cells", *Journal of cellular physiology,* .

Kobayashi, C.I. & Suda, T. 2011b, "Regulation of reactive oxygen species in stem cells and cancer stem cells", *Journal of cellular physiology,* .

Kodaman, P.H., Aten, R.F. & Behrman, H.R. 1994, "Lipid hydroperoxides evoke antigonadotropic and antisteroidogenic activity in rat luteal cells", *Endocrinology,* vol. 135, no. 6, pp. 2723-2730.

Koh, C.M., Bieberich, C.J., Dang, C.V., Nelson, W.G., Yegnasubramanian, S. & De Marzo, A.M. 2010, "MYC and Prostate Cancer", *Genes & cancer,* vol. 1, no. 6, pp. 617-628.

Kohle, C. & Bock, K.W. 2007, "Coordinate regulation of Phase I and II xenobiotic metabolisms by the Ah receptor and Nrf2", *Biochemical pharmacology,* vol. 73, no. 12, pp. 1853-1862.

Korenchuk, S., Lehr, J.E., MClean, L., Lee, Y.G., Whitney, S., Vessella, R., Lin, D.L. & Pienta, K.J. 2001a, "VCaP, a cell-based model system of human prostate cancer", *In vivo (Athens, Greece),* vol. 15, no. 2, pp. 163-168.

Korenchuk, S., Lehr, J.E., MClean, L., Lee, Y.G., Whitney, S., Vessella, R., Lin, D.L. & Pienta, K.J. 2001b, "VCaP, a cell-based model system of human prostate cancer", *In vivo (Athens, Greece),* vol. 15, no. 2, pp. 163-168.

Kumar, B., Koul, S., Khandrika, L., Meacham, R.B. & Koul, H.K. 2008, "Oxidative stress is inherent in prostate cancer cells and is required for aggressive phenotype", *Cancer research,* vol. 68, no. 6, pp. 1777-1785.

Lee, S.Y., Gong, E.Y., Hong, C.Y., Kim, K.H., Han, J.S., Ryu, J.C., Chae, H.Z., Yun, C.H. & Lee, K. 2009, "ROS inhibit the expression of testicular steroidogenic enzyme genes via the suppression of Nur77 transactivation", *Free radical biology & medicine,* vol. 47, no. 11, pp. 1591-1600.

Leonarduzzi, G., Vizio, B., Sottero, B., Verde, V., Gamba, P., Mascia, C., Chiarpotto, E., Poli, G. & Biasi, F. 2006, "Early involvement of ROS overproduction in apoptosis induced by 7-ketocholesterol", *Antioxidants & redox signaling,* vol. 8, no. 3-4, pp. 375-380.

Li, T., Su, Y., Mei, Y., Leng, Q., Leng, B., Liu, Z., Stass, S.A. & Jiang, F. 2010, "ALDH1A1 is a marker for malignant prostate stem cells and predictor of prostate cancer patients' outcome", *Laboratory investigation; a journal of technical methods and pathology,* vol. 90, no. 2, pp. 234-244.

Lindros, K.O., Oinonen, T., Kettunen, E., Sippel, H., Muro-Lupori, C. & Koivusalo, M. 1998, "Aryl hydrocarbon receptor-associated genes in rat liver: regional coinduction of aldehyde dehydrogenase 3 and glutathione transferase Ya", *Biochemical pharmacology,* vol. 55, no. 4, pp. 413-421.

Locke, J.A., Guns, E.S., Lubik, A.A., Adomat, H.H., Hendy, S.C., Wood, C.A., Ettinger, S.L., Gleave, M.E. & Nelson, C.C. 2008, "Androgen levels increase by intratumoral de novo steroidogenesis during progression of castration-resistant prostate cancer", *Cancer research,* vol. 68, no. 15, pp. 6407-6415.

Magni, M., Shammah, S., Schiro, R., Mellado, W., Dalla-Favera, R. & Gianni, A.M. 1996, "Induction of cyclophosphamide-resistance by aldehyde-dehydrogenase gene transfer", *Blood,* vol. 87, no. 3, pp. 1097-1103.

Mahon, K.L., Henshall, S.M., Sutherland, R.L. & Horvath, L.G. 2011, "Pathways of chemotherapy resistance in castration-resistant prostate cancer", *Endocrine-related cancer,* vol. 18, no. 4, pp. R103-23.

Mimeault, M. & Batra, S.K. 2011, "Frequent Gene Products and Molecular Pathways Altered in Prostate Cancer- and Metastasis-Initiating Cells and their Progenies and Novel Promising Multitargeted Therapies", *Molecular medicine (Cambridge, Mass.)* .

Mori, K., Shibanuma, M. & Nose, K. 2004, "Invasive potential induced under long-term oxidative stress in mammary epithelial cells", *Cancer research,* vol. 64, no. 20, pp. 7464-7472.

Nebert, D.W., Roe, A.L., Dieter, M.Z., Solis, W.A., Yang, Y. & Dalton, T.P. 2000, "Role of the aromatic hydrocarbon receptor and [Ah] gene battery in the oxidative stress response, cell cycle control, and apoptosis", *Biochemical pharmacology,* vol. 59, no. 1, pp. 65-85.

Ohtake, F., Fujii-Kuriyama, Y. & Kato, S. 2009, "AhR acts as an E3 ubiquitin ligase to modulate steroid receptor functions", *Biochemical pharmacology,* vol. 77, no. 4, pp. 474-484.

Pani, G., Galeotti, T. & Chiarugi, P. 2010, "Metastasis: cancer cell's escape from oxidative stress", *Cancer metastasis reviews,* vol. 29, no. 2, pp. 351-378.

Pelicano, H., Carney, D. & Huang, P. 2004, "ROS stress in cancer cells and therapeutic implications", *Drug resistance updates : reviews and commentaries in antimicrobial and anticancer chemotherapy,* vol. 7, no. 2, pp. 97-110.

Pfeiffer, M.J., Smit, F.P., Sedelaar, J.P. & Schalken, J.A. 2011, "Steroidogenic Enzymes and Stem Cell Markers Are Upregulated during Androgen Deprivation in Prostate Cancer", *Molecular medicine (Cambridge, Mass.),* vol. 17, no. 7-8, pp. 657-664.

Pinthus, J.H., Bryskin, I., Trachtenberg, J., Lu, J.P., Singh, G., Fridman, E. & Wilson, B.C. 2007, "Androgen induces adaptation to oxidative stress in prostate cancer: implications for treatment with radiation therapy", *Neoplasia (New York, N.Y.),* vol. 9, no. 1, pp. 68-80.

Rigas, B. & Sun, Y. 2008, "Induction of oxidative stress as a mechanism of action of chemopreventive agents against cancer", *British journal of cancer,* vol. 98, no. 7, pp. 1157-1160.

Sarkar, F.H., Li, Y., Wang, Z. & Kong, D. 2008, "NF-kappaB signaling pathway and its therapeutic implications in human diseases", *International reviews of immunology,* vol. 27, no. 5, pp. 293-319.

Savouret, J.F., Antenos, M., Quesne, M., Xu, J., Milgrom, E. & Casper, R.F. 2001, "7-Ketocholesterol is an Endogenous Modulator for the Arylhydrocarbon Receptor", *The Journal of biological chemistry,* vol. 276, no. 5, pp. 3054-3059.

Sharifi, N., Gulley, J.L. & Dahut, W.L. 2010, "An update on androgen deprivation therapy for prostate cancer", *Endocrine-related cancer,* vol. 17, no. 4, pp. R305-15.

Shibutani, S., Takeshita, M. & Grollman, A.P. 1991, "Insertion of specific bases during DNA synthesis past the oxidation-damaged base 8-oxodG", *Nature,* vol. 349, no. 6308, pp. 431-434.

Sophos, N.A. & Vasiliou, V. 2003, "Aldehyde dehydrogenase gene superfamily: the 2002 update", *Chemico-biological interactions,* vol. 143-144, pp. 5-22.

Stocco, D.M., Wells, J. & Clark, B.J. 1993, "The effects of hydrogen peroxide on steroidogenesis in mouse Leydig tumor cells", *Endocrinology,* vol. 133, no. 6, pp. 2827-2832.

Sun, Y., Huang, L., Mackenzie, G.G. & Rigas, B. 2011, "Oxidative stress mediates through apoptosis the anticancer effect of phospho-NSAIDs: Implications for the role of oxidative stress in the action of anticancer agents", *The Journal of pharmacology and experimental therapeutics,* .

Sung, S.Y., Kubo, H., Shigemura, K., Arnold, R.S., Logani, S., Wang, R., Konaka, H., Nakagawa, M., Mousses, S., Amin, M., Anderson, C., Johnstone, P., Petros, J.A., Marshall, F.F., Zhau, H.E. & Chung, L.W. 2006, "Oxidative stress induces ADAM9 protein expression in human prostate cancer cells", *Cancer research,* vol. 66, no. 19, pp. 9519-9526.

Swanson, T.A., Krueger, S.A., Galoforo, S., Thibodeau, B.J., Martinez, A.A., Wilson, G.D. & Marples, B. 2011, "TMPRSS2/ERG fusion gene expression alters chemo- and radio-responsiveness in cell culture models of androgen independent prostate cancer", *The Prostate,* .

Szatrowski, T.P. & Nathan, C.F. 1991, "Production of large amounts of hydrogen peroxide by human tumor cells", *Cancer research,* vol. 51, no. 3, pp. 794-798.

Tam, N.N., Gao, Y., Leung, Y.K. & Ho, S.M. 2003, "Androgenic regulation of oxidative stress in the rat prostate: involvement of NAD(P)H oxidases and antioxidant defense machinery during prostatic involution and regrowth", *The American journal of pathology,* vol. 163, no. 6, pp. 2513-2522.

Tannock, I.F., de Wit, R., Berry, W.R., Horti, J., Pluzanska, A., Chi, K.N., Oudard, S., Theodore, C., James, N.D., Turesson, I., Rosenthal, M.A., Eisenberger, M.A. & TAX 327 Investigators 2004, "Docetaxel plus prednisone or mitoxantrone plus prednisone for advanced prostate cancer", *The New England journal of medicine,* vol. 351, no. 15, pp. 1502-1512.

Toyokuni, S., Okamoto, K., Yodoi, J. & Hiai, H. 1995, "Persistent oxidative stress in cancer", *FEBS letters,* vol. 358, no. 1, pp. 1-3.

Tsai, S.C., Lu, C.C., Lin, C.S. & Wang, P.S. 2003, "Antisteroidogenic actions of hydrogen peroxide on rat Leydig cells", *Journal of cellular biochemistry,* vol. 90, no. 6, pp. 1276-1286.

Vainio, P., Gupta, S., Ketola, K., Mirtti, T., Mpindi, J.P., Kohonen, P., Fey, V., Perala, M., Smit, F., Verhaegh, G., Schalken, J., Alanen, K.A., Kallioniemi, O. & Iljin, K. 2011, "Arachidonic acid pathway members PLA2G7, HPGD, EPHX2, and CYP4F8 identified as putative novel therapeutic targets in prostate cancer", *The American journal of pathology,* vol. 178, no. 2, pp. 525-536.

van Bokhoven, A., Varella-Garcia, M., Korch, C., Johannes, W.U., Smith, E.E., Miller, H.L., Nordeen, S.K., Miller, G.J. & Lucia, M.S. 2003, "Molecular characterization of human prostate carcinoma cell lines", *The Prostate,* vol. 57, no. 3, pp. 205-225.

van den Hoogen, C., van der Horst, G., Cheung, H., Buijs, J.T., Lippitt, J.M., Guzman-Ramirez, N., Hamdy, F.C., Eaton, C.L., Thalmann, G.N., Cecchini, M.G., Pelger, R.C. & van der Pluijm, G. 2010, "High aldehyde dehydrogenase activity identifies tumor-initiating and metastasis-initiating cells in human prostate cancer", *Cancer research,* vol. 70, no. 12, pp. 5163-5173.

Vrzal, R., Ulrichova, J. & Dvorak, Z. 2004, "Aromatic hydrocarbon receptor status in the metabolism of xenobiotics under normal and pathophysiological conditions", *Biomedical papers of the Medical Faculty of the University Palacky, Olomouc, Czechoslovakia,* vol. 148, no. 1, pp. 3-10.

Wang, J., Cai, Y., Shao, L.J., Siddiqui, J., Palanisamy, N., Li, R., Ren, C., Ayala, G. & Ittmann, M.M. 2010, "Activation of NF-kB by TMPRSS2/ERG fusion isoforms through Toll-like receptor-4", *Cancer research,* .

Yoshida, A., Rzhetsky, A., Hsu, L.C. & Chang, C. 1998, "Human aldehyde dehydrogenase gene family", *European journal of biochemistry / FEBS,* vol. 251, no. 3, pp. 549-557.

Yossepowitch, O., Pinchuk, I., Gur, U., Neumann, A., Lichtenberg, D. & Baniel, J. 2007, "Advanced but not localized prostate cancer is associated with increased oxidative stress", *The Journal of urology,* vol. 178, no. 4 Pt 1, pp. 1238-43; discussion 1243-4.

Yu, C., Yao, Z., Dai, J., Zhang, H., Escara-Wilke, J., Zhang, X. & Keller, E.T. 2011, "ALDH Activity Indicates Increased Tumorigenic Cells, But Not Cancer Stem Cells, in Prostate Cancer Cell Lines", *In vivo (Athens, Greece),* vol. 25, no. 1, pp. 69-76.

Zhang, M., Shoeb, M., Goswamy, J., Liu, P., Xiao, T.L., Hogan, D., Campbell, G.A. & Ansari, N.H. 2009a, "Overexpression of aldehyde dehydrogenase 1A1 reduces oxidation-induced toxicity in SH-SY5Y neuroblastoma cells", *Journal of neuroscience research,* .

Zhang, Q., Helfand, B.T., Jang, T.L., Zhu, L.J., Chen, L., Yang, X.J., Kozlowski, J., Smith, N., Kundu, S.D., Yang, G., Raji, A.A., Javonovic, B., Pins, M., Lindholm, P., Guo, Y., Catalona, W.J. & Lee, C. 2009b, "Nuclear factor-kappaB-mediated transforming growth factor-beta-induced expression of vimentin is an independent predictor of biochemical recurrence after radical prostatectomy", *Clinical cancer research : an official journal of the American Association for Cancer Research,* vol. 15, no. 10, pp. 3557-3567.

Permissions

All chapters in this book were first published by InTech Open; hereby published with permission under the Creative Commons Attribution License or equivalent. Every chapter published in this book has been scrutinized by our experts. Their significance has been extensively debated. The topics covered herein carry significant findings which will fuel the growth of the discipline. They may even be implemented as practical applications or may be referred to as a beginning point for another development.

The contributors of this book come from diverse backgrounds, making this book a truly international effort. This book will bring forth new frontiers with its revolutionizing research information and detailed analysis of the nascent developments around the world.

We would like to thank all the contributing authors for lending their expertise to make the book truly unique. They have played a crucial role in the development of this book. Without their invaluable contributions this book wouldn't have been possible. They have made vital efforts to compile up to date information on the varied aspects of this subject to make this book a valuable addition to the collection of many professionals and students.

This book was conceptualized with the vision of imparting up-to-date information and advanced data in this field. To ensure the same, a matchless editorial board was set up. Every individual on the board went through rigorous rounds of assessment to prove their worth. After which they invested a large part of their time researching and compiling the most relevant data for our readers.

The editorial board has been involved in producing this book since its inception. They have spent rigorous hours researching and exploring the diverse topics which have resulted in the successful publishing of this book. They have passed on their knowledge of decades through this book. To expedite this challenging task, the publisher supported the team at every step. A small team of assistant editors was also appointed to further simplify the editing procedure and attain best results for the readers.

Apart from the editorial board, the designing team has also invested a significant amount of their time in understanding the subject and creating the most relevant covers. They scrutinized every image to scout for the most suitable representation of the subject and create an appropriate cover for the book.

The publishing team has been an ardent support to the editorial, designing and production team. Their endless efforts to recruit the best for this project, has resulted in the accomplishment of this book. They are a veteran in the field of academics and their pool of knowledge is as vast as their experience in printing. Their expertise and guidance has proved useful at every step. Their uncompromising quality standards have made this book an exceptional effort. Their encouragement from time to time has been an inspiration for everyone.

The publisher and the editorial board hope that this book will prove to be a valuable piece of knowledge for researchers, students, practitioners and scholars across the globe.

List of Contributors

Marnix G.E.H. Lam
Department of Radiology and Nuclear Medicine, The Netherlands

Bernard A. Zonnenberg
Department of Radiology and Nuclear Medicine, The Netherlands
Department of Internal Medicine University Medical Center Utrecht, The Netherlands

Umberto Maestroni and Francesco Ziglioli
Department of Urology, University Hospital of Parma, Parma, Italy

Philipp Wolf
Department of Urology, University Medical Centre Freiburg Germany

Zsuzsanna Tabi, Lisa K. Spary and John Staffurth
Department of Oncology, School of Medicine, Cardiff University, Cardiff United Kingdom

Jorge Rioja, Carlos Blanco and Jorge Aranda
Dept Urology, University Hospital Miguel Servet, Zaragoza Spain

Tatjana Arsenijević, Kata Dabić Stanković, Miodrag Aćimović and Ljiljana Radošević Jelić
Institute for Oncology and Radiology of Serbia, Institute for Urology Serbia

Margareth Santos Zanchetta
Ryerson University, Faculty of Community Services, Daphne Cockwell School of Nursing, Toronto, ON, Canada

Margot Kaszap
University Laval, Faculty of Education, Quebec, QC, Canada

Marko Monteiro
State University of Campinas, Dept. of Science and Technology Policy, Campinas, SP, Brazil

Franklin Gorospe IV
Humber Institute of Technology and Advanced Learning, School of Health Sciences, Nursing Program & University Health Network - Toronto General Hospital, Toronto, ON, Canada

Roger Pilon
Laurentian University, School of Nursing, Sudbury, ON, Canada

Tine Hajdinjak
Center UROL Maribor Department of Surgery, General Hospital Murska Sobota, Medical Faculty, University of Maribor, Slovenia

Moshe Rogosnitzky and Rachel Danks
MedInsight Research Institute Israel

Kirsi Ketola and Kristiina Iljin
Medical Biotechnology, VTT Technical Research Centre of Finland and University of Turku, Turku, Finland

Anu Vuoristo and Matej Orešič
VTT Technical Research Centre of Finland, Espoo, University of Helsinki, Finland

Olli Kallioniemi
Institute for Molecular Medicine, Finland (FIMM), University of Helsinki, Finland

Index

www.ingramcontent.com/pod-product-compliance
Lightning Source LLC
LaVergne TN
LVHW080614210926
848485LV00003B/159